Chronic physical illness:
self-management and
behavioural interventions

Chronic physical illness: self-management and behavioural interventions

Editors

Stanton Newman, Liz Steed and Kathleen Mulligan

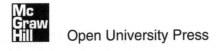 Open University Press

Open University Press
McGraw-Hill Education
McGraw-Hill House
Shoppenhangers Road
Maidenhead
Berkshire
England
SL6 2QL

email: enquiries@openup.co.uk
world wide web: www.openup.co.uk

and Two Penn Plaza, New York, NY 10121—2289, USA

First published 2009

A catalogue record of this book is available from the British Library

ISBN-10: 0-335-21786-9 (pb) 0-335-21787-7 (hb)
ISBN-13: 978-0-335-21786-1 (pb) 978-0-335-21787-8 (hb)

Typeset by Kerrypress, Luton, Bedfordshire
Printed and bound in the UK by Bell and Bain Ltd., Glasgow

Fictitious names of companies, products, people, characters and/or data that may be used herein (in case studies or in examples) are not intended to represent any real individual, company, product or event.

The **McGraw·Hill** Companies

Contents

About the editors   vi
List of contributors   vii
Introduction   ix

PART I CONTEXT

1   The health profile of ageing populations   3
2   Changing attitudes to the role of patients in health care   28

PART II DELIVERY

3   Self-management and behaviour change: theoretical models   47
4   Different types and components of self-management interventions   64
5   Delivery of self-management interventions   78
6   Training and quality assurance of self-management interventions   98
7   Facilitating self-management through telemedicine and interactive
    health communication applications   120

PART III EVALUATION

8   Development and evaluation of self-management interventions   135
9   Outcomes of self-management interventions   148

PART IV SELF-MANAGEMENT IN SPECIFIC CONDITIONS

10 Diabetes   169
11 Rheumatoid arthritis   189
12 Asthma   204
13 Coronary artery disease   224
14 Heart failure   238
15 Chronic obstructive pulmonary disease (COPD)   254
16 Hypertension   271

PART V CONCLUSION

17 Conclusion: The integration of self-management into
    routine healthcare   289

Index   299

About the editors

Stanton Newman D.Phil is Professor of Health Psychology and Head of the Centre for Behavioural and Social Sciences at University College London. He is a Chartered Health and Clinical Psychologist and has published widely and continues to research on the impact, cognitions and coping with chronic illness. He has developed and evaluated interventions to improve chronic illness self-management in a range of conditions.

Liz Steed PhD is a Chartered Health Psychologist working at the Royal Brompton Hospital, London, where she has a specialist interest in patients with respiratory and cardiac conditions. In addition, she is an Honorary Research Associate at University College London. Current research includes self-management in diabetes and difficult-to-control asthma.

Kathleen Mulligan PhD is a Chartered Health Psychologist and a Research Fellow at University College London. Her research interests are in factors that influence how people cope with chronic illness and in the development of interventions to improve chronic illness self-management.

Contributors

Susan J. Blalock PhD is Associate Professor at the School of Pharmacy, University of North Carolina, USA.

Debbie Cooke is a Research Fellow at Royal Free & University College Medical School Centre for Behavioural & Social Sciences in Medicine, UK.

Angela Coulter PhD is Chief Executive of Picker Institute Europe.

Karina W. Davidson PhD is Associate Professor at the Department of Medicine Columbia University, USA.

Robert F. DeVellis PhD is Professor at the Department of Health Behavior & Health Education School of Public Health at the University of North Carolina, USA.

Jo Ellins is a Research Fellow at the Health Services Management Centre, University of Birmingham, UK.

Maarten J. Fischer MA is a Researcher at Leiden University, The Netherlands.

Wendy Hardeman MSc is Senior Research Associate at the General Practice and Primary Care Research Unit, Department of Public Health and Primary Care, Institute of Public Health, University of Cambridge, UK.

Eric S. Hart Psy.D is the Clinical Assistant Professor at the Department of Health Psychology, University of Missouri, USA.

Paul Higgs is a Reader in Medical Sociology at the Centre for Behavioural Social Sciences in Medicine, Division of Medicine, University College London, UK.

Martin Hyde is Senior lecturer in Sociology at Sheffield Hallam University, UK.

Ad A. Kaptein PhD is Professor of Medical Psychology at Leiden University, The Netherlands.

Kate Lorig is Professor of Medicine and Director of the Patient Education Researcher Center at Stanford University School of Medicine, USA.

Patrick McGowan PhD is an Associate Professor at the Centre on Aging & Faculty of Social Sciences, University of Victoria, Victoria, British Columbia, Canada.

Susan Michie is a Professor of Health Psychology at University College London, UK.

Debra K. Moser DNSc RN FAAN is Professor and Gill Endowed Chair at the Center for Biobehavioral Research in Self-Care University of Kentucky, USA. She is also Editor of *The Journal of Cardiovascular Nursing*, and Co-Director of the RICH Heart Program.

Serap Osman is a Health Psychology Researcher at the Centre for Behavioural and Social Sciences in Medicine, UCL, UK.

Jerry C. Parker PhD is the Associate Dean for Research at the School of Medicine, University of Missouri, USA.

Sheetal Patel is an Honorary Research Assistant at Royal Free & University College London Medical School Centre for Behavioural & Social Sciences in Medicine, UK.

Nina Rieckmann PhD is Assistant Professor at the Department of Psychiatry, Mount Sinai School of Medicine, USA.

Margreet Scharloo PhD is Lecturer in Medical Psychology at Leiden University, The Netherlands.

Nancy E. Schoenberg PhD is the Marion Pearsall Professor of Behavioral Science and Associate Editor of *The Gerontologist* at the University of Kentucky, USA.

Anna Serlachius Researcher, Deakin University, Australia

Timothy C. Skinner is helping to establish a fruit farm in Scotland while writing academic papers and learning to make Native American flutes.

Jane R. Smith is a Lecturer in Health Psychology at the School of Medicine, Health Policy & Practice, University of East Anglia, UK.

Lucia Snoei MA is a Researcher at Leiden University, The Netherlands.

Frank J. Snoek is Professor of Medical Psychology at the Diabetes Psychology Research Group, VU University Medical Centre, The Netherlands.

Stephen Sutton PhD is Professor of Behavioural Science at the University of Cambridge, UK.

John Weinman PhD is a Professor at the Health Psychology Section, King's College London, UK.

Manuel Paz Yepez Department of Psychiatry, Mount Sinai School of Medicine, USA.

Introduction

It has increasingly become recognized that the self-management of physical health conditions is an important aspect of today's health care systems. Yet, despite a growing body of work, there are few attempts to bring together in a single volume a comprehensive picture of the area that presents the background, context, theory and compares and contrasts what is known about self-management in different illness areas. The current book aims to address this need. The book is organized in five parts. Part I addresses the social and cultural context which makes self-management a central issue in today's health care. Part II presents the theoretical underpinnings and guidance on development. Part III presents the issues on the evaluation of self-management interventions. Part IV examines the literature of self-management in a number of illness areas. Part V contains the concluding chapter that examines the future of self-management.

In presenting evidence on the state of self-management, the first essential task is to be clear on what is meant by the term self-management. A lack of consistency in the use of the term can only serve as a barrier to progression of the field. At best it increases inconsistencies in interventions and at worst there is a danger of self-management becoming a term that is used to re-badge activity with little real change in practice.

In this book we have used the single, albeit wide-ranging definition of self-management given by Barlow et al. (2002). This is:

> Self-management refers to the individual's ability to manage the symptoms, treatment, physical and psychosocial consequences and lifestyle changes inherent in living with a chronic condition. Efficacious self-management encompasses ability to monitor one's condition and to effect the cognitive, behavioural and emotional responses necessary to maintain a satisfactory quality of life. Thus, a dynamic and continuous process of self-regulation is established.

This definition highlights that self-management of a chronic illness is not solely concerned with managing the medical aspects of the illness, such as self-monitoring of symptoms or taking medication, but also involves dealing with the broader impact of the illness on daily life. Self-management extends beyond behaviour change to also encompass the emotional and social adjustments that people have to make to cope with a chronic illness. An important aspect of this book is to examine the extent to which interventions address all or only some of these aspects of self-management. Within the chapters on specific conditions, authors have been requested to reflect on the extent that interventions meet this definition, even where the label may have been used differently within the literature.

To appreciate the field of self-management, one first must understand the socio-cultural context within which self-management has taken on a growing importance. Part I addresses two important contextual areas. Chapter 1 (Hyde et al.) starts the debate by presenting evidence on the demographic and social changes in recent years which have led to a context where the traditional approaches to the management of chronic illnesses have and are being questioned. Of particular importance is the role of the ageing population where one prevalent view suggests that the increasing proportion of older people will lead to an increase in chronic illness that is likely to become unmanageable with current health practices. While this view is not without its critics, it is one premise that has led to self-management interventions as positing an additional important aspect of chronic disease management.

Chapter 2 reflects on how changing attitudes to and of patients within health care have enabled a self-management approach to take place. In this chapter Coulter and Ellins highlight the importance of a more critical and demanding patient who has a desire for a more interactive role within their health care through joint decision-making with their health care professionals.

Key issues concerning the development and delivery of self-management interventions are covered in Part II. In Chapter 3 Serlachius and Sutton describe those theories that have been most prevalent in the field of self-management and discuss the relative benefits of these different approaches to behaviour change. There is some evidence to suggest that where interventions are based on sound theoretical principles, they tend to have greater efficacy. However, these theoretical approaches are to be contrasted with the later illness-based chapters, which indicate that to date, many interventions have little theoretical perspective and tend to take a more pragmatic approach. Such pragmatic approaches are often driven by clinical agendas that see the need for change in practice but have paid less attention to deriving these interventions from theory. While this pragmatism can be understood from a clinical perspective, it can in some circumstances serve to limit progress.

To appreciate the multifaceted nature of many self-management interventions and the global nature of the term, Mulligan et al. (Chapter 4) present common components that comprise these interventions. By examining the components, it becomes clear the variety of approaches that come under a self-management banner. In addition, although components are presented as well defined, this is rarely the case in self-management interventions. To understand any such intervention, it is important to identify the components and this leads directly to a need for typography of components. This chapter also discusses the relationship between self-management interventions and other approaches such as cognitive behavioural interventions and cognitive behavioural therapy.

Following the chapter on components, the issue of delivery of self-management interventions is discussed in Chapter 5 by McGowan and Lorig. They present the relative benefits of issues such as group versus individual interventions, and who should deliver such interventions. They also discuss approaches to encourage self-management within the routine consultation and other novel ways of delivery such as through telephone- or computer-based programmes. The issue of intervention delivery and specifically the training of facilitators is further explored in Chapter 6 by Hardeman and Michie who consider that not only the overall approach but also many of the components of self-management interventions are outside of the traditional training of health care professionals (or lay leaders) and that an adequate investment in training in this arena is essential if self-management is to be delivered in anything more than name. Further, they highlight that to understand the extent that interventions are delivered as anticipated, checks on treatment fidelity become essential. Such analysis should be seen as a central part of the design and evaluation of self-management interventions and Steed picks up this point in Chapter 8.

The final chapter (Cooke et al.) in this second part of the book looks to the potential role of technology in the evolution of self-management. It highlights that the issues in the widespread adoption of technology in this area of health care extend beyond their efficacy and include the attitudes of people with the condition, as well as professionals using the technology, and the system to cope with new ways of working.

Part III addresses the issues of research and evaluation of self-management interventions. Chapter 8 (Steed et al.) illustrates how linking underlying theory to evaluation may not only be reflected in the efficacy of interventions but may also lead to greater understanding of which mechanisms are active and most fruitful in self-management. Such systematic analysis will address the current criticism that is often levelled at self-management interventions that although they may show some efficacy, what works for whom and at what time points is often not elucidated. A model of intervention development based on the UK's MRC development of complex interventions is presented as a guiding principle. They highlight the need for such interventions to go through an integrative process using feedback from early feasibility studies to refine the intervention before formal assessment. Crucial to the evaluation of self-management interventions is a clear understanding of the types of outcome used to assess efficacy and their properties. This topic is explored by De Vellis and Blaylock in Chapter 9.

Part IV presents overviews of self-management interventions within a range of chronic illnesses. The current state of self-management for each condition is reflected upon by experts within each area. While the conditions presented in this section are not an exhaustive coverage of conditions where self-management interventions have been applied, conditions were selected which were either most developed or where self-management is particularly central as management of the condition involves a variety of behaviours and pressures on the person. In Chapters 10–16 the conditions covered include many of the major chronic illnesses and include diabetes (Snoek et al.), arthritis (Parker et al.), asthma (Smith), coronary artery disease (Schoenberg et al.), heart failure (Mulligan), COPD (Kaptein et al.) and hypertension (Rieckmann et al.).

It is important to point out that some conditions with high prevalence are not covered. These include the work that has evolved from neurorehabilitation such as stroke and head injury, as well as newly developed interventions such as those in lower urinary tract symptoms. These are primarily excluded because although self-management is pertinent to these conditions, too few studies have been conducted to legitimize review. In addition, in the case of stroke, the focus of interventions has primarily been in reducing disability through rehabilitation as opposed to through a self-management approach. It is hoped that this section will illustrate the differences in the nature and evolution of self-management in the conditions covered and how the symptoms, treatment and nature of the disease has served to drive the development of self-management interventions.

The final chapter of the book (Chapter [17]) concludes by considering the future of self-management. It focuses on how research evidence can be translated into practice and looks at barriers to this process and finally concludes with suggested directions for the future practice of self-management.

Stanton Newman
Liz Steed
Kathleen Mulligan

Part I

Context

1 The health profile of ageing populations

Martin Hyde, Paul Higgs and Stanton Newman

Introduction

Populations are ageing and life expectancy continues to increase throughout most of the world as both death rates at older ages and fertility rates decline. Although many rightly celebrate these achievements in the extension of human life, others are asking whether present and future cohorts of older people will be healthier than previous generations or whether increased longevity comes with deteriorating health, an increased risk of disability or poor quality of life. Disability and chronic illness are connected concepts insofar as the former represents an objective assessment of physical limitations, while, according to Armstrong (2005) the latter corresponds to the development of long-term health conditions that may or may not have an impact on assessments of disability. Their relationship to quality of life is linked to the growing significance of the patient's perspective of the impact of chronic conditions and/or disability (Armstrong 2005). By charting changes in life expectancy and rates of chronic illness and disability, we are able to provide a better basis for understanding the changing circumstances in which chronic illness occurs and is treated. This provides a backdrop for considering the potential role and importance of self-management.

Epidemiological transitions

Writers such as Wesndorp (2006) have argued that human genes are programmed for early survival, hence for reproduction, not ageing. Therefore, although the risk of early mortality has been successively reduced, through improvements in the occupational environment and advances in medicine, health remains determined by this genetic heritage and the human body is unable to cope with ageing itself. Conversely, others have argued that there is no natural limit to human lifespan (Kirkwood 1999; Wilmoth et al. 2000). Crimmins (2004) situates this debate between the 'failure of success' model and the 'compression of morbidity' thesis. The argument that increased longevity might lead to higher rates of morbidity and/or disability, the 'failure of success' can be seen as part of a general set of theories that raise concerns about the impact of modern medicine on human ageing.

Notable are the arguments that industrial societies have passed through a third (or fourth or even a fifth) epidemiological transition which, by eliminating many acute and occupational illnesses, has shifted the burden of disease onto chronic conditions in later life (Dubos 1965; Antonovsky 1968; Omran 1971; Olshansky and Ault 1986; Olshansky et al. 1997; Smallman-Raynor and Phillips 1999). Related to this is the success of medical interventions in the treatment and management of children with chronic disorders which enable them to survive into early adulthood and even beyond (Gruenberg 1977). Finally, other writers have argued that increases in medical expenditure are mainly focused on very intensive and expensive medical care to preserve life in elderly, very ill, disabled persons but which only result in limited levels of additional and relatively poor quality life (Waidmann and Manton 1998).

However, these positions have become increasingly challenged. Some commentators have argued that linking industrialization with chronic disease is based largely on the historically and culturally localized instances of increased risk of male coronary heart disease found in the USA and the UK during decades following World War II (Kaplan and Keil 1993). Other researchers have produced evidence that the health of older people has been improving for a considerable time in parts of the industrialized world (Lanska and Mi 1993; Fogel 1994; Perutz 1998; Padiak 2005). Thus, contrary to the argument that increased life expectancy comes at the cost of an 'expansion of morbidity', writers such as James Fries have proposed a thesis built around a 'compression of morbidity' (Fries 1980; Fries et al. 1989; Fries 2003). Simply stated, the argument holds that, even with increasing longevity, the proportion of life that is spent in ill health, that is with morbid conditions, will be concentrated into an ever shorter period prior to death. As Olshansky et al. (1990) make clear, mortality and morbidity are linked through changes in the exposure to risk factors. Thus, if ill health in later life is connected to the main causes of death, then an increase in the age of death will lead to a compression of morbidity. But if morbidity is unrelated to mortality then there will be an expansion of morbidity.

Manton (1982) has proposed a third model – the 'dynamic equilibrium model' – which is commonly seen as a mid-point between the expansion and compression of morbidity arguments. His model assumes that (population) ageing will result in a greater incidence of disease and chronic illness but that these will be less severe. For example, data from the Medicare Beneficiary Survey (MCBS) in the USA show that there has been an increase in some cardiovascular diseases but that these are less disabling than in the past (Crimmins 2004).

However, the debate on the health of older people has suffered from argument at cross purposes. Different studies use different definitions and/or dimensions of health and illness. Furthermore, although most studies have focused on disability as this accounts for a large share of health and social care expenditure, it is important to note that not all older people will necessarily pass through the same stages and some can actually move out of poor health states (Crimmins 2004). In addition, some conditions that affect health care usage, such as diabetes and hypertension (see Chapters 10, 16), do not result in disability in the early stages of the condition but, in the context of this book, have implications for self-management interventions, which are designed to limit the impact of a chronic condition.

Yet the arguments about the health of older people are not merely questions of scholarly interest. A better understanding of the (future) health of older people is of crucial policy importance as it affects public expenditure on the income, health and long-term care needs of the ageing populations and the potential importance of self-management to limit the complications and costs associated with some chronic conditions. In ageing societies these costs will have critical implications for the future financial stability of national budgets. There are two main areas of concern; labour market participation rates of older workers (often crudely referred to as dependency ratios) and projected health care expenditure. Labour force participation rates among older workers have been falling drastically (Kohli and Rein 1991; Guillemard and Rein 1993; Gruber and Wise 1998; Yeandle 2003; Laczko and Phillipson 2004). Although much attention has rightly been given to the increase in early voluntary labour market exit, it ought not to be forgotten that poor health is still a major factor in forcing older workers out of the labour market (Emmerson and Tetlow 2005; Beatty and Fothergill 2003).

However, it is generally concern about future pressures on health care use that has generated the most alarm. It is certainly true that older people are relatively heavy users of (primary) health care. In England data for 2002/3 showed that although those aged 65 years and over made up only 16 per cent of the population, they accounted for 47 per cent of total hospital and community health spending. Over the same period around 20 per cent of the English population aged 50 years and over had consulted a GP and 10 per cent had seen a practice nurse in the previous fortnight. One in five older people had attended an outpatient or casualty department in the previous year and one in ten had had a hospital inpatient stay (Evandrou 2005).

Turning to a consideration of disability and dependency, the projections from the Wanless report in the UK, based on the prevalence of ADL and Instrumental Activities of Daily Living (IADL) limitations in the 1998/9 General Household Survey, have shown that there will be a 57 per cent rise in the number of dependent older people between 2001–2031. The report's authors argue, based on these figures, places in residential care will need to expand from around 400,000 in 1996 to 450,000 by 2010 and 670,000 by 2031. This represents an increase of about 65 per cent over the period. In addition, the number of home care hours provided will have to increase from just below 2 million hours per week in 1996 to around 2.9 million per week by 2031, an increase of 48 per cent. Overall this would correspond to a rise, in real terms, of around 148 per cent in expenditure on long-term care which would mean an increase from around £9.8b in 1996 to around £24.3b in 2031 (Wittenberg et al. 2001; Comas-Herrera et al. 2003). To the extent that improved management techniques are available to keep people in their own homes and managing their own condition, this expansion in costs may be able to be contained.

However, the real costs of population ageing will depend on the actual health of future cohorts of older people (Cutler 2001a; Cutler 2001b), as present-day evidence demonstrates health care utilization is highly influenced by the health of older people. For example, only 16 per cent of those aged between 65–74 living in England who did not have a limiting long-standing illness (LLI) visited a GP in the last two weeks. Yet for those in the same age group who did have a LLI, the figure was double that at 32 per cent. Similarly, only 10 per cent of those without a LLI visited a practice nurse compared to 15 per cent of those with a LLI (Evandrou 2005). Therefore, when assessing the utility of their projections Wittenberg et al. (2001:13) conclude that *'past trends may not provide reliable estimates of future trends* [and] *much may depend on the future management of disabling conditions'*.

Trends in life expectancy and lifespan

Over the last half of the twentieth century, we have witnessed gains in life expectancy across the majority of the world's regions. As can be seen from the data on selected countries presented in Figure 1.1, there has been a substantial rise in life expectancy at birth throughout the Organization for Economic Co-operation and Development (OECD). On average life expectancy increased by 9.2 years for the OECD 30 from

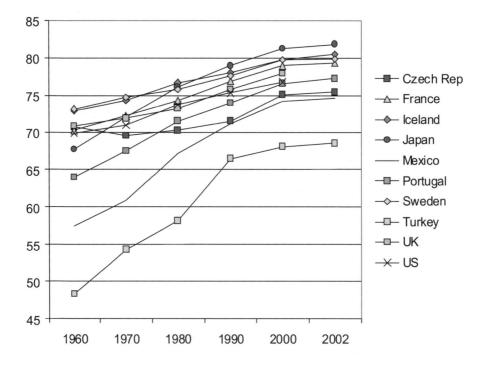

Source: OECD (2004).

Figure 1.1 Life expectancy at birth for selected OECD countries: 1960–2002

1960 to 2002. However, some countries recorded much greater increases. For example, life expectancy in Japan rose by 14 years, an average of a third of a year per year, while in Turkey life expectancy rose by 20 years, an average of nearly half a year per year over this period. What is remarkable about these improvements is that, especially, although not exclusively, in the advanced industrial economies, they are due to gains in life expectancy from mid-life rather than those produced by combating infant mortality as was witnessed at the beginning of the last century (Vaupel and Jeune 1994; Manton and Vaupel 1995). As the data in Figures 1.2 and 1.3 show, the rise in life expectancy at age 65 has been rising for both men and women, although somewhat steeper for women, since the 1960s.

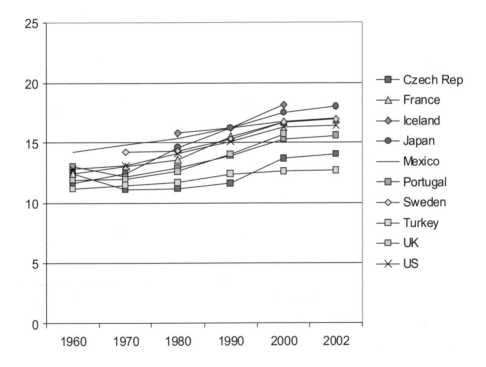

Source: OECD (2004).

Figure 1.2 Male life expectancy at age 65 for selected OECD countries: 1960–2002

As an alternative to life expectancy, which is based on the average age of death for a cohort, some researchers have been looking at the maximum lifespan to test the assertion that there is a fixed limit to human life. Swedish data on the oldest achieved age of any recorded individual show that this has risen from 101 years in 1850 to 108 years in the 1990s. This increase has been more marked over the latter decades of the period. Lifespan rose by 0.44 years per decade from 1850 to 1969 and by 1.1 years per

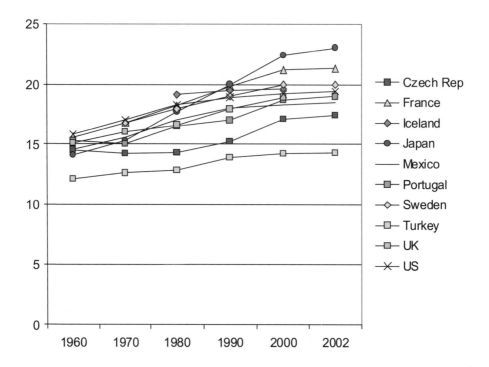

Source: OECD (2004).

Figure 1.3 Female life expectancy at age 65 for selected OECD countries: 1960–2002

decade from then up to the end of the 1990s. Seventy per cent of this increase was found to be attributable to a reduction in mortality rates among those aged 70 years and over (Wilmoth et al. 2000).

These developments are not restricted to the advanced industrialized economies. The gap in life expectancy between the developing and the developed world narrowed considerably over the latter half of the last century. In 1960 those in the more developed countries could expect to live an average of 22 years longer than their counterparts in the developing world. By 2000 this has been reduced to a difference of 12 years. However, the gap between men in the developing world and the developed world today is much less than that for women, being 9 years and 14 years, respectively (UN 2001).

However, some writers have argued that these trends may slow, stagnate or even reverse. Olshansky et al. (1990) calculated that for life expectancy at birth to reach 85 years in the USA, mortality rates from all causes of death would need to decline by 55 per cent for all ages or by 60 per cent among those aged 50 years and over. Hence, they concluded that 'barring major advances in the development and use of life extending technologies in the alteration of human aging at the molecular level, the period of rapid increases in life expectancy in the developed nations has come to an end' (Olshansky et al. 1990: 634).

Many have predicted the emergence of an 'obesity epidemic' which may reverse this upward trend and may lead to new patterns of chronic illness. Olshansky et al. (2005) argue that current trends in obesity in the USA may result in a decline in life expectancy for future cohorts. Based on current rates of death associated with obesity, they predict that life expectancy will be reduced by between one-third and three-quarters of a year. A study from the Netherlands appears to offer empirical evidence for these claims. Janssen et al. (2003) found a sudden reversal of old age mortality decline in 1980. Increases in smoking-related cancers and pulmonary disease were found to be chiefly responsible for this reversal. One may conclude from these studies that health behaviour (as opposed to technology) appears to be the greatest influence on declines in life expectancy. This has implications for developing strategies to tackle any future health problems within an ageing population and might suggest that greater research on, and investment in, behaviour modifying programmes is warranted.

Population ageing

Notwithstanding these arguments, the general trends towards longer life, coupled with falling fertility rates throughout many parts of the world, have resulted in greater proportions of the global population entering older age. By 2050 it is estimated that there will be almost 2 billion people aged 60 years or over throughout the world. If these projections are correct then there will be more older people than children on the planet, which in and of itself will mark an unprecedented event in human history. Although these demographic trends have been the subject of much discussion, this has mainly been in relation to the trends in Europe and north America. Less well discussed is that in the near future the largest number of older people are actually expected to be found in the developing world. As Figures 1.4–1.7 show population ageing has become a truly global phenomenon. Although only 12 per cent of the population in the developing world is expected to be aged over 60 by 2025, compared to 25 per cent in the developed world, they will number around 860 million representing approximately 71 per cent of the world's older population (Mboya 2003; Wisnesale 2003). In 2002 there were around 40 million people aged over 60 years in Africa and although life expectancy is expected to decline slightly in the first decade of the twenty-first century, mainly due to the impact of AIDS/HIV mortality, by 2025 Africans can expect to live to 71 years on average which will be only six years less than the life expectancy of those living in the developed world. In the former Soviet states of east and central Europe, there are around 70 million older people and, although this is expected to decline somewhat, by 2010 the proportion of the population aged over 60 years will also be greater than the proportion of children in this region. It is, however, Asia that dominates the present and future scenario of an ageing global population. Today, just over half of those aged over 60 years and over live in Asia, the largest numbers of, some 130 million, which are in China. This group as a whole is expected to rise to around two-thirds of the global aged population (Allen et al. 2002).

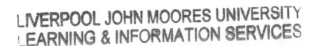

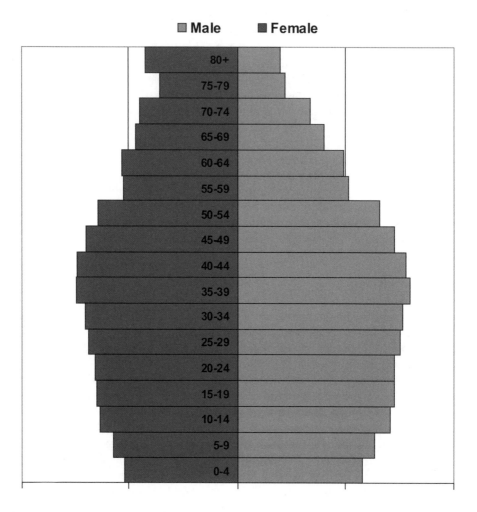

Source: www.census.gov/cgi-bin/ipc/agggen.

Figure 1.4 Population pyramid for the more developed world region: 2000

Trends in chronic illnesses among older people

Population ageing raises a whole series of serious concerns for health as many chronic illnesses, such as cardiovascular disease, arthritis and diabetes, rise with age. For example, congestive heart failure (HF) currently afflicts 4.7 million Americans, with 550,000 new cases diagnosed each year. The burden of HF is greatest in the older population, with 80 per cent of HF hospitalizations and 90 per cent of HF-related deaths occurring among those aged 65 years and older (Harlan et al. 2000). Indeed, heart failure is the single most frequent reason for hospitalization among the elderly

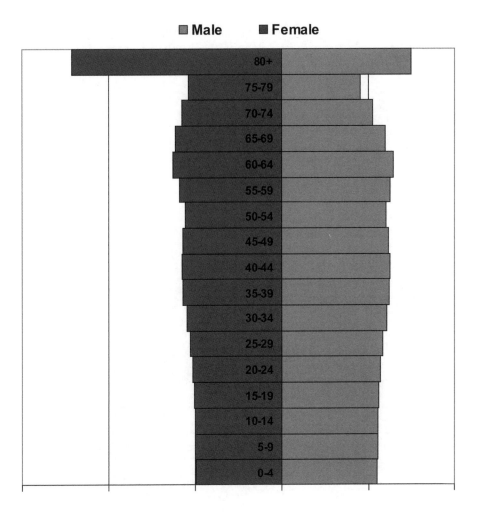

Source: www.census.gov/cgi-bin/ipc/agggen.

Figure 1.5 Projected population pyramid for the more developed world region: 2050

population. In turn, higher rates of hospitalization and more intensive care unit days have also been shown to be associated with higher health care costs. Data on 4860 older participants from the National Heart, Lung and Blood Institute Cardiovascular Study to Medicare from 1992 to 2003 reveal that mean medical costs over the 10-year period were significantly higher among older Americans with HF than those without (Liao et al. 2007).

However, getting reliable longitudinal or cross-national data on the rates of chronic illness among older people is often difficult (Kupari et al. 1997). For example, despite the tremendous methodological and statistical effort invested in reporting the prevalence of chronic illnesses and disability from the Global Burden of Disease study,

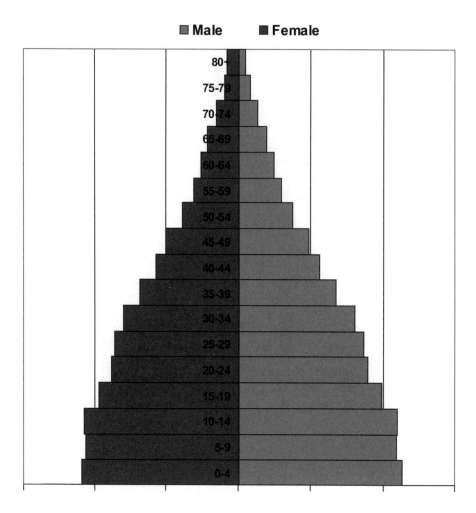

Source: www.census.gov/cgi-bin/ipc/agggen.

Figure 1.6 Population pyramid for the less developed world region: 2000

Lopez et al. (2006) do not show any data on those aged 60 years or over. What data does exist is largely confined to the advanced industrial high-income countries. This fact reflects both the population age structure and the development of data collection agencies and surveys in these countries relative to less developed parts of the world. Despite this every effort has been made to present data on as wide a range of countries as possible. However, this means that the number of chronic conditions that are covered are not as extensive as they could be. Instead, they are restricted to those that are most routinely recorded. These are inevitably those which pose the greatest burden of disease in the population (as a whole). Based on the Global Burden of Disease ischemic heart failure and cerebrovascular diseases were the two most

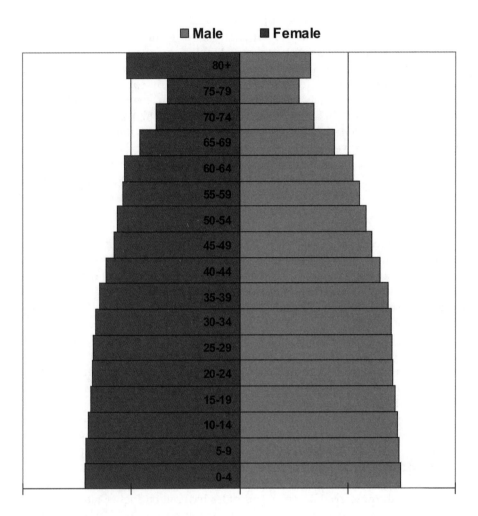

■ Male   ■ Female

Source: www.census.gov/cgi-bin/ipc/agggen.

Figure 1.7 Projected population pyramid for the less developed world region: 2050

important causes of death in the world in 1990 and are predicted to remain so by 2020 (Murray and Lopez 1997). Given the age-associated decrements in cardiovascular performance (Oxenham and Sharpe 2003), trends and patterns in coronary illness are a major focus of this section.

Cardiovascular and coronary heart disease

According to the World Health Organization (WHO), globally 16.7 million people died in 2003 from cardiovascular disease (CVD). This represents close to 30 per cent of all worldwide deaths. In addition, there were 7.22 million deaths from CHD and around 15 million people each year suffer strokes of whom around 5.5 million die and a further 5 million are left permanently disabled.

Cardiovascular illness among older people is a major concern in the USA. A congressional budget report found that Americans with congestive heart failure, coronary artery disease or diabetes are much more likely to be in the top 25 per cent of Medicare beneficiaries (Congressional Budget Office (CBO) 2005). Data from the National Health Interview Survey (USA) in 2000/1 found that 31.1 per cent of respondents aged 65 years and over reported some form of heart disease and 49.2 per cent said that they had been diagnosed with hypertension (NCHS Data on Aging). The rates of hypertension, stroke and CHD among older Americans have remained relatively stable since 1997. There is, however, evidence of an increase in diabetes. In 1997 around 13 per cent of the over 65s had diabetes. By 2004 this had risen to nearly 17 per cent.

Similar concerns are shared in Canada where CVD accounts for more deaths than any other disease; 34 per cent of male deaths and 36 per cent of female deaths. This costs the Canadian economy $18.4b annually. As the number of older Canadians has been increasing, the number of deaths due to stroke and CHD is also predicted to increase. However, a study of data from the National Population Health Survey, 1994/5 on the health status of older people found that the 'profile of this [elderly] population ... is in many respects not much different from that of the remaining adult population until the age of 75 years' (Rosenburg and Moore 1997: 1025). However, after the age of 75 people were much more likely to experience cardiovascular helth prohlems. This was found to be associated with an increased use of health care services (Rosenburg and Moore 1997).

In Europe data from the Survey for Health, Ageing and Retirement in Europe (SHARE) show that national variations in the prevalence of heart disease are evident although not dramatic (see table 4). For example, among those aged between 50 and 64 years, the proportion who have high blood pressure ranges from 22 per cent in The Netherlands to 30 per cent in Italy. However, age differences are starker. In each country studied, those aged 65 years and older have much higher rates of all heart diseases, often by a considerable margin. For example 8 per cent of Swedes aged 50 to 64 reported having been diagnosed with a heart attack compared with 26 per cent of those aged 65 years and over. Similar figures are found elsewhere. Estimates from the Helsinki Ageing Study show that around 54 per cent of Finns aged 75–86 experience hypertension, 54 per cent reported ischemic heart disease and 8 per cent suffered congestive heart failure (Kupari et al. 1997). The prevalence of cardiovascular disorders among those aged over 65 years in Estonia ranged from 63.2 per cent who had been diagnosed with hypertension, 56.5 per cent with CHD, 41.4 per cent with heart failure and 9.8 per cent with MI. However, the prevalence of CHD was much higher in those aged 85 and over (Saks et al. 2003). Models based on data drawn from the General Practice Registry Database (GPRD) in the UK found that the number of cases of coronary heart disease is predicted to increase by 44 per cent to 3,900,000 in 2031 leading to an increase of 32 per cent, to 265,000, in the number of hospital admissions. In addition, the number of cases of heart failure is predicted to increase by 54 per cent to 1,303,000 in 2031 and the number of admissions is predicted to rise by 55 per cent to 124,000. Finally, the number of cases of atrial fibrillation is predicted to increase by 46 per cent to 1,093,000 with a corresponding rise in the number of hospital admissions by 39 per cent to 85,000 (Majeed and Aylin 2005).

These concerns are not restricted to the advanced industrial economies. Data from the INTERHEART study showed that rates of CVD have risen greatly in low- and middle-income countries with about 80 per cent of the global burden of disease occurring in these countries (Lancet 2004: 364, 937–52). About 140m people in the Americas suffer from hypertension. The prevalence of hypertension in Latin America and the Caribbean has been estimated at between 8–30 per cent. In Africa the prevalence of hypertension is estimated at 20 million people. Some 250,000 deaths are estimated to have been preventable through effective case management. Projections suggest that in China hypertension will increase from 18.6 per cent to 25 per cent between 1995–2025. In India the equivalent figures are 16.3 per cent and 19.4 per cent.

Diabetes is also a global health concern and not restricted to the developed economies of Europe and north America. Some authors have already begun to talk about a global 'diabetes epidemic'. When one considers the predictions such terminology is understandable. Estimates from the Diabetes Atlas show that the number of people worldwide with diabetes is expected to rise from 194 million in 2003 to 333 million in 2025. Much of this increase is assumed to be caused by population ageing dynamics. Given the association between age and the presence of diabetes this appears well founded. Rates of type 2 diabetes rise from almost zero among the under 19s to around 12 per cent among 60 to 64-year-olds and around 14 per cent for over 80-year-olds (Wild et al. 2000). If, as the data above suggest, the proportion of the population aged over 80 years experience the greatest increase over the coming decades, then this might have serious implications for the rates of diabetes in the population. Wild et al. (2004) used data from around 40 countries to extrapolate the age-specific prevalence of diabetes in all 191 WHO member states. Assuming that associated risk factors such as obesity remain stable, they predict that the prevalence of diabetes for all age groups will rise from 2.8 per cent in 2000 to 4.4 per cent in 2030. They argue that the most important factor in this predicted increase will be the growth in the number of people aged 65 years and over. Their data show that in the developed world the greatest number of people will be aged 65 years and over, with nearly twice as many as those aged 45 to 64. In the developing world it will be the middle-aged group which will have the greatest number of people with diabetes. Yet in this region the greatest relative rise will be among the over 65s, from just over 20 million to around 80 million. However, another study, based on prevalence data from Finland and Samoa, found that 'improved life expectancy … and population demographic changes could explain no more than 20–25% of the total increase in the prevalence of diabetes' (Colagiuri et al. 2005).

Underpinning these projected increases in diabetes is the assumption that rates of obesity will remain unchanged. The evidence seems to suggest an accelerated obesity increase. The Centre for Disease Control reports that in 1990 in the USA, of those states participating in the Behavioral Risk Factor Surveillance System, 10 states had a prevalence of obesity of less than 10 per cent and no states had prevalence equal to or greater than 15 per cent. This had changed by 1998, where no state had a prevalence of obesity of less than 10 per cent, seven states had a prevalence of obesity between 20–24 per cent, and no state had prevalence equal to or greater than 25 per cent. In 2006 yet further dramatic increases in obesity were found. At that time only four states had a prevalence of obesity of less than 20 per cent and twenty-two states had a prevalence equal or greater than 25 per cent (Mokdad 1999, 2001; CDC 2006). Rates of obesity in Europe vary significantly by country but the general trend shows a clear increase in numbers. This is most noticeable in the UK where rates of obesity in women more than doubled to 20 per cent between 1908–1998 (Petersen et al. 2005).What is important about the impact of obesity is that it is directly linked to behaviours that are under voluntary control. It is clear that dietary and exercise behaviours, targets of self-management interventions, can have an impact on the projected increase of diabetes and resulting complications in those who develop the condition.

Trends in functioning and disability among older people

Although the prevalence of chronic illness among the older population is a major research and policy focus, especially in relation to interventions to reduce the impact of chronic conditions, an important related issue is older individuals' functioning and disability. This is perhaps to be expected given the importance that these have for welfare expenditure. It is also unsurprising that, as entitlement to Medicare starts at age 65, the majority of data available in this area comes from the USA.

In the 1970s data from the National Health Interview Survey (NHIS) showed increasing proportions of older adults classifying themselves as limited in certain activities of daily living. Despite concerns raised over methodological and conceptual problems with these data (Wilson and Drury 1984), many researchers concluded that the health of older people deteriorated in the 1970s (Colvez and Blanchet 1981; Verbrugge 1984, 1989; Chirikos 1986; Crimmins 1990; Crimmins and Ingegneri 1993, 1994; Crimmins et al. 1997). However, the NHIS trend in self-reported disability rates changed dramatically during the 1980s. Between 1983–1993 the data showed statistically significant declines in the prevalence of disabilities related to routine needs (Waidmann et al. 1995). These patterns have been observed in a series of other US studies. Possibly the main source of information on the health of older Americans is the National Long Term Care Survey (NLTCS). Analyses of the NLTCS have consistently shown downward trends in the prevalence of chronic disability. For the 12-year period between 1982–1994, for example, NLTCS data show that the proportion of the 65 to 74-year-olds free from chronic disability increased by 2.6 percentage points while the corresponding proportion of the 75 to 84-year-olds rose by 5.4 percentage points (Manton et al. 1997b). The proportion of those with only IADL impairments fell by nearly one-quarter for those aged 65–84 years and the proportion of those who were either ADL-impaired or institutionalized fell significantly for all age groups. These declines have been confirmed using multivariate analyses applied to a broader range of disability measures which included a series of physical performance assessments (Manton et al. 1998b). More recently Manton and Land have returned to these data to estimate active life expectancy (ALE), which they define as the period of life free from difficulties with ADL tasks. Their analyses revealed longer periods of ALE than had previously been estimated (Manton and Land 2000).

Another longitudinal study that has been used is the Survey of Income and Program Participation (SIPP). A comparison of data using several measures of physical function, such as reading a newspaper, lifting and carrying a package weighing 10 pounds, for the 1984 and 1993 panels found statistically significant declines in functional limitation for several measures over the nine-year period (Freedman and Martin 1997a). Data from the Longitudinal Study of Aging (LSOA) from 1986, 1988 and 1990 found no evidence of significant declines in ADL disability (Waidmann and Manton 1998). However, recent analyses of LSOA data that controlled for changes in the age and sex composition of the non-institutionalized population found that the disability prevalence rate fell by 2 percentage points between 1982 and 1993 (Crimmins et al. 1997). Similarly, preliminary analysis of the Medicare Current Beneficiary Survey (MCBS) , which controlled for demographic shifts in age, ethnic group, educational qualifications, marital status, and gender, found significant declines in both ADL and IADL disability and in measures of functional limitation (Waidmann and Liu 1998). Figures 1.8 and 1.9 show the rates of ADL and IADL limitation in the MCBS sample. As can be seen the prevalence of limitations in almost all ADL and IADL tasks has dropped although for some, such as walking or doing heavy housework, the decline is more noticeable.

However, some commentators have raised concerns about these findings. Firstly, some studies have revealed socio-economic differences in the prevalence of disability. Data from a sample of 149,000 men and 186,675 women aged 55 years and over, taken from the US Census 2000 Supplementary Survey, showed a clear gradient in limiting long-standing illness and household income with those in the most advantageous economic position reporting the lowest rates of long-standing illness (Minkler et al. 2006). Although time series data from the NHIS from 1982 to 2002 show that all groups experienced declines in the age and gendered adjusted prevalence of disability over this 20-year period, the average annual percentage declines were smaller for the least advantaged socio-economic groups (Schoeni 2005). Similarly, other studies have found a smaller decline in disability rates for those with lower educational qualifications and for African Americans (Clark et al. 1996; Manton et al. 1997b; Manton et al. 1998).

Others have raised concerns over the survey methodologies and the (different) ways in which disability and/or functional limitation have been operationalized in the different surveys and across time. Waidmann and Manton (1998) identify five possible threats to the validity of these data: differences in the survey methodology, that is whether the sample includes the institutionalized population, how the data are collected and what form the questions take; changes or differences in the proxy rates, that is Dorevitch et al. (1992) found that proxy respondents are more likely to report disability than sample members themselves; non-random attrition (for longitudinal surveys); environmental changes; and socio-economic changes.

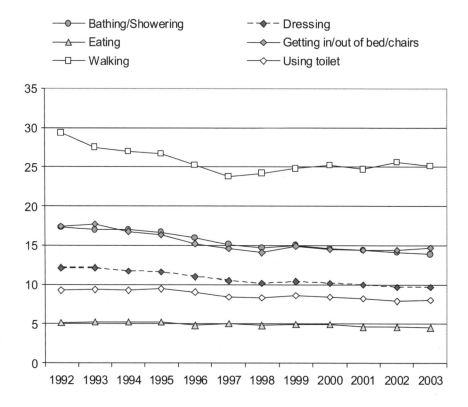

Source: Medicare Beneficiary Survey.

Figure 1.8 Difficulty performing activities of daily living among those aged 65 years and over in the USA: 1992–2003

A working group set up to evaluate these trends drew attention to the different wording used in different studies to measure functional limitation. For example, some studies ask whether the respondent finds it difficult to perform the task, while others ask whether they require help to perform the task (Freedman et al. 2004). In order to address this Wolf et al. (2005) re-analysed the data from the NLTCS. They restricted the analyses to those aged between 65–69 in order to be able to handle the different ways in which ADLs have been asked in the studies. Their findings show a more gradual decline than previous analyses. A systematic review of 16 articles (selected from over 800) which shows a reduction in disability among older people in the USA of about 1.55 per cent and 0.92 per cent per annum from the 1980s and reductions in IADLs of between 2.74–0.40 per cent offers considerable support for these findings (Freedman et al. 2002). Thus, methodological considerations notwithstanding, there seems to be a general consensus that 'overall the weight of evidence suggests large disability reductions as reported in the NLTCS' (Cutler 2001a).

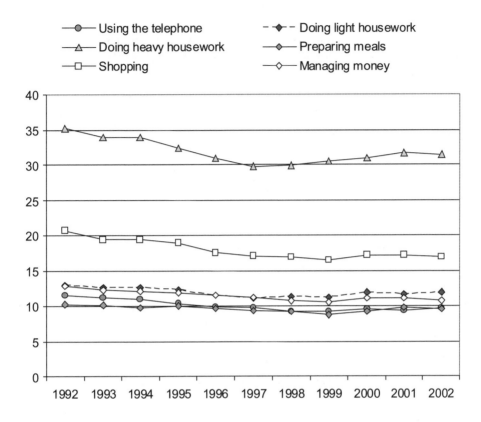

Source: Medicare Beneficiary Survey.

Figure 1.9 Difficulty performing instrumental activities of daily living among those aged 65 years and over in the USA: 1992–2002

Although most of the data has come from the USA, there are some studies from Europe and the rest of the world which have been used to explore these trends as well. In the mid-1990s Bone (1995) published data on the rates of limiting long-standing illness in the older British population. Although she had expected to find increasing rates of dependency (an expansion of morbidity), she reported fairly stable trends over the two decades. For the purpose of this chapter we have updated these findings. As Figure 1.10 shows there has been a rise in the proportions reporting a long-standing illness for both age groups (although more so for those aged 65–74 years). However, in line with Bone's original findings, rates of limiting long-standing illness are stable across the period for both age groups.

The Burden of Disease Network Project (2004) reported that approximately 20 per cent of people aged 70 years and older and 50 per cent of people 85 and over living in the EU report difficulties in such basic activities of daily living as bathing

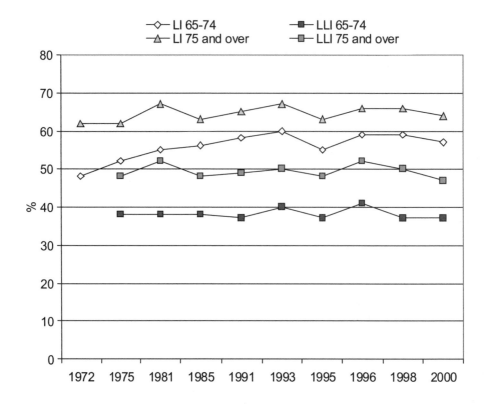

Source: General Household Survey.

Figure 1.10 The proportion of those aged 65–74 and those aged 75 and over reporting a long-standing illness (LI) and reporting a limiting long-standing illness (LLI) in the UK: 1972–2000

and dressing. Furthermore, according to the Evergreen project about 8 per cent of people aged 75 years and 28 per cent of people aged 85 were not able to move outdoors without assistance.

Cross-national data from SHARE on selected activities of daily living show relatively low rates of impairment across the region as well as national differences, with rates in Spain and France higher than those in the other countries. Similar trends are evident from other studies in France (Robine et al. 1998), Italy (Minicuci and Noale 2005), Australia (Mathers 1994), Taiwan (Tu and Chen 1994) and the Caribbean (Reyes-Ortiz et al. 2006).

One further caveat needs to be added to the summary of trends in disability and functioning in later life and this can be drawn from the considerable literature on the sociology of chronic illness that has emerged over the past few decades and which has focused on the experience of chronic conditions. Work by Mike Bury, among others, have pointed out the need to locate the understanding of disabling conditions and chronic illnesses within the accounts given by those living with the conditions (Bury 1997). They suggest that while disability prevalence rates may be decreasing, their individual and social significance may be changing as expectations of health change and the social definitions of ordinary life begin to cover wider and wider arenas. Evandrou and Falkingham (2000) point out that younger cohorts of older people report more limiting long-standing illness than did their predecessors at similar ages. This may reflect a greater propensity for all cohorts to report ill health or it may reflect real health differences between cohorts. While it is difficult to disentangle such period effects, the importance of this work is that perceptions and reporting of health, chronic illness and disability must be viewed in the contexts that people give them as well as from more detached vantage points.

Conclusion

This chapter has investigated the relationship between an ageing population and chronic health conditions and disability. The evidence is that alongside increases in longevity there have also been increases in some chronic conditions within older populations. It is against these data that the attempts to devise and demonstrate the efficacy and effectiveness of different methods of the management of chronic conditions need to be considered. The projected increase in chronic conditions with an ageing population is exacerbated by lifestyle and in particular diet and obesity. The abilities of people to self-manage their condition may be related to their physical capacities. Therefore, it is important that the evidence with regard to those conditions resulting in disability is that for older people these rates are showing some evidence of decline. The implication of these data is that while health care costs may increase through increased absolute numbers of people with chronic conditions, levels of disability associated with ageing may not be as great a burden on the costs of social and health services as has often been assumed. The issues surrounding chronic illness are maybe more complicated but also more receptive to the interventions described in the rest of this book.

Bibliography

Allen et al. (2002). The state of the world's older people 2002. HelpAge; London.

Antonovsky, A. (1968). Social class and the major cardiovascular diseases. *Journal of Chronic Diseases* 21:65–106.

Armstrong, D. (2005) Chronic Illness: Epidemiological or social explosion, *Chronic Illness*, 1: 26–7.

Beatty, C. and Fothergill, S. (2003) The detached male labour force, in P. Alcock, C. Beatty, S. Fothergill, R. Macmillan and S. Yeandle (eds) *Work to Welfare: How Men became Detached from the Labour Market*. Cambridge: Cambridge University Press.

Bone, M. (1995) *Trends in Dependency among Older People in England*. London: OPCS.

Burden of Disease Network Project (2004) *Disability in Old Age: Final Report, Conclusions and Recommendations*. Finland: University of Jyväskylä, (www.jyu.fi/BURDIS).

Bury, M. (1997) *Health and Illness in a Changing Society*. London: Routledge.

CDC (2006) State-specific prevalence of obesity among adults – United States, 2005, *Morbidity and Mortality Weekly Report (MMWR)*, 55(36): 985–8.

Chirikos, TN: Accounting for the historical rise in work-disability prevalence. *Milbank Quarterly* 64:271–301, 1986.

Colagiuri, S., Borch-Johnsen, K., Glümer, C. and Vistisen, D. (2005) There really is an epidemic of type 2 diabetes, *Diabetologic*, 48: 1459–63.

Colvez, A and Blanchet, M: Disability trends in the United States population 1966–76: Analysis of reported causes. *American Journal of Public Health* 71(5):464–471, 1981.

Comas-Herrera, A., Pickard, L., Wittenberg, R., Davies, B. and Daton, R. (2003) *Future Demands for Long Term Care 2001–2031: Projections of Demand for Long Term Care for Older People in England*. London: Personal Social Services Research Unit (PSSRU).

Congressional Budget Office (2005) *High Cost Medicare Beneficiaries*. Washington: Congress Budget Office.

Crimmins, EM: Are Americans healthier as well as longer-lived? *Journal of Insurance Medicine* 22: 89–92, 1990.

Crimmins, E.M. (2004) Trends in the health of the elderly, *Annual Review of Public Health*, 25: 79–98.

Crimmins, EM and Ingegneri, DG : Trends in health among the American population. In *Demography and Retirement*: The 21st Century, eds. D. Bartlett and A.M. Rappaport. Westport, CT: Praeger, 1993.

Crimmins, EM and Ingegneri, DG: Trends in health of the U.S. population: 1957–1989. In *The State of Humanity*, ed. Julian Simon. Cambridge, MA: Blackwell, 1994.

Crimmins, EM, Saito, Y and Reynolds, SL: Further evidence on recent trends in the prevalence and incidence of disability among older Americans from two sources: the LSOA and the NHIS. *Journals of Gerontology, Series B, Psychological Sciences & Social Sciences* 52(2):S59-S71, 1997.

Cutler, D.M. (2001a) The reduction in disability among the elderly, *Proceedings of the National Academy of Sciences (PNAS)*, 98: 6546–7.

Cutler, D.M. (2001b) Declining disability among the elderly, *Health Affairs*, 20: 11–27.

Dorevitch, MI, Cossar, RM, Bailey, FJ, Bisset, T, Lewis, SJ, Wise, LA and MacLennan, WJ: The accuracy of self and informant ratings of physical functional capacity in the elderly. *Journal of Clinical Epidemiology* 45(7):791–798, 1992.

Dubos, R. (1965). *Man Adapting*. Yale University Press: New Haven and London.

Emmerson, C. and Tetlow, G. (2005) Labour market transitions, in J. Banks, E. Breeze, C. Lessof and J. Nazroo *Retirement, Health and Relationships Of The Older Population in England: The 2004 English Longitudinal Study of Ageing (Wave 2)* (pp. 41–64). London: Institute for Fiscal Studies.

Evandrou, M. (2005) Health and social care, *Focus on Older People* (pp. 51–66). London: Her Majesty's Stationery Office (HMSO).

Evandrou, M. and Falkingham, J. (2000) Looking back to look forward: lessons from four birth cohorts for ageing in the 21st century, *Population Trends*, 99: 21–30.

Fogel, R.W: Economic growth, population theory and physiology: The bearing of long-term processes on the making of economic policy. *American Economic Review* 84(3): 369–395, 1994.

Freedman, V.A., Martin, L.G. and Schoeni, R.F. (2002) Recent trends in disability and functioning among older adults in the United States: a systematic review, *Journal of the American Medical Association*, 3137–46.

Freedman VA, Crimmins E, Schoeni RF, Spillman BC, Aykan H, Kramarow E, Land K, Lubitz J, Manton K, Martin L, Shinberg D & Waidmann T. (2004). *Resolving Inconsistencies In Trends In Old-Age Disability: Report From A Technical Working Group*. Demography, 41, 417–441

Freedman, VA and Martin, LG: Changing patterns of functional limitations among older Americans. *American Journal of Public Health*, 1997a.

Fries, J.F. (1980) Aging, natural death and the compression of morbidity, *New England Journal of Medicine*, Volume 1, 303: 130–5.

Fries, J.F. (2003) Measuring and monitoring success in compressing morbidity, *Annals of Internal Medicine*, 139: 455–9.

Fries, J.F., Green, L.W. and Levine, S. (1989) Health promotion and the compression of morbidity, *The Lancet* 481–3.

Gee, E. (2000) Voodoo demography, population aging and social policy, in E. Gee and G. Gutman (eds) *The Overselling of Population Aging*. Oxford: Oxford University Press.

Gruber, J. and Wise, D. (1998). Social security program and retirement around the world. *NBER working paper No. 6134*.

Gruenberg, RM. (1977). The failure of success. *Milbank Memorial Fund Quarterly* 55:3–24.

Guillemard, A.M. and Rein, M. (1993) Comparative patterns of retirement: recent trends in developed societies, *Annual Review of Sociology*, 19: 469–503.

Harlan, M., Krumholz, H.M., Baker, D.W., Ashton, C.M., Dunbar, S.B., Friesinger, C.G., Havranek, E.P., Hlatky, M.A., Konstam, M., Ordin, D.L., Pina, I.L., Pitt, B. and Spertus, J.A. (2000) Evaluating quality of care for patients with heart failure, *Circulation*, 101: 122.

Janssen, F., Nusselder, W.J., Looman, C.W.N., Mackenbach, J.P. and Kunst, A.E. (2003) Stagnation in mortality decline among elders in the Netherlands, *The Gerontologist*, 43: 722–34.

Kaplan, GA & Keil, JE. (1993). Socioeconomic factors and cardiovascular disease: A review of the literature. *Circulation* 88(4):1973–1998.

Kirkwood T. (2001). The end of age. Why everything about ageing is changing. Profile Books. London

Kohli, M. and Rein, M. (1991) *The changing balance of work and retirement*, in M. Kohli, M. Rein, A.M. Guillemard and H. Van Gunsteren (eds) *Time for Retirement: Comparative Studies of Early Exit from the Labor Force* (pp. 1–35). Cambridge: Cambridge University Press.

Kupari, M., Lindroos, M., Iivanainen, A.M., Heikkilä, J. and Tilvis, R. (1997) Congestive heart failure in old age: prevalence, mechanisms, and 4-year prognosis in the Helsinki Ageing study, *Journal of Internal Medicine*, 241: 387–94.

Laczko, F. and Phillipson, C. (2004) *Changing Work and Retirement*. Milton Keynes: Open University Press.

Lanska, DJ & Mi, X. (1993). Decline in US stroke mortality in the era before antihypertensive therapy. *Stroke* 24(9):1382–1388.

Liao, L., Anstrom, K.J., Gottdiener, J.S., Pappas, P.A., Whellan, D.J., Kitzman, D.W., Aurigemma, G.P., Mark, D.B., Schulmann, K.A. and Jollis, J.G. (2007) *American Heart Journal*, 153: 245–52.

Lopez, A., Mathers, C., Ezzati, M., Jamison, D. and Murray, C. (2006) *Global and regional burden of disease and risk factors, 2001: systematic analysis of population health data, The Lancet*, 367: 1747–57.

Majeed, M. and Aylin, P. (2005) *Dr Foster's case notes: the ageing population of the United Kingdom, BMJ*, 331: 1362.

Manton KG.(1982). Changing concepts of morbidity and mortality in the elderly population. Milbank Quartlery, 60:183–244.

Manton, K.G. and Land, K.C. (2000) Active life expectancy estimates for the U.S. elderly population: a multidimensional continuous-mixture model of functional change applied to competed cohorts, *Demography*, 37: 253–65.

Manton, K.G., Stallard, E. and Corder, L: Education specific estimates of life expectancy and age specific disability in the U.S. elderly population: 1982 to 1991. *Journal of Aging and Health*. 9:419–450, 1997.

Manton, KG, Stallard, E and Corder, L: Education specific estimates of life expectancy and age specific disability in the U.S. elderly population: 1982 to 1991. *Journal of Aging and Health*. 9:419–450, 1997.

Manton, KG, Stallard, E and Corder, L: The dynamics of dimensions of age related disability 1982 to 1994 in the U.S. elderly population. *Journal of Gerontology: Biological Sciences* 53A(1):B59-B70, 1998.

Manton, KG & Vaupel, JW. (1995). Survival after the age of 80 in the United States, Sweden, France, England, and Japan. *New England Journal of Medicine* 333, 1232–1235.

Manton KG.(1982). Changing concepts of morbidity and mortality in the elderly population. Milbank Quartlery, 60:183–244.

Mathers, CD. (1994). New calculations: Health expectancies in Australia 1993: Preliminary results. In: *Advances in Health Expectancies*. Australian Institute of Health and Welfare: Canberra, Australia: 198–212, 1994.

Minicuci, N. and Noale, M. for the ILSA group (2005) Influence of level of education on disability free life expectancy by sex: the ILSA study, *Experimental Gerontology*, 40: 997–1003.

Minkler, M., Fuller-Thomson, E. and Guralnik, J.M. (2006) Gradient of disability across the socio-economic spectrum in the United States, *New England Journal of Medicine*, 355: 695–703.

Mokdad, A.H. et al. (1999) The spread of the obesity epidemic in the United States, 1991–1998, *JAMA* 282, 16, 1519–22.

Mokdad, A.H., et al. (2001) The continuing epidemics of obesity and diabetes in the United States, *JAMA*, 286: 10, 1519–22.

Murray, C. and Lopez, A. (1997) Alternative projections of mortality and disability by cause 1990–2020 Global Burden of Disease Study, *The Lancet*, 349: 1498–504.

Olshansky, S.J. and Ault, A.B. (1986) The fourth stage of the epidemiologic transition: the age of delayed degenerative diseases, *Milbank Memorial Fund Quarterly*, 64: 355–91.

Olshansky, S.J., Carnes, B.A. and Cassel (1990) In search of Methuselah: estimating the upper limits to human longevity, *Science*, 250: 634–40.

Olshansky, S.J., Carnes, B., Rogers, R.G. and Smith, L. (1997) Infectious diseases Ð new and ancient threats to world health, *Population Bulletin*, Volume 52, pp. 2–8.

Olshansky, S.J., Passaro, D.I., Hershaw, R.C., Layden, J., Carnes, B.A., Broody, J., Hayflick, L., Bulter, R.N., Allinson, D.B. and Ludwig, D.S. (2005) A potential decline in life expectancy in the United States in the 21st century, *New England Journal of Medicine*, 352: 1138–45.

Omran, A. (1971). The Epidemiologic Transition: A theory of the epidemiology of population change. *Milbank Memorial Quarterly* XLIX: 509–538.

Organization for Economic Co-operation and Development (2004) *Health Data 2004* (1st edn). Paris: OECD (www.oecd.org/health/healthdata).

Oxenham, H. and Sharpe, N. (2003) Cardiovascular aging and heart failure, *The European Journal of Heart Failure*, 5: 427–34.

Padiak, J. (2005) The role of morbidity in the mortality decline of the nineteenth century: evidence from the military population of Gibraltar, *Journal of the History of Medicine and Allied Sciences*, 60: 73–95.

Perutz, M: And they all lived happily ever after. *The Economist*, 82–83, 1998.

Petersen, S., Peto, V., Rayner, M., Leal, J., Luengo-Fernandez, R. and Gray, A. (2005) *European Cardiovascular Disease Statistics*. London: British Heart Foundation.

Reyes-Ortiz, C.A., Ostir, G.V., Pelaez, M. and Ottenbacher, K.J. (2006) Cross-national comparison of disability in Latin American and Caribbean persons aged 75 and older. *Archives of Gerontology and Geriatrics*, 42: 21–33.

Robine, JM, Mormiche, P and Sermet, C: Examination of the Causes and Mechanisms of the Increase in Disability-Free Life Expectancy. *Journal of Aging and Health* 10(2):171–191, 1998.

Rosenburg, M.W. and Moore, E.G. (1997) The health of Canada's elderly population: current status and future implications, *Canadian Medical Association Journal*, 157: 1025–32.

Saks, K., Kolk, H., Soots, A., Takker, U. and Vask, M. (2003) Prevalence of cardiovascular disorders among the elderly in primary care in Estonia, *Scandinavian Journal of Primary Health Care*, 21: 106–9.

Schoeni, R.F. (2005) Persistent and growing socioeconomic disparities in disability among the elderly: 1982–2002, *American Journal of Public Health*, 95, 2065–70.

Smallman-Raynor, M. and Phillips, D. (1999) Late stages of epidemiological transition: health status in the developed world, *Health and Place*, 5: 209–22.

Swinburn, B. et al. *Prevalence of obesity, adults, by sex, 1981–1998, selected European countries*. Geneva: World Health Organization Report.

Tu, EJC & Chen, K. (1994). Health expectancies in the Middle East and Asia: Recent changes in active life expectancy in Taiwan. In: *Advances in Health Expectancies*. Australian Institute of Health and Welfare: Canberra, Australia: 367–382.

UN (2001) *World Aging 1959–2050*. Geneva: United Nations (UN) Population Division.

UN (2005) *Living Arrangements of Older Persons around the World*. Geneva: United Nations (UN) Department of Economic and Social Affairs/Population Division.

Vaupel, JW & Jeune, B. (1994). The emergence and proliferation of centenarians. Aging Research Unit, Odense University, Medical School, Odense, Denmark.

Verbrugge, L: Longer life but worsening health? Trends in health and mortality of middle-aged and older persons. *Milbank Memorial Fund Quarterly* 62:475–519, 1984.

Verbrugge, L, Lepkowski, J and Imanaka, Y: Comorbidity and its impact on disability. *Milbank Quarterly* 67:450–484, 1989.

Waidmann TA and Liu KB. (2000). *Disability trends among elderly persons and implications for the future.* Journals of Gerontology Series B-Psychological Sciences and Social Sciences. 55. 298–307

Waidmann, T.A. and Manton, K.G. (1998) *International Evidence on Disability Trends among the Elderly.* The Urban Institute: www.aspe.hhs.gov/daltcp/home.htm.

Waidmann, T, Bound, J and Schoenbaum, M: The illusion of failure: Trends in the self-reported health of the U.S. elderly. *Milbank Quarterly* 73(2):253–287, 1995.

Wesndorp, R.G.J. (2006) What is healthy aging in the 21st century? *American Journal of Clinical Nutrition*, 83: 404S–9S.

Wild, S., Roglic, G., Green, A., Sicree, R., & King, H. (2004) Global Prevalence of Diabetes: Estimates for the year 2000 and projections for 2030. Diabetes Care, 27 (5): 1047–1053.

Wild, S., Sicree, R., Roglic, G., King, H. and Green, A. (2004) *Diabetes Care*, 27: 1047–53.

Wilmoth, J.R., Deegan, L.J., Lundström, H. and Horiuchi, S. (2000) Increase in the maximum life span in Sweden 1861–1999, *Science*, 289: 2366–8.

Wilson, R.Q. and Drury, T.F: Interpreting trends in illness and disability: health statistics and health status. In *Annual Review of Public Health 5*. Palo Alto, CA: Annual Reviews, 1984.

Wilson, RW and Drury, TF: Interpreting trends in illness and disability: health statistics and health status. In *Annual Review of Public Health* 5. Palo Alto, CA: Annual Reviews, 1984.

Wittenberg, R; Pickard, L.; Comas-Herrera, A.; Davies, B & Darton, R. (2001). *Demand for Long-term Care for Older People in England to 2031.* Health Statistics Quarterly 12, 5–17.

Wolf, D.A., Hunt, K. and Kuickman, J. (2005) Perspectives on the recent decline in disability at older ages, *The Millbank Quarterly*, 83: 365–95.

Yeandle, S. (2003) The international context, in P. Alcock, C. Beatty, S. Fothergill, R. Macmillan and S. Yeandle, (eds) *Work to Welfare: How Men became Detached from the Labour Market.* Cambridge: Cambridge University Press.

Yusuf S, Hawken S, Ôunpuu S, Dans T, Avezum A, Lanas F, McQueen M, Budaj A, Pais P, Varigos J & L on behalf of the INTERHEART Study Investigators. (2004). *Effect of potentially modifiable risk factors associated with myocardial infarction in 52 countries (the INTERHEART study): case-control study.* The Lancet; 364, 937–952

2 Changing attitudes to the role of patients in health care

Angela Coulter and Jo Ellins

Clinician–patient relationships

It used to be assumed that doctors and patients shared the same goals, but only the doctor was sufficiently informed and experienced to decide on the most appropriate course of treatment and how to manage the patient's condition. Patients were seen as ignorant and incompetent in medical matters, so they were expected to trust the doctor and follow medical advice without question. In 1932, American physician Walton H. Hamilton, summarized the prevailing view as follows:

> The art of medicine is intricate; the relation of the treatment of the sick to results obtained cannot be appraised by a layman; in medicine, almost more certainly than anywhere else, the patient has not the knowledge requisite for judgment. (Dissenting Opinion on the Report of the Committee on American Medicine, 1932)

However, this view began to be challenged by patients, clinicians and social scientists who recognized that in certain circumstances the patient might play a different, more active role. As early as the 1950s Szasz and Hollender described three basic models of the doctor–patient relationship: activity-passivity, guidance-cooperation and mutual participation (Szasz and Hollender 1956). In the first of these the patient is an entirely passive recipient of the doctor's actions; for example when suffering severe injury or a similar emergency. In the second model, guidance-cooperation, the patient plays a more active role but they are expected to cooperate in whatever action the doctor deems appropriate without argument. The third model, mutual participation, assumes that both doctor and patient have mutual roles and responsibilities. In this case the relationship is a partnership in which the doctor helps the patient to help him/herself, for example, in the management of chronic illness. The doctor, and other clinicians such as nurses or therapists, must act as educators, facilitators and supporters, helping patients themselves to play the main role in day-to-day monitoring and management of symptoms and impairments resulting from chronic illness.

Several terms are used to describe an individual's role in looking after their own health. Self-care refers to all the things that a person, healthy or ill, can do to maintain their health. This may include, for example, adopting healthy behaviours or lifestyles, understanding symptoms and taking appropriate action, selecting appropriate treatments, taking medicines and monitoring their treatment. Self-management is a subset of self-care strategies, usually used to refer specifically to actions taken by people with chronic illnesses, in particular applying actions that are likely to have been recommended by health professionals. Self-help, on the other hand, is often used to describe health actions taken without any input from health professionals, but often with the active support and encouragement of other people with the same condition.

Helping patients to participate actively in their health care requires strategies to improve health literacy, to engage patients in decision-making, and to strengthen their capacity to undertake effective health promotion and self-management of long-term conditions. If they are to fulfil this role effectively, patients need to work with clinicians who recognize and actively support their contribution and are willing to engage with them as health care partners.

Unfortunately, many patients do not receive the help they need. An analysis of data from the Commonwealth Fund's international health policy surveys carried out in 2004 and 2005 in Australia, Canada, Germany, New Zealand, the UK and the USA found that while most patients gave positive reports of the manner in which health professionals communicated with them, provision of advice on health behaviours was poor (Coulter 2006). Furthermore, less than half of those surveyed felt they were sufficiently involved in treatment decisions and among people with chronic conditions less than a third had been given self-management plans.

We now look at each of these areas in turn to examine the evidence on patients' support needs and the various ways in which these are being addressed.

Information needs and health literacy

The key to greater patient engagement lies in building health literacy and ensuring that clinicians help patients to help themselves. Health literacy has been defined as 'the ability to make sound health decisions in the context of everyday life – at home, in the community, at the workplace, the health care system, the market place and the political arena' (Kickbusch et al. 2005). The concept broadly encompasses the skills of obtaining, understanding and using health information, both written and verbal. Health literacy does not necessarily equate to basic literacy. Some people with relatively high levels of basic literacy may lack understanding of how their body works and what to do when they experience symptoms, while others who struggle to read and write may be perfectly capable of managing health problems. Most people can recognize minor illnesses, such as colds, flu or stomach upsets, and these are often treated and managed without recourse to professional help. Indeed, in looking after themselves and their family members, lay people provide a far greater quantity of health care than do health professionals (Hannay 1979).

In the USA it has been estimated that 90 million adults have inadequate health literacy (Ad Hoc Committee on Health Literacy for the Council on Scientific Affairs 1999). Although health literacy does not directly correlate with other inequalities in health, low health literacy appears to be particularly prevalent among lower socio-economic groups, the elderly, ethnic minority groups and those with chronic medical conditions or disabilities (Andrus and Roth 2002; Sihota and Lennard 2004). Inadequate health literacy can have profound health and financial consequences, leading to impaired ability to self-care, poorer health status, higher rates of hospital admission, lower rates of adherence to treatments, less use of preventive services and weaker understanding of health-promoting behaviours.

Failures in communication about illness and treatment are the most frequent source of patient dissatisfaction (Grol et al. 2000; Coulter and Cleary 2001). Currently, there is plenty of evidence that patients expect clinicians to respect their autonomy, to listen to them, to inform them, to take account of their preferences, to involve them in treatment decisions, and to support their efforts in self-care (Coulter 2002). This includes taking action to prevent the occurrence or recurrence of disease, understanding the causes of illness and the treatment options, being involved in treatment decisions, monitoring symptoms and treatment effects, and learning to manage the symptoms of chronic disease.

For example, studies indicate that patients want more information than they currently receive and health professionals frequently overestimate the amount of information they supply (Richards 1998). Patients' information needs are very diverse. They are shaped by demographic characteristics including age, gender and socio-economic status, as well as by the patient's particular circumstances, beliefs, preferences and styles of coping. There are also important differences due to patients' skills and abilities, with particular needs arising from low literacy skills, auditory or visual impairment, and for those who do not speak English. The type of information that is sought by an individual patient is likely to change during the course of their illness. For example, in the initial stages following diagnosis there is a preference for practical information to support care decisions, including information on treatment options and their likely outcomes. More in-depth and specific information needs emerge later, when the patient's focus often turns to issues of self-care and long-term prognosis.

There has been a marked proliferation of consumer health information in recent years. Above all, this has been driven by the rapid expansion of the internet as an information source. Surveys of American internet users report that 80 per cent have searched online for information on at least one major health topic (Fox 2006). Numerous internet and computer-based information tools have been developed for consumer use; in some cases combining information delivery with additional services such as decision aids or virtual support groups. The potential of the internet to effectively disseminate consumer health information is limited, however, by disparities in both access to and ability to use computer technology. A 'digital divide' has been widely documented, with rates of computer (and internet) use highest among the young, affluent and employed and far lower in low income, low literacy and ethnic minority groups and among disabled and older people. Rather than facilitating the empowerment of new categories of health care consumer, the internet appears to be largely reinforcing existing patterns of information-seeking behaviour (Wilkins and Navarro 2001). This is taken as further evidence of the operation of an 'inverse information law', whereby those with the greatest need for health information are least able to access it. The gap may diminish as internet access becomes more widespread, but in the meantime various attempts are being made to tackle inequalities in access to information and knowledge.

Strategies for tackling low health literacy have focused on three key objectives: enhancing health knowledge, skills and behaviours by providing health information; encouraging appropriate use of health services by means of media campaigns; and reducing health inequalities by targeting information and education at disadvantaged groups. Research has demonstrated the limitations of traditional methods (e.g. health education leaflets) and pointed to the particular value of visually enhanced and interactive information materials. The evidence suggests that written information used as an adjunct to professional consultation and advice can help to improve health knowledge and recall, particularly when it is personalized to the individual. In comparison to generalized information, tailored materials tend to produce better health- and service-related outcomes and are more highly valued by patients themselves (Bull et al. 1999; Jones et al. 1999). Computer-based systems are one means by which a tailored approach may be achieved and internet-based educational programmes have been shown to produce positive effects (Bessell et al. 2002). Information booklets or computer packages can enhance knowledge, but information alone appears to be less effective than information used as part of an educational package (McPherson et al. 2001; Forster et al. 2005).

Initiatives designed specifically to target low-literacy groups have had mixed results, with some studies showing beneficial effects on health behaviour, but there have been relatively few attempts to test the effect of these on reducing health inequalities. However, there is some evidence that disadvantaged groups can achieve greater benefit from well-designed computer-based educational packages than those in advantaged groups (Gustafson et al. 2002).

Participation in medical decisions

As we have seen, the traditional model of decision-making assumed that only the doctor was sufficiently informed and experienced to decide what should be done, and that patient involvement should be confined to giving or withholding consent to treatment. However, this paternalistic approach now seems seriously outdated. Many, if not most patients nowadays expect to be given information about their condition and the treatment options, and they want clinicians to take account of their preferences. Some expect to go further: to be actively engaged in the decision-making process, or even to take the decisions themselves. This type of partnership or patient-led approach is known as shared decision-making.

Shared decision-making has been defined as 'a process in which patients are involved as active partners with the clinician in clarifying acceptable medical options and in choosing a preferred course of clinical care' (Sheridan et al. 2004). In modern clinical practice there are often multiple options for treating a problem and the best choice depends on how an individual patient values the potential benefits and harms of the alternatives. In these situations it makes sense to involve the patient in deciding on the best course of action. In shared decision-making the intention is that both the process of decision-making and the outcome – the treatment decision – will be shared. This is a partnership approach based on the notion that two types of expertise are involved. The doctor is, or should be, well informed about diagnostic techniques, the causes of disease, prognosis, treatment options and preventive strategies. Yet only the patient knows about his or her experience of illness, social circumstances, habits and behaviour, attitudes to risk, values and preferences. Both types of knowledge are needed to manage illness successfully, so both parties should be prepared to share information and take decisions jointly. Shared information is an essential prerequisite, but the process also depends on a commitment from both parties to engage in a negotiated decision-making process. There may be resistance to this process on the part of both patients and clinicians, dependent on a range of characteristics and circumstances, as discussed below.

The desire on the part of patients to participate in clinical decision-making has been found to vary by age, educational status and disease severity. An age-related trend has been found in a number of studies – younger and better-educated people are more likely to want to play an active role (Krupat et al. 2000; Robinson and Thomson 2001; O'Connor et al. 2003). Despite the association between age and decision-making preferences, age on its own is not a reliable predictor of a patient's preferred role (Kennelly and Bowling 2001). Older people are particularly likely to suffer from the presumption that they are incapable of taking decisions or unwilling to face choices about their medical care. Care of patients at the end of life is a case in point. National guidance requires that do-not-resuscitate orders should not be applied without first discussing the issue with patients and/or their relatives, yet there is evidence that this does not happen in two-thirds of cases (Bowling and Ebrahim 2001).

People's preferences may vary according to the stage in the course of a disease episode and the severity of their condition. Surveys of healthy populations tend to elicit much more positive responses about involvement in decision-making than surveys of people with life-threatening conditions. For example, an Australian population survey found that more than 90 per cent preferred an active role in decisions about diagnostic tests or treatments (Davey et al. 2002), whereas a British study of the decision-making role preferences of cancer patients found that 48 per cent of those with breast cancer and only 22 per cent of those with colorectal cancer wanted to be involved (Beaver et al. 1999).

There may also be important cultural differences. A population survey carried out in eight European countries found significant variations in response to a question about who should take the lead in making treatment choices (Coulter and Magee 2003). While 91 per cent of respondents from Switzerland, 87 per cent of those from Germany and 74 per cent of those from the UK felt the patient should have a role in treatment decisions, either sharing responsibility for decision-making with the doctor or being the primary decision-maker, the proportion of Polish patients who felt the same way was only 59 per cent and in Spain it was only 44 per cent.

A review of studies exploring the extent to which patients wanted to participate in decisions confirmed the variations but concluded that patients should always be informed of treatment alternatives and given the opportunity to express their preferences when more than one effective alternative exists (Guadagnoli and Ward 1998). The only way to find out patients' preferred role is to ask them, but their responses may be influenced by previous experience. Some patients may assume a passive role because they have never been encouraged to participate and remain unaware of alternatives. There is also an apparent illogicality about asking patients to indicate their preferred role in decision-making before they have been informed about the nature of the choices they face (Elwyn et al. 1999), so the argument for informing everyone about treatment options has some force.

The evidence suggests that true shared decision-making is not widely practised by clinicians (Stevenson et al. 2004). Doctors often fail to explore patients' values and preferences, and risk communication is often poorly expressed by doctors and not well understood by patients. Braddock and colleagues studied 1057 audio-taped encounters among 59 primary care physicians and 65 general and orthopaedic surgeons in the USA, during the course of which 3552 clinical decisions were taken (Braddock et al. 1999). Only 9 per cent of these met accepted standards of completeness for informed decision-making. Among the elements of the decision process studied, discussion of the nature of the intervention occurred in 71 per cent of cases and patients' preferences were discussed in 21 per cent, but alternative treatments were mentioned in only 11 per cent of consultations, risks and benefits of the alternatives in 6 per cent, uncertainties associated with the decision in 4 per cent, and assessment of the patient's level of understanding took place in only 1.5 per cent of the consultations.

Stevenson and her colleagues reviewed 134 papers reporting observational studies of communication between patients and practitioners about medicine-taking (Stevenson et al. 2004). They were specifically interested to find out if patients were encouraged to share their beliefs, experiences and preferences and if a truly two-way communication took place. They found that most patients were happy to discuss their concerns, but health professionals did not always encourage them to do so. Patients often failed to disclose to professionals that they had not taken the medicines as recommended. Doctors tended to dominate discussion in the consultation and patients usually took a passive role. When providing information, doctors rarely assessed patients' understanding of it, despite an awareness of the importance of doing so. Overall they found scant evidence of shared decision-making.

When challenged to explain why they fail to engage patients more actively in decisions about their care, doctors frequently refer to time pressures and the belief that their patients do not want to play an active role. However, it is clear that there are often deeper fears that allowing patients to have a say in decision-making will unleash a demand for treatments that clinicians feel are inappropriate. For example, a survey of primary care physicians in Canada found a high level of concern about dealing with patients who wanted something (e.g. a test, prescription or referral) that the doctor did not think was appropriate or necessary (Towle and Godolphin 2001). The problems that they found most challenging were those that involved negotiating such decisions and resolving conflict.

Despite these fears that encouraging involvement in decisions will lead to an increase in demand for inappropriate medical treatments, research evidence suggests that shared decision-making often has the opposite effect. When patients are provided with appropriate information and encouraged to express their preferences, they often choose less invasive and less expensive options. For example, a large randomized trial of decision support for patients with menorrhagia carried out in the west of England resulted in a reduction in hysterectomy rates. As a result, the intervention, which included a booklet for patients setting out the treatment options and outcomes, a video and nurse counselling, led to lower service costs (Kennedy et al. 2002). The collective evidence on the effects of this and other patient decision aids shows that they improve knowledge, enable patients to play an active role in choosing appropriate treatments, and improve agreement between patients' values and the treatments chosen (O'Connor et al. 2002). Decision aids that provide individualized risk information generally increase uptake of screening, except for prostate cancer screening where it is appropriately reduced (Whelan et al. 2002; Edwards et al. 2003; Briss et al. 2004).

Other initiatives to promote greater patient involvement in decisions that have been evaluated include coaching and decision prompts and provision of audio-tapes or summaries of consultations (McDonald et al. 2002; Harrington et al. 2004). While most studies show benefits in terms of improvements in patients' knowledge and understanding of treatment effects, there is little evidence of direct effects on health status. There has been considerable debate in the literature about the goals of shared decision-making and the relative importance of various outcomes. Many investigators now agree that the primary goal is to ensure that treatment choices are consistent with patients' values (Sepucha et al. 2004). An appropriate measure of decision quality would focus on the extent to which patients acquire relevant knowledge and on the level of agreement between their relative preferences for the salient outcomes of each treatment option and the treatment or management plan they eventually choose.

Support for self-care

Self-care encompasses all the things individuals can do to protect their health and manage or ameliorate the effects of disease. It includes actions that people take to prevent ill health: for example avoiding unhealthy behaviours and adopting healthy ones; drawing on knowledge and experience to interpret symptoms, making a self-diagnosis and taking effective action; self-monitoring to assess the course of an illness and deciding if or when professional intervention is required; self-medicating with over-the-counter preparations; taking prescribed medicines and other treatments effectively and appropriately; and self-managing long-term conditions such as diabetes, asthma or arthritis. In short, the term covers everything to do with people's active involvement in their own health care and that of their families.

There is nothing new about self-care. Before the advent of national health systems, most people were forced to rely on their own efforts or those of their family for much of the care they needed. Nowadays, it is still the case that in looking after themselves and their family members lay people provide a far greater quantity of health care than do health professionals. Health professionals, even those working in 'first contact' care such as general practice, see only a small fraction of the afflictions that could potentially trigger a consultation and they are in direct contact with each individual for only a tiny proportion of the duration of their illness. Research also suggests that people would like more involvement in their care; a 2005 survey of the population in England, for example, found that 87 per cent of people with chronic illnesses were interested in more actively managing their health condition (Department of Health 2005).

What *is* new, however, is the recognition that self-care is the crucial underpinning of an effective health system and as such it requires active support. Instead of ignoring or taking for granted the key role played by individuals and communities in health care provision, the new approach calls for explicit acknowledgement of the fact that active engagement of individuals and families and promotion of more effective self-care can lead to more appropriate and cost-effective utilization of health services and better health outcomes. In a review of future funding needs for the health service carried out on behalf of the UK Treasury, Derek Wanless called for a new focus on moderating demand by investing in effective health promotion and supporting self-care (Wanless 2002). Wanless believed that patient engagement should be a key component of the strategy to keep future health care spending within manageable limits. In other words, the sustainability of the NHS will depend on the effectiveness of efforts to eliminate the unhealthy paternalism that still characterizes patient–professional relationships in the British health system. This theme was echoed in a recent White Paper on community services, which promised to help patients to take responsibility for their health, support their independence, put them in control and focus on the promotion of health and well-being (Secretary of State for Health 2006).

Support for self-management

Chronic illnesses constitute the major proportion of the burden of ill health, so helping people to care for themselves wherever possible, coupled with proactive monitoring and intensive targeted support for those who need it most, should be a more effective way to manage scarce health care resources than the current system of reactive, paternalistic care. Management of chronic diseases usually depends on patients playing an active role and people with long-term health problems often become quite expert in managing their treatment. For example, people with type 1 diabetes have to monitor their blood sugar levels and give themselves regular injections; people with asthma must become knowledgeable about inhalers and use them appropriately; and people on long-term medication must take their pills at regular intervals. They also have to adapt their lifestyles to cope with long-term symptoms. We would not expect health professionals to take on these responsibilities without education and training, but patients have often been expected to do it with little support.

Influenced by research evidence on the scope for improving management of chronic illnesses (Bodenheimer et al. 2002a; Bodenheimer et al. 2002b), self-management education has been adopted as a key element of the policy response in a number of countries. For example, some health care providers in north America have moved towards a model of care that explicitly recognizes and encourages active patient participation. The approach developed by an American health maintenance organization, Kaiser Permanente, considers patients to be co-producers of their health and health care, rather than simply consumers of health services. Kaiser has sought to encourage patients to become more actively involved in, and educated about their healthcare by offering self-management education programmes in chronic illness and pain management.

This approach is beginning to be enshrined in legislation in the USA. For example, as of December 2005 46 states had some type of law requiring health insurance coverage to include treatment for diabetes, including the costs of equipment and supplies used by patients in their own homes (www.ncsl.org/programs/health/diabetes.htm). To improve care for patients with chronic disease, the Medicare Modernization Act (passed in 2003) established a disease management model entitled Medicare Health Support (www.cms.hhs.gov/CCIP). The programme aims to increase adherence to evidence-based care, reduce unnecessary hospital stays and emergency room visits, and help participants avoid costly and debilitating complications. The organizations operating the programmes are required to assist participants in managing their health holistically, including all co-morbidities, relevant health care services, and medication in a manner that is responsive to the particular needs of individual patients.

In Australia, the Sharing Health Care Initiative established a series of demonstration projects to test a range of chronic condition self-management models (www.chronicdisease.health.gov.au/sharing.htm) and a similar initiative entitled Supporting Self-Care ran for five years in Canada (www.hc-sc.gc.ca/hcs-sss/hhr-rhs/collabor/self-auto/index_e.html). The Department of Health in England is now promoting service delivery models designed to improve the quality, coordination and efficiency of care for chronically ill patients (Department of Health 2004). As well as promoting proactive case management for people with complex health problems and coordinated disease management for those at high risk, the government has been active in developing and promoting self-care initiatives, principally through the establishment of the Expert Patient Programme (Department of Health 2001). The centrepiece of this is a series of community-based self-management courses, modelled on a programme developed at Stanford University, California.

The goal of self-management support is to enable patients to perform three sets of tasks: medical management of their illness (e.g. taking medication, adhering to a special diet); coping with the effects of their illness or impairment and carrying out normal roles and activities; and managing the emotional impact (Lorig and Holman 1993). While the original self-management courses developed at Stanford were disease-specific (focused on coping with arthritis), the model now being promoted is generic, in other words designed for any patient with a long-term condition. A tenet of the programme is that the educational interventions should be 'lay-led'; in other words people with experience of living with chronic diseases are trained to lead the groups, based on a self-help model. However, while many such groups have been established with active involvement from patient organizations, in practice group leaders have often come from the ranks of health professionals.

The strong emphasis on lay-led, generic programmes promoted under the Expert Patient banner is, however, not well supported by the research evidence (Barlow et al. 1998; Lorig et al. 1999; Lorig et al. 2001a; Lorig et al. 2001b; Lorig et al. 2002; Lorig et al. 2004; Kennedy et al. 2007). Although it has been claimed that self-management education of this type improves health outcomes, the current evidence for its effects on health status is weak (Newman et al. 2004). Sustaining the lay-led groups has sometimes proved problematic, and GPs and other health professionals have been slow to refer their patients to the programmes. Furthermore, the few studies that have measured outcomes beyond six months have found that the effects were not sustained.

The Expert Patient Programme is focused on promoting community-based group approaches to education for self-management, but professionally-led one-to-one patient education may be more appropriate for the majority of patients with chronic conditions (Coulter and Ellins 2006). Evaluations have focused on a fairly narrow range of clinical conditions (in particular diabetes, asthma and arthritis) and a limited range of clinical settings. The evidence is mixed, but studies of disease-specific educational programmes have tended to produce more positive results than generic approaches (Hampson 2001; Gibson et al. 2003; NICE 2003; Riemsma 2003; Wolf 2003).

While self-management programmes play an important role in encouraging self-care, other initiatives also broadly support greater patient involvement in the process of care. Moves to reclassify certain prescription-only products to pharmacist-prescribed or general sales list (which can be sold in any retail outlet) is improving patients' access to medicines and their ability to self-medicate for less serious ailments. A self-help guide has been produced by NHS Direct, providing information and advice about how to treat common health problems at home. Developments in information technology are also playing a role; NHS HealthSpace, for example, is an online service for storing and accessing personal health information. It is intended that patients will eventually be able to gain electronic access to their own medical records via this service. Many patients welcome the idea of having access to and even ownership of their medical records (Health Which? and National Programme for Information Technology 2003), and there is some evidence that patient-held records increase patients' sense of control (Brown and Smith 2004). Cooke and Newman discuss the issues of technology in health care in more detail in Chapter 7.

In common with all efforts to support self-care, effective clinician–patient communication is critical to the management of chronic conditions (Hasman et al. 2006). If patients' beliefs and fears are not fully addressed in clinical consultations, there is a strong likelihood that problems will be missed and treatment may be ineffective. For example, if the doctor does not understand the patient's attitude to medicine-taking or does not adequately communicate the reasons for prescribing a particular drug, the patient may fail to take the prescription as recommended, reducing its efficacy. The quality of clinical communication can have an effect on outcome (Di Blasi et al. 2001). Patients who are well informed about prognosis and treatment options, including benefits, harms and side-effects, are more likely to adhere to treatments, leading to better health outcomes (Marinker et al. 1997). They are also less likely to accept ineffective or risky procedures (Wolf et al. 1996). Patients want the doctor to listen to their concerns, but failure to address the patient's agenda is common (Barry et al. 2000). Meanwhile, patients often fail to take medicines as prescribed, resulting in a significant waste of resources and possible health risks. The necessary skills for achieving a true partnership can be taught and a number of intervention studies have demonstrated that progress is possible (Lewin et al. 2002). When clinicians encourage participation and listen attentively to patients' views, patients are more likely to adhere to recommended regimes and health outcomes improve (Haynes et al. 2000).

Conclusion

Many patients nowadays expect to play an active role in managing their own health care. A growing body of evidence shows that people who are actively involved in protecting their health and managing their health care have better health outcomes. In order to be fully engaged, patients require help from clinicians who recognize and actively support their contribution and are willing to work with them as health care partners. They may also benefit from interacting with other patients who share their problems, so self-help groups and voluntary organizations have a role to play. And public policy should support their efforts by investing in information and education and by ensuring that regulatory procedures give due recognition to the need to support the patient's role.

Health professionals and policy-makers should be encouraged to recognize their responsibility to promote health literacy, to involve patients in treatment decisions, and to support self-care and self-management. Clinicians may need to develop new skills and competences, including knowing how to guide patients to appropriate sources of information on health and health care, how to educate patients about protecting their health and preventing occurrence and recurrence of illness, how to elicit and understand patients' preferences, how to communicate information on risk and probability, how to share treatment decisions, and how to provide support for self-care and self-management.

Certain groups require more intensive support; for example older people, those with less education and the chronically ill (Ellins and Coulter 2005). These people can benefit from interventions designed to improve their capacity for self-care, through improving their knowledge and building their self-confidence to take control of their health care. In addition to educating patients about how to monitor and manage their health problems, ownership of health care is encouraged through patients' active involvement in clinical decisions and collaborative relationships with health professionals. Encouraging patients to express their preferences and improving opportunities for shared decision-making will underscore the transition to more effective self-care.

References

Ad Hoc Committee on Health Literacy for the Council on Scientific Affairs, A.M.A. (1999) Health literacy: report of the Council on Scientific Affairs, *Journal of the American Medical Association*, 281(6): 552–57.

Andrus, M.R. and Roth, M.T. (2002) Health literacy: a review, *Pharmacotherapy*, 22(3): 282–302.

Barlow, J.H., Turner, A.P. and Wright, C.C. (1998) Long-term outcomes of an arthritis self-management programme, *British Journal of Rheumatology*, 37(12): 1315–19.

Barry, C.A., Bradley, C.P., Britten, N., Stevenson, F.A. and Barber, N. (2000) Patients' unvoiced agendas in general practice consultations: qualitative study, *British Medical Journal*, 320: 1246–250.

Beaver, K., Bogg, J. and Luker, K.A. (1999) Decision-making role preferences and information needs: a comparison of colorectal and breast cancer, *Health Expectations*, 2: 266–76.

Bessell, T.L., McDonald, S., Silagy, C.A., Anderson, J.N., Hiller, J.E. and Sansom, L.N. (2002) Do internet interventions for consumers cause more harm than good? A systematic review, *Health Expectations*, 5(1): 28–37.

Bodenheimer, T., Wagner, E.H. and Grumbach, K. (2002a) Improving primary care for patients with chronic illness, *JAMA*, 288(14): 1775–79.

Bodenheimer, T., Wagner, E.H. and Grumbach, K. (2002b) Improving primary care for patients with chronic illness: the Chronic Care Model, Part 2, *JAMA*, 288(15): 1909–14.

Bowling, A. and Ebrahim, S. (2001) Measuring patients' preferences for treatment and perceptions of risk, *Quality in Health Care*, 10(Suppl. 1): i12–8.

Braddock, C.H., Edwards, K.A., Hasenberg, N.M., Laidley, T.L. and Levinson, W. (1999) Informed decision making in outpatient practice: time to get back to basics, *Journal of the American Medical Association*, 282(24): 2313–20.

Briss, P., Rimer, B., Reilley, B., Coates, R.C., Lee, N.C., Mullen, P., Corso, P., Hutchinson, A.B., Hiatt, R., Kerner, J., George, P., White, C., Gandhi, N., Saraiya, M., Breslow, R., Isham, G., Teutsch, S.M., Hinman, A.R. and Lawrence, R. (2004) Promoting informed decisions about cancer screening in communities and healthcare systems, *American Journal of Preventive Medicine*, 26(1): 67–80.

Brown, H.C. and Smith, H.J. (2004) Giving women their own case notes to carry during pregnancy, *Cochrane Database of Systematic Reviews*, Issue 2, No. CD002856.

Bull, F.C., Kreuter, M.W. and Scharff, D.P. (1999) Effects of tailored, personalized and general health messages on physical activity, *Patient Education and Counseling*, 36: 181–92.

Coulter, A. and Ellins, J. (2006), *Patient-focused Interventions: A Review of the Evidence.* London: *The Health Foundation.*

Coulter, A. (2006) *Engaging Patients in their Healthcare: How is the UK Doing Relative to Other Countries?*, Oxford: Picker Institute Europe.

Coulter, A. and Cleary, P.D. (2001) Patients' experiences with hospital care in five countries, *Health Affairs*, 20(3): 244–52.

Coulter, A. and Magee, H. (2003), *The European Patient of the Future.* Maidenhead: Open University Press.

Davey, H.M., Barratt, A.L., Davey, E., Butow, P.N., Redman, S., Houssami, N., and Salkeld, G.P. (2002) Medical tests: women's reported and preferred decision-making roles and preferences for information on benefits, side-effects and false results, *Health Expectations*, 5(4): 330–40.

Department of Health (2001) *The Expert Patient: A New Approach to Chronic Disease Management for the 21st Century.* London: Department of Health.

Department of Health (2004) *Improving Chronic Disease Management.* London: Department of Health.

Department of Health (2005) *Public Attitudes to Self Care: Baseline Survey.* London: Department of Health.

Di Blasi, Z., Harkness, E., Ernst, E., Georgiou, A. and Kleijnen, J. (2001) Influence of context effects on health outcomes: a systematic review, *Lancet*, 357: 757–62.

Edwards, A., Unigwe, S., Elwyn, G. and Hood, K. (2003) Personalised risk communication for informed decision making about entering screening programs, *The Cochrane Database of Systematic Reviews*, Issue 1, No. CD001865.

Ellins, J. and Coulter, A. (2005) *How Engaged are People in their Healthcare? Findings of a National Telephone Survey.* Oxford: Picker Institute.

Elwyn, G., Edwards, A., Gwyn, R. and Grol, R. (1999) Towards a feasible model for shared decision making: focus group study with general practice registrars, *British Medical Journal*, 319: 753–56.

Forster, A., Smith, J., Young, J., Knapp, P., House, A. and Wright, J. (2005) Information provision for stroke patients and their caregivers, *Cochrane Database of Systematic Reviews*, CD page CD001919 Issue 3.

Fox, S. (2006) *Online Health Search 2006.* Washington: Pew Internet and American Life Project.

Gibson, P.G., Powell, H., Coughlan, J., Wilson, A.J., Abramson, M., Haywood, P., Bauman, A., Hensley, M.J. and Walters, E.H. (2003) Self-management education and regular practitioner review for adults with asthma. *The Cochrane Database of Systematic Reviews*, Issue 1, No. CD001117.

Grol, R., Wensing, M., Mainz, J., Jung, H.P., Ferreira, P., Hearnshaw, H., Hjortdahl, P., Olesen, F., Reis, S., Ribacke, M. and Szecsenyi, J. (2000) Patients in Europe evaluate general practice care: an international comparison, *British Journal of General Practice*, 50: 882–87.

Guadagnoli, E. and Ward, P. (1998) Patient participation in decision-making, *Social Science & Medicine*, 47(3): 329–39.

Gustafson, D.H., Hawkins, R.P., Boberg, E.W., McTavish, F., Owens, B., Wise, M., Berhe, H. and Pingree, S. (2002) CHESS: 10 years of research and development in consumer health informatics for broad populations, including the underserved, *International Journal of Medical Informatics*, 65: 169–77.

Hamilton W. H. Dissenting opinion. Medical care for the American people. The final report of the Committee on the Costs of Medical Care. Chicago: The University of Chicago Press, 1932.

Hampson, S.E. (2001) Effects of educational and psychosocial interventions for adolescents with diabetes mellitus: a systematic review, *Health Technology Assessment*, 5(10): 1–79.

Hannay, D.R. (1979) *The Symptom Iceberg: A Study of Community Health*. London: Routledge and Kegan Paul.

Harrington, J., Noble, L. and Newman, S. (2004) Improving patients' communication with doctors: a systematic review of intervention studies, *Patient Education and Counseling*, 52(1): 7–16.

Hasman, A., Coulter, A. and Askham, J. (2006) *Education for Partnership: Developments in Medical Education*. Oxford: Picker Institute Europe.

Haynes, R.B., Montague, P., Oliver, T., McKibbon, K.A., Brouwers, M.C. and Kanani, R. (2000) Interventions for helping patients to follow prescriptions for medications (Cochrane Review). *Cochrane Library* [4]. Oxford: Update Software.

Health Which? and National Programme for Information Technology (2003) *The Public View on Electronic Health Records*. London: Which?

Jones, R., Pearson, J., McGregor, S., Cawsey, A.J., Barrett, A., Craig, N., Atkinson, J.M., Gilmour, W.H. and McEwen, J. (1999) Randomised trial of personalised computer based information for cancer patients, *British Medical Journal*, 319: 1241–47.

Kennedy, A., Reeves, D., Bower, P., Lee, V., Middleton, E., Richardson, G., Gardner, C., Gately, C. and Rogers, A. (2007) The effectiveness and cost effectiveness of a national lay-led self care support programme for patients with long-term conditions: a pragmatic randomised controlled trial, *Journal of Epidemiology and Community Health*, 61(3): 254–61.

Kennedy, A.D.M., Sculpher, M.J., Coulter, A., Dwyer, N., Rees, M., Abrams, K.R., Horsley, S., Cowley, D., Kidson, C., Kirwin, C., Naish, C. and Stirrat, G. (2002) Effects of decision aids for menorrhagia on treatment choices, health outcomes, and costs, *Journal of the American Medical Association*, 288: 2701–08.

Kennelly, C. and Bowling, A. (2001) Suffering in deference: a focus group study of older cardiac patients' preferences for treatment and perceptions of risk, *Quality in Health Care*, 10(Suppl. 1): i23–8.

Kickbusch, I., Maag, D. and Saan, H. (2005) Enabling healthy choices in modern health societies, Paper presented at the 8th European Health Forum Badgastein, 5–8 October.

Krupat, E., Rosenkranzz, S.L., Yeager, C.M., Barnard, K., Putnam, S.M. and Inui, T.S. (2000) The practice orientations of physicians and patients: the effect of doctor-patient congruence on satisfaction. *Patient Education and Counseling*, 39: 49–59.

Lewin, S.A., Skea, Z.C., Entwistle, V., Zwarenstein, M. and Dick, J. (2002) Interventions for providers to promote a patient centred approach in clinical consultations (Cochrane Review). *Cochrane Library* [1]. Oxford: Update Software.

Lorig, K. and Holman, H. (1993) Arthritis self-management studies: a twelve year review, *Health Education Quarterly*, 20(1): 17–28.

Lorig, K.R., Bodenheimer, T., Holman, H. and Grumbach, K. (2002) Patient self-management of chronic disease in primary care, *Journal of the American Medical Association*, 288(19): 2469–75.

Lorig, K., Ritter, P., Laurent, D. and Fries, J. (2004) Long-term randomized controlled trials of tailored-print and small-group arthritis self-management interventions, *Medical Care*, 42(4): 346–54.

Lorig, K.R., Ritter, P.L., Stewart, A.L., Sobel, D.S., Brown, B.W., Bandura, A., Gonzalez, V.M., Laurent, D.D. and Holman, H.R. (2001a) Chronic disease self-management program: 2-year health status and health care utilization outcomes, *Medical Care*, 39(11): 1217–23.

Lorig, K.R., Sobel, D.S., Ritter, P.L., Laurent, D. and Hobbs, M. (2001b) Effect of a self-management program on patients with chronic disease, *Effective Clinical Practice*, 4: 256–62.

Lorig, K.R., Sobel, D.S., Stewart, A.L., Brown, B.W., Bandura, A., Ritter, P., Gonzalex, V.M., Laurent, D.D. and Holman, H.R. (1999) Evidence suggesting that a chronic disease self-management program can improve health status while reducing utilization and costs: a randomized trial, *Medical Care*, 37(1): 5–14.

Marinker, M. et al. (1997) *From Compliance to Concordance: Achieving Shared Goals in Medicine Taking*. London: Royal Pharmaceutical Society of Great Britain.

McDonald, H.P., Garg, A.X. and Haynes, R.B. (2002) Interventions to enhance patient adherence to medication prescriptions, *Journal of the American Medical Association*, 288(22): 2868–79.

McPherson, C.J., Higginson, I.J. and Hearn, J. (2001) Effective methods of information in cancer: a systematic literature review of randomized controlled trials, *Journal of Public Health Medicine*, 23(3): 227–34.

Newman, S. (2004) Self-management interventions for chronic illness, *Lancet*, 364(9444): 1523–37.

NICE (2003) *Guidance on the Use of Patient-education Models for Diabetes*. London: National Institute for Clinical Excellence.

O'Connor, A., Drake, E.R., Wells, G.A., Tugwell, P., Laupacis, A. and Elmslie, T. (2003) A survey of the decision-making needs of Canadians faced with complex health decisions, *Health Expectations*, 6(2): 97–109.

O'Connor, A.M., Stacey, D., Rovner, D., Holmes-Rovner, M., Tetroe, J., Llewellyn-Thomas, H., Entwistle, V., Rostom, A., Fiset, V., Barry, M. and Jones, J. (2002) Decision aids for patients facing health treatment or screening decisions (Cochrane Review). *Cochrane Library* [1]. Oxford: Update Software.

Richards, T. (1998) Partnership with patients, *British Medical Journal*, 316: 85–86.

Riemsma, R.P. (2003) Patient education for adults with rheumatoid arthritis, *Cochrane Database of Systematic Reviews*, Issue 2, No. CD003688.

Robinson, A. and Thomson, R. (2001) Variability in patient preferences for participating in medical decision making: implications for the use of decision support tools, *Quality in Health Care*, 10(Suppl. I): i34–8.

Secretary of State for Health (2006) *Our Health, Our Care, Our Say*. London: The Stationery Office.

Sepucha K. R, Fowler F. J, Mulley A. G. Policy support for patient-centred care: the need for measurable improvements in decision quality. Health Affairs 2004, Oct 7, web exclusive.

Sheridan, S.L., Harris, R.P. and Woolf, S.H. (2004) Shared decision making about screening and chemoprevention: A suggested approach from the U.S. Preventive Services Task Force, *American Journal of Preventive Medicine*, 26(1): 56–66.

Sihota, S. and Lennard, L. (2004) *Health Literacy: Being Able to Make the Most of Health*. London: National Consumer Council.

Stevenson, F.A., Cox, K., Britten, N. and Dundar, Y. (2004) A systematic review of the research on communication between patients and health care professionals about medicines: the consequences for concordance, *Health Expectations*, 7(3): 235–45.

Szasz, T.S. and Hollender, M.H. (1956) A contribution to the philosophy of medicine: the basic models of the doctor-patient relationship, *Archives of Internal Medicine*, 97: 585–92.

Towle, A. and Godolphin, W. (2001) Education and training of health care professionals, in A. Edwards and G. Elwyn (eds) *Evidence-based Patient Choice* (pp. 245–69). Oxford: Oxford University Press.

Wanless, D. (2002) *Securing our Future Health: Taking a Long-term View (Final Report)*. London: HM Treasury.

Whelan, T.M., O'Brien, M.A., Villasis-Keever, M., Robinson, P., Skye, A., Gafni, A., Brouwers, M., Charles, C., Baldassarre, F. and Gauld, M. (2002) *Impact of Cancer-related Decision Aids*. Rockville, MD: Agency for Healthcare Research and Quality.

Wilkins, S.T. and Navarro, F.H. (2001) has the web really empowered health care consumers?, *Marketing Health Services* Volume 21, Issue 3, pp. 5–9.

Wolf, A.M.D., Nasser, J.F., Wolf, A.M. and Schorling, J.B. (1996) The impact of informed consent on patient interest in prostate-specific antigen screening, *Archives of Internal Medicine*, 156: 1333–36.

Wolf, F.M. (2003) Educational interventions for asthma in children, *Cochrane Database of Systematic Reviews*, Issue 1, No. CD000326.

PART II

Delivery

3 Self-management and behaviour change: theoretical models

Anna Serlachius and Stephen Sutton

Behaviour and behaviour change are central aspects of the self-management of chronic disease. According to Barlow and colleagues, for example, 'Self-management refers to the individual's ability to manage the symptoms, treatment, physical and psychosocial consequences and life style changes inherent in living with a chronic condition' (Barlow et al. 2002: 178). The particular behaviours that are important in self-management differ between different chronic conditions. In asthma, relevant behaviours may include self-monitoring of peak flow rates, taking daily medication and avoiding exposure to stimuli that may trigger an asthma attack. Taking medication is also a relevant behaviour in the case of type 2 diabetes but lifestyle changes such as increasing physical activity are also important to reduce the risk of complications, including heart disease. To give a third example, self-management of arthritis may involve the use of strategies to control pain (see also Chapter 4).

This chapter focuses on the use of theory to develop interventions to increase self-management behaviours among patients with chronic disease. There are many different theories that have been or could be applied to self-management behaviours. We have selected four theories that have been used in this context: the self-regulation or common sense model; social cognitive theory; the theory of planned behaviour; and the transtheoretical ('stages of change') model. Theories are useful in intervention development because they specify determinants of behaviour that are potentially amenable to change. Thus, theories inform us which variables should be targeted in interventions – which variables we should try to change in order to produce the desired change in behaviour. These are also the variables that we should measure (along with the target behaviour) when evaluating the impact of an intervention. In particular, it is important to assess whether an intervention that is designed to target behavioural determinants such as self-efficacy or attitude actually produces changes in these variables. If it does not, this provides one plausible reason for a lack of an intervention effect on behaviour.

For each of the four theories, we provide an outline of the theory and describe a study in which it has been used as the basis for a behaviour change intervention. We then briefly compare the theories and their potential to guide the development of interventions to change self-management behaviours. We conclude by making a number of recommendations for the use of theories in intervention development.

The self-regulation model

The self-regulation model, also referred to as the common sense model (CSM), describes how an individual comes to understand their illness and how they develop coping strategies to manage their illness. This theory views the patient as an 'active problem-solver' and emphasizes the role of both cognitive and emotional processes in influencing illness perceptions and coping strategies, including self-management behaviours (Leventhal et al. 1984, 1992, 2001).

The CSM specifies three phases: representation, coping and appraisal (Figure 3.1). In the first phase, the person develops mental representations of their illness in response to illness stimuli which include 'lay' information already assimilated by the individual from previous social communication and cultural knowledge about the illness, information from external sources in the social environment such as a doctor or relatives and information derived from current experience with the illness including symptoms. In addition to an emotional representation of the illness (e.g. anger and anxiety generated by the illness) five attributes of cognitive illness representations have been identified: identity (how the person describes or labels their illness); timeline (beliefs about the duration of the illness), cause (beliefs regarding what caused the illness); controllability (the extent to which the person believes that their illness is manageable and possible to control); and consequences of the disease (beliefs about how the illness will impact on the person's life).

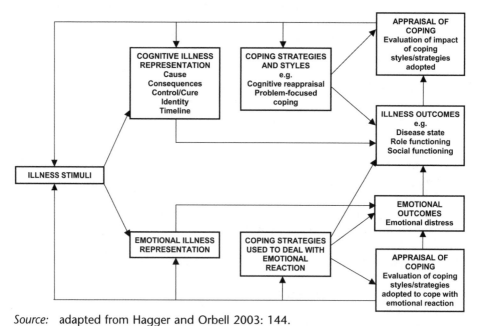

Source: adapted from Hagger and Orbell 2003: 144.

Figure 3.1 The common sense model of illness representation

According to the CSM, illness representations influence the coping process, during which the individual adopts coping strategies to manage both the illness and their emotional well-being. In some cases, a coping strategy may serve both purposes; for example, increasing physical activity may help to manage the health threat (by reducing the perceived risk of experiencing future physical deterioration or complications) and at the same time reduce anxiety. In other cases, a coping strategy may achieve one purpose at the expense of the other as, for example, when the individual attempts to maintain their emotional well-being by denying or minimizing the threat, for example, of the long-term consequences of an illness. The coping strategies adopted will influence outcomes such as social functioning and emotional distress. In the final phase (appraisal), the patient evaluates their coping strategy and decides whether to continue or to try another strategy. Key features of the model are the assumption of two parallel processes representing cognitive and emotional responses to illness and the presence of feedback loops representing a dynamic self-regulatory process in which the individual adopts coping strategies, appraises progress and revises strategies accordingly.

The CSM is a rich and complex theory that has the potential for increasing our understanding of many aspects of chronic disease self-management. In practice, researchers have used simplified versions of the model in which measures of cognitive illness representations (e.g. causes, timeline) are used to predict coping responses, including self-management behaviours, in cross-sectional or prospective designs. Many studies have used the Illness Perception Questionnaire (IPQ) (Weinman et al. 1996), which measures five dimensions of illness perceptions corresponding to the five cognitive attributes listed earlier. For example, Horne and Weinman (2002) used the IPQ to measure beliefs about asthma as potential predictors of self-reported adherence to medication. A revised version of the IPQ has since been published by Moss-Morris et al. (2002) and a brief version of this scale by Broadbent et al. (2006).

The CSM implies that changing illness perceptions may lead to changes in relevant self-management behaviours. However, to date, few studies have used the model to develop behaviour change interventions. One study that did was reported by Petrie et al. (2002). Petrie and colleagues developed a brief psychological hospital-based intervention designed to change inaccurate and negative illness perceptions among patients with their first myocardial infarction (MI). It consisted of three 30- to 40-minute intervention sessions conducted by a psychologist in addition to the standard care delivered by rehabilitation nurses. The content of the intervention was tailored to patients' responses on the IPQ, and aimed to modify maladaptive beliefs concerning MI as well as to educate patients about MI. For example, in the second session the patients' scores on the consequences and timeline subscales of the IPQ were used to target negative beliefs (e.g. a consequence of having a MI is that you must stop all physical activity) and the patient was encouraged to develop a personalized action plan of exercise, dietary change and return to work. The intervention was evaluated against standard care in a randomized controlled trial among 65 first-time MI patients aged under 65 who were consecutive admissions to Auckland Hospital, New Zealand over a 12-month period.

The intervention produced significant changes in patients' beliefs about their illness. At the time of discharge from hospital, there were significant differences between the groups on four of the five IPQ subscales, indicating that participants in the intervention group had a more positive view of the duration and consequences of their illness, as well as whether their illness could be controlled. Timeline and control/cure beliefs remained significantly different at the three-month follow-up. At this time, participants in the intervention group reported a significantly lower rate of angina symptoms than control participants ($p < 0.05$). The intervention group subsequently returned to work at a significantly faster rate than the control group ($p < 0.05$); however, there were no significant differences in rehabilitation attendance between the two groups.

This study suggests that an intervention designed to change patients' illness perceptions can lead to improved functional outcome after MI. However, a limitation of the study is that, although the intervention targeted exercise, dietary change, smoking and medication adherence, measures of these self-management behaviours were not included as outcomes.

The evidence for a causal link between illness perceptions and self-management behaviours is weak. In a meta-analysis of mainly cross-sectional studies of the relationship between illness representations (consequences, control/cure, identity and timeline) and coping behaviours, Hagger and Orbell (2003) found that only the control/cure dimension yielded a significant correlation with the category of outcomes they called 'problem-focused coping–specific', which included self-management behaviours ($r = 0.12, p < 0.05$), suggesting that beliefs about treatment or beliefs about behaviour may be more important than beliefs about the illness. A practical implication is that future interventions that aim to change self-management behaviours should target control/cure beliefs in preference to the other illness perceptions, although the correlation reported in the meta-analysis still suggests that the relationship is rather weak.

Social cognitive theory

Another highly influential model that has been applied to self-management behaviours in chronic disease is social cognitive theory (SCT) (Bandura 1986, 1997). According to SCT, behaviour is influenced directly by goals and self-efficacy expectations and indirectly by self-efficacy, outcome expectations and sociostructural factors (Figure 3.2). Goals are similar to intentions in other theories of health behaviour; they determine the amount of effort that the individual invests in changing their behaviour and serve as guides to action. Self-efficacy refers to a person's belief in their ability to perform a specific action in a particular situation. Outcome expectations are beliefs regarding the consequences (positive and negative) of performing the behaviour. The theory distinguishes between different kinds of outcome expectation. For example, social outcome expectations might include anticipated approval or disapproval from one's partner, whereas self-evaluative outcome expectations refer to anticipated feelings arising from internal standards such as pride in having achieved a change in one's behaviour. Finally, the theory incorporates perceived opportunities and barriers which are assumed to influence goals.

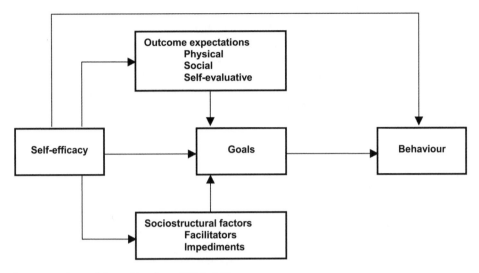

Source: adapted from Bandura 2000: 121.

Figure 3.2 Social cognitive theory

Although SCT includes a number of constructs, the majority of empirical applications of the theory focus on self-efficacy. There is a large body of evidence from observational studies showing that self-efficacy expectations consistently predict behaviour (Luszczynska and Schwarzer 2005). The theory has also been used as the basis for behaviour change interventions, again focusing almost exclusively on self-efficacy. According to Bandura (1997), there are several ways of enhancing self-efficacy. These include: mastery experiences, in which the person gains confidence by achieving a modest goal; observation of someone similar to themselves successfully performing a behaviour, known as modelling or vicarious learning; and verbal persuasion.

As an example of an intervention study that was partly based on SCT, we consider Steed et al.'s (2005) trial of a self-management programme for adults with type 2 diabetes. The intervention was a group-based programme consisting of five sessions held weekly over a five-week period and facilitated by trained health professionals. It incorporated techniques that were designed to increase self-efficacy such as problem-solving and goal-setting. The intervention was evaluated by comparison with a control group that did not receive any additional education or attention apart from measurement. One-hundred and twenty-four participants with type 2 diabetes and microalbuminuria were recruited from outpatient clinics at two inner-city hospitals and alternately allocated to control or intervention group. Participants in both groups were assessed at baseline, immediately post-intervention (six weeks) and three-month follow-up using a range of outcome measures. Self-management behaviours were assessed by a revised version of the Summary of Diabetes Self-Care Activities scale (Toobert and Glasgow 1994; Toobert et al. 2000), and self-efficacy for each of the behaviours by a subscale of the Multidimensional Diabetes Scale (Talbot et al. 1997).

At three-month follow-up, the intervention group had significantly higher scores on the measures of a diabetes-specific diet ($p < 0.001$), exercise and blood glucose monitoring ($p < 0.05$) compared with the control group. Self-efficacy for glucose monitoring and for exercise were also significantly higher in the intervention group compared with controls at three months ($p < 0.05$). However, there were no differences in self-efficacy between the groups immediately post-intervention, which may suggest that behaviour change led to change in self-efficacy rather than vice versa.

The theory of planned behaviour

The theory of planned behaviour (TPB) (Ajzen 1991, 2002b), an extension of the theory of reasoned action (Ajzen and Fishbein 1980), is widely used to study the cognitive determinants of health behaviours (Sutton 2004; Conner and Sparks 2005). According to the theory, behaviour is determined by the strength of the person's intention to perform that behaviour and the amount of actual control that the person has over performing the behaviour. According to Ajzen, intention is:

> 'the cognitive representation of a person's readiness to perform a given behaviour, and ... is considered to be the immediate antecedent of behavior', and actual behavioural control '... refers to the extent to which a person has the skills, resources and other prerequisites needed to perform a given behavior.'
>
> (Ajzen 2002b)

Perceived behavioural control, similar to Bandura's (1986) construct of self-efficacy, refers to the person's perceptions of their ability to perform the behaviour and is assumed to reflect actual behavioural control more or less accurately. To the extent that perceived behavioural control is an accurate reflection of actual behavioural control, it can, together with intention, be used to predict behaviour.

The strength of a person's intention is determined by three factors: their attitude towards the behaviour, that is, their overall evaluation of performing the behaviour; their subjective norm, that is, the extent to which they think that important others would want them to perform it; and their perceived behavioural control. Attitude, subjective norm and perceived behavioural control are each held to be determined by sets of salient (also called accessible) beliefs about the behaviour, that is, beliefs that are 'top of the mind' and most likely to be elicited in response to open-ended questions such as 'What would be the advantages for you of performing behaviour X?'. Attitude towards the behaviour is determined by behavioural beliefs about the personal consequences of performing the behaviour; subjective norm by normative beliefs about the views of important others; and perceived behavioural control by control beliefs about the presence of factors that may facilitate or impede performance of the behaviour (Figure 3.3).

The TPB has been widely used in observational studies to predict and explain intentions and behaviour. Meta-analyses of these studies show that, on average, the

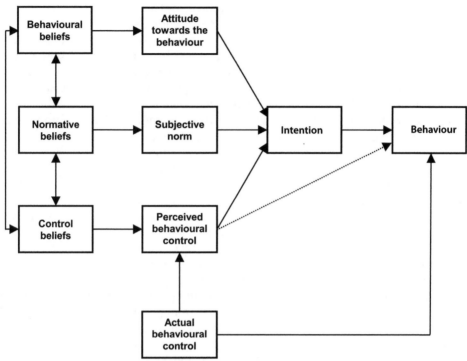

Figure 3.3 The theory of planned behaviour

TPB explains between 35–50 per cent of the variance in intentions and 26–35 per cent of the variance in behaviour (Sutton 2004). However, to date the theory has not been widely used to develop behaviour change interventions (Hardeman et al. 2002). In one of the few studies of TPB-based interventions in the self-management domain, Wyer et al. (2001) developed letters that were designed to influence MI patients' attitudes, subjective norm and perceived behavioural control with respect to attending a cardiac rehabilitation programme and evaluated their effectiveness in a randomized controlled trial. The 87 participants were patients admitted to a district hospital for acute MI and referred to a cardiac rehabilitation programme. Patients were randomly assigned to one of two groups: experimental and control. At three days post-MI, all participants were handed a sealed envelope containing a nominal letter thanking them for agreeing to take part in the study. Half of the envelopes also contained an intervention letter which was designed to increase attitude, subjective norm and perceived behavioural control.

For example, the letter attempted to increase subjective norm with the statement: 'The medical and nursing professions recommend that people who have had a heart attack should attend a cardiac rehabilitation programme.', and to increase attitude towards the behaviour with the following statements: 'This is because those who attend such a programme are more likely to recover sooner and better than those who do not attend. In addition, research has shown that attendance can reduce the chances of dying from another heart attack' (p. 156). The cardiac rehabilitation nurse then saw all participants for routine assessment and to invite them to join the rehabilitation programme. Three weeks post-MI, a second intervention letter was sent to those in the experimental group who had accepted the offer of cardiac rehabilitation. Those in the experimental group who had declined the offer were sent a letter wishing them well and informing them that they were still welcome to contact the team. Accepters in both groups were sent a letter giving details of the course dates.

The findings showed evidence for the effectiveness of the intervention letters. Compared with those in the control group, those in the experimental group were significantly more likely to accept the invitation to attend the cardiac rehabilitation programme (86% v. 70%, $p < 0.039$) and were also significantly more likely to attend (86% v. 59%, $p < 0.0025$).

It is important to appreciate that, according to the TPB, attitude, subjective norm and perceived behavioural control are determined by the individual's salient beliefs about the behaviour and therefore that, in order to change attitude, subjective norm and perceived behavioural control, it is necessary to change the corresponding sets of salient beliefs. There are three strategies for achieving this aim: change existing salient beliefs; make existing non-salient beliefs salient; or create new salient beliefs. In developing a TPB-based intervention, it is recommended that researchers or practitioners conduct an elicitation study to identify salient beliefs with respect to the target behaviour in a sample of people drawn from the target population. Those beliefs that are elicited first in response to open-ended questions such as 'What do you see as the advantages for you of attending a cardiac rehabilitation programme?' are assumed to be salient for the individual and could be used to inform an individually tailored TPB-based intervention. Those beliefs elicited most frequently in the sample are designated the modal salient beliefs and can be used to guide a generic TPB-based intervention in which all participants receive the same intervention (as in the study by Wyer et al. 2001). A limitation of the TPB and similar theories is that it does not specify how to change beliefs, only that belief change requires provision of information, broadly conceived to include not just written information of the kind used by Wyer and colleagues but also direct experience with the target behaviour and observation of others performing the behaviour.

In addition to changing attitude, subjective norm and perceived behavioural control through changing salient beliefs, the TPB also implies that behaviour change can be facilitated directly by increasing the individual's actual control over the behaviour, for example, by increasing his/her skills or opportunities to perform the behaviour. We are not aware of any intervention studies that have used the TPB in this way.

For a detailed discussion of the steps involved in developing TPB-based interventions and some of the problems and assumptions involved, see Sutton (2002b).

The transtheoretical ('stages of change') model

Stage theories of health behaviour assume that behaviour change involves movement through a sequence of discrete stages, that different factors influence the different stage transitions, and therefore that interventions should be matched to a person's stage (Weinstein et al. 1998; Sutton 2005). The transtheoretical model (TTM) (Prochaska et al. 1992; Prochaska and Velicer 1997) is the dominant stage model in the field. The model has been used in a large number of studies of smoking cessation, but it has also been applied to a wide range of other health behaviours (Prochaska et al. 1994). Although it is often referred to simply as the stages of change model, the TTM includes several additional constructs: the pros and cons of changing (together known as decisional balance); confidence and temptation; and the processes of change (Table 3.1). The TTM was an attempt to integrate these different constructs drawn from different theories of behaviour change and systems of psychotherapy into a single coherent model; hence the name transtheoretical.

The stages of change provide the basic organizing principle. The most widely used version of the model specifies five stages: precontemplation, contemplation, preparation, action and maintenance. The first three stages are pre-action stages and the last two stages are post-action stages (although preparation is sometimes defined partly in terms of behaviour change). People are assumed to move through the stages in order, but they may relapse from action or maintenance to an earlier stage. People may cycle through the stages several times before achieving long-term behaviour change.

The pros and cons are the perceived advantages and disadvantages of changing one's behaviour. They were originally derived from Janis and Mann's (1977) model of decision-making, though similar constructs occur in most theories of health behaviour. Confidence is similar to Bandura's (1986) construct of self-efficacy. It refers to the confidence that one can carry out the recommended behaviour across a range of potentially difficult situations. The related construct of temptation refers to the temptation to engage in the unhealthy behaviour across the same range of difficult situations.

Finally, the processes of change are the covert and overt activities that people engage in to progress through the stages. Ten processes that appear to be common to different behaviours have been identified: five experiential (or cognitive-affective) processes and five behavioural processes (Table 3.1).

Table 3.1 The TTM constructs

Construct	Description
Stages of change	
Precontemplation	Has no intention to take action within the next six months
Contemplation	Intends to take action within the next six months
Preparation	Intends to take action within the next 30 days and has taken some behavioural steps in this direction
Action	Has changed overt behaviour for less than six months
Maintenance	Has changed overt behaviour for more than six months

Construct	Description
Decisional balance	
Pros	The benefits of changing
Cons	The costs of changing
Self-efficacy	
Confidence	Confidence that one can engage in the healthy behaviour across different challenging situations
Temptation	Temptation to engage in the unhealthy behaviour across different challenging situations
Processes of change	
Experiential processes	
Consciousness raising	Finding and learning new facts, ideas and tips that support the healthy behaviour change
Dramatic relief	Experiencing the negative emotions (fear, anxiety, worry) that go along with unhealthy behavioural risks
Self-re-evaluation	Realizing that the behaviour change is an important part of one's identity as a person
Environmental re-evaluation	Realizing the negative impact of the unhealthy behaviour or the positive impact of the healthy behaviour on one's proximal social and physical environment
Self-liberation	Making a firm commitment to change
Behavioural processes	
Helping relationships	Seeking and using social support for the healthy behaviour change
Counter-conditioning	Substituting healthier alternative behaviours and cognitions for the unhealthy behaviour
Reinforcement management	Increasing the rewards for the positive behaviour change and decreasing the rewards of the unhealthy behaviour
Stimulus control	Removing reminders or cues to engage in the unhealthy behaviour and adding cues and reminders to engage in the healthy behaviour
Social liberation	Realizing that the social norms are changing in the direction of supporting the healthy behaviour change

Source: adapted from Prochaska et al. (2002).

In stage theories, the transitions between adjacent stages are the dependent variables, and the other constructs are variables that are assumed to influence these transitions – the independent variables. The processes of change, the pros and cons of changing, and confidence and temptation are all independent variables in this sense (Figure 3.4).

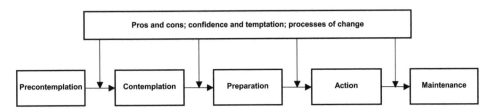

Figure 3.4 The transtheoretical model

The TTM implies that interventions should be matched to the participant's stage by targeting the variables that are assumed to influence the transition from that stage to the next. Some TTM-based interventions not only match materials to the participant's stage but also individually tailor the information on the basis of the other TTM variables. The Pathways To Change (PTC) intervention is a useful example of this approach in the self-management domain. The effectiveness of the PTC intervention in producing change in three diabetes self-care behaviours was evaluated in a randomized trial conducted in Canada: the Diabetes Stages of Change (DiSC) study (Jones et al. 2001, 2003). The three behaviours targeted in the intervention were frequency of self-monitoring of blood glucose (SMBG), healthy eating and smoking cessation. The study aimed to recruit individuals from the general diabetes population who were in a pre-action stage for any of the relevant behaviours (defined as performing SMBG fewer than four times a day if treated with insulin or less often than twice a day if treated with oral antihyperglycaemic agents alone, or having a BMI > 27 kg/m^2, or smoking cigarettes). The PTC intervention consisted of stage-matched personalized assessment reports, self-help manuals, newsletters and individual telephone counselling, with monthly contact over 12 months. A total of 1029 individuals with type 1 or type 2 diabetes were randomly allocated to the PTC intervention or usual care.

The findings were encouraging. For healthy eating, PTC produced more movement to action and maintenance over 12 months than usual care (32.5% v. 25.8%, $p < 0.001$ on a 1-tailed test). There were also significant intervention effects for SMBG ($p < 0.001$, 1-tailed test) and smoking cessation ($p = 0.03$, 1-tailed test). This was a pragmatic trial and, as the authors acknowledge, it is possible that repeated contact in the intervention condition rather than its basis in the TTM was responsible for the effect.

The descriptions of the PTC intervention in Jones et al. (2001, 2003) do not specify which variables were targeted at each stage. Similarly, expositions of the TTM do not clearly specify which variables influence which stage transitions. It would be helpful if the developers of the theory were to provide a full specification of the model that (a) stated the variables that influence each of the main transitions and (b) specified the causal relationships among the pros and cons, confidence and temptation, and processes of change.

Although the TTM is still enormously popular, it has attracted a lot of criticism in recent years, culminating in a call for the model to be abandoned (West 2005). In particular, there are fundamental problems with the definition and operationalization of the stages: they are defined using arbitrary time periods, suggesting that they are not real stages, and some of the staging algorithms contain logical flaws (Sutton 2001, 2005). In our view, the TTM cannot be recommended in its present form.

Comparison of theories

The four theories we have considered differ in important ways. The CSM differs from the other three theories in that it includes beliefs about the illness (e.g. beliefs about the causes of the disease). Although the model does include beliefs about possible coping responses (e.g. personal control), it does not incorporate beliefs about particular target behaviours. By contrast, the other three theories focus on beliefs about the target behaviour. If the aim is to predict, explain and change particular self-management behaviours (e.g. frequency of blood glucose monitoring), the CSM may be less appropriate than, for example, SCT or the TPB. On the other hand, the CSM includes aspects of a patient's response to chronic illness that are not covered by the other theories; for example, emotional representations of illness and may be useful if the focus is on the broader aspects of self-management rather than just change in behaviour.

A second important distinction is that between stage theories such as the TTM and non-stage (also called 'continuum') theories such as SCT and the TPB (Weinstein et al. 1998; Sutton 2005). These two types of theory have different formal structures and different implications for intervention. According to stage theories, different interventions should be developed for each stage; these should target the variables that are postulated to influence transition to the next stage. By contrast, continuum models imply that the interventions should target the determinants of the behaviour; for example, a TPB-based intervention should aim to change behavioural beliefs, normative beliefs, control beliefs and actual behavioural control over the behaviour (see Figure 3.3).

The theories also differ in the extent to which the constructs and the causal relationships among them are clearly specified. Of the four, the TPB is the most highly specified (though there are still some ambiguities; see Sutton 2004). Another advantage of the TPB is that there exist clear recommendations for how the constructs should be operationalized (Ajzen 2002a). The other theories lack clarity in important respects. In the case of the TTM, for example, it is not possible to develop stage-matched interventions unless an intervention developer is willing to make additional assumptions about the variables that influence each stage transition, in other words to further specify the theory.

The four theories also differ in degree of empirical support. Our reading of the literature is that SCT (self-efficacy in particular) and the TPB have relatively strong empirical support whereas the TTM and the CSM have relatively weak empirical support. However, the vast majority of studies using these theories have employed observational rather than experimental designs. For a theory to be useful as the basis for a behaviour change intervention, ideally there should be evidence that the behavioural determinants specified by the theory are causally related to behaviour. In this sense, interventions should be not only theory-based but also evidence-based. However, drawing causal inferences from non-experimental data requires several strong assumptions (Sutton 2002a). Thus, intervention developers have to make a leap of faith from evidence that a particular theoretical construct predicts behaviour in observational studies to the assumption that modifying this construct in an intervention will lead to behaviour change.

Finally, the four theories differ in the extent to which they specify how the constructs in the theory – the behavioural determinants – can be changed. SCT scores highly in this respect: there are clear recommendations for how to enhance self-efficacy (Bandura 1997). Given the similarity between the two constructs, these techniques could in principle be used to increase perceived behavioural control in interventions based on the TPB.

Conclusions and recommendations

We conclude by making a number of recommendations about the use of theory in the development of interventions to change self-management behaviours.

First, interventions should be explicitly based on theory. The rationale for this recommendation is straightforward: theories of behaviour change identify the factors that need to be changed in order to produce a desired change in behaviour. A theory of behaviour change can be embedded in a larger causal model that specifies the hypothesized causal relationships between the components of the proposed intervention (including the proposed behaviour change techniques), the determinants of the target behaviour, the behaviour itself and consequent clinical and health outcomes (Hardeman et al. 2005). Drawing a causal model is a useful early step in the process of planning and designing an intervention. Such a model also helps in designing the evaluation of the intervention. In particular, it informs decisions about what should be measured; for example, measures of the theoretical determinants of the target behaviour can be included as intermediate outcomes. It also guides the analysis of the data; for example, if measures of the theoretical determinants are included, mediation analysis can be used to test hypotheses about causal pathways (see Chapter 8). This causal modelling approach to intervention development is consistent with the influential Medical Research Council (MRC) Framework for the Development and Evaluation of Complex Interventions (Campbell et al. 2000), which is currently being revised.

Second, intervention developers need to be aware of the differences between different theories of behaviour change and should select a theory only after careful consideration of the alternatives available. We have mentioned several important criteria in the preceding section. The ideal theory would be: (1) well specified with clear definitions of constructs and clear specifications of the causal relationships among them; (2) have substantial empirical support, including evidence that the putative behavioural determinants do influence behaviour; and (3) specify how the behavioural determinants can be modified. No existing theory satisfies all three criteria, so intervention developers will need to make compromises and trade-offs between the different criteria for theory selection.

Third, and related to the previous point, intervention developers should think carefully before combining theories. The common practice of 'picking and mixing' components from several different theories (or what Bandura 1997: 285, calls 'cafeteria-style theorizing') is not recommended, unless a strong case can be made for the coherence of the new hybrid theory. Stage and continuum theories are incompatible and should not be combined.

Fourth, in reporting an intervention study, the content of the intervention should be described in detail showing how it maps onto the guiding theory, so that readers can assess the fidelity of this translation process. Given the limitations on journal space, this is likely to require supplementary, online documents. Manuals, protocols and materials should also be made available. This recommendation extends existing recommendations on improving the reporting quality of randomized (Davidson et al. 2003) and non-randomized (Des Jarlais et al. 2004) evaluations of behavioural interventions, neither of which currently refer to the theoretical basis of interventions.

Finally, although we have argued that theories of behaviour change are useful in intervention development, developers need to be aware that there are many aspects of an intervention that such theories cannot inform. For example, theories of behaviour change provide no guidance on: the ideal number or schedule of sessions whether the intervention should be one-to-one or administered in small or large groups; whether role-play or audio-visual aids should be used, and so on (see Chapter 5). Thus, interventions can never be entirely theory-based and to some extent a pragmatic approach to some factors will need to be used.

References

Ajzen, I. (1991) The theory of planned behavior, *Organizational Behavior and Human Decision Processes*, 50: 179–211.

Ajzen, I. (2002a) *Constructing a TpB Questionnaire: Conceptual and Methodological Considerations* (www.people.umass.edu/aizen: accessed 1 February 2007).

Ajzen, I. (2002b) *The Theory of Planned Behavior* (www.people.umass.edu/aizen: accessed 1 February 2007).

Ajzen, I. and Fishbein, M. (1980) *Understanding Attitudes and Predicting Social Behavior*. Englewood Cliffs, NJ: Prentice Hall.

Bandura, A. (1986) *Social Foundations of Thought and Action: A Social Cognitive Theory*. Englewood Cliffs, NJ: Prentice Hall.

Bandura, A. (1997) *Self-efficacy: The Exercise of Control*. New York: Freeman.

Bandura, A. (2000) Cultivate self-efficacy for personal and organizational effectiveness, in E.A. Locke (ed.) *The Blackwell Handbook of Principles of Organizational Behaviour* (pp. 120–136). Oxford: Blackwell.

Barlow, J., Wright, C., Sheasby, J., Turner, A. and Hainsworth, J. (2002) Self-management approaches for people with chronic conditions: a review, *Patient Education and Counseling*, 48: 177–87.

Broadbent, E., Petrie, K.J., Main, J. and Weinman, J. (2006) The Brief Illness Perception Questionnaire (BIPQ), *Journal of Psychosomatic Research*, 60: 631–37.

Campbell, M., Fitzpatrick, R., Haines, A. et al. (2000) Framework for the design and evaluation of complex interventions to improve health, *British Medical Journal*, 321: 694–96.

Conner, M. and Sparks, P. (2005) Theory of planned behaviour and health behaviour, in M. Conner and P. Norman (eds) *Predicting Health Behaviour: Research and Practice with Social Cognition Models* (2nd edn, pp. 170–222). Maidenhead: Open University Press.

Davidson, K.W., Goldstein, M., Kaplan, R.M. et al. (2003) Evidence-based behavioral medicine: what is it and how do we achieve it?, *Annals of Behavioral Medicine*, 26: 161–71.

Des Jarlais, D.C., Lyles, C., Crepaz, N. and the TREND Group (2004) Improving the reporting quality of nonrandomized evaluations of behavioral and public health interventions, *American Journal of Public Health*, 94: 361–66.

Hagger, M.S. and Orbell, S. (2003) A meta-analytic review of the common-sense model of illness representations, *Psychology and Health*, 18: 141–84.

Hardeman, W., Johnston, M., Johnston, D. et al. (2002) Application of the theory of planned behaviour in behaviour change interventions: a systematic review, *Psychology and Health*, 17: 123–58.

Hardeman, W., Sutton, S., Griffin, S. et al. (2005) A causal modelling approach to the development of theory-based behaviour change programmes for trial evaluation, *Health Education Research*, 20: 676–87.

Horne, R. and Weinman, J. (2002) Self-regulation and self-management in asthma: exploring the role of illness perceptions and treatment beliefs in explaining non-adherence to preventer medication, *Psychology and Health*, 17: 17–32.

Janis, I.L. and Mann, L. (1977) *Decision Making: a psychological analysis of conflict, choice and commitment*. New York: Free Press.

Jones, H., Edwards, L., Vallis, T.M. et al. (2003) Changes in diabetes self-care behaviors make a difference in glycemic control: the Diabetes Stages of Change (DiSC) Study, *Diabetes Care*, 26: 732–37.

Jones, H., Ruggiero, L., Edwards, L. et al. (2001) Diabetes Stages of Change (DISC): methodology and study design, *Canadian Journal of Diabetes Care*, 25: 97–107.

Leventhal, H., Diefenbach, M. and Leventhal, E.A. (1992) Illness cognition: using common sense to understand treatment adherence and affect cognition interactions, *Cognitive Therapy and Research*, 16: 143–63.

Leventhal, H., Leventhal, E.A. and Cameron, L. (2001) Representations, procedures, and affect in illness self-regulation: a perceptual-cognitive model, in A. Baum, T.A. Revenson and J.E. Singer (eds) *Handbook of Health Psychology* (pp. 19–47). Mahwah, NJ: Lawrence Erlbaum Associates, Inc.

Leventhal, H., Nerenz, D.R. and Steele, D.J. (1984) Illness representations and coping with health threats, in A. Baum, S.E. Taylor and J.E. Singer (eds) *Handbook of Psychology and Health: social psychological aspects of health*, Vol. 4 (pp. 219–52). Hillsdale, NJ: Lawrence Erlbaum Associates, Inc.

Luszczynska, A. and Schwarzer, R. (2005) Social cognitive theory, in M. Conner and P. Norman (eds) *Predicting Health Behaviour: Research and Practice with Social Cognition Models* (2nd edn, pp. 127–69). Maidenhead: Open University Press.

Moss-Morris, R., Weinman, J., Petrie, K.J. et al. (2002) The revised Illness Perception Questionnaire (IPQ-R), *Psychology and Health*, 17: 1–16.

Petrie, K.J., Cameron, L.D., Ellis, C.J., Buick, D. and Weinman, J. (2002) Changing illness perceptions after myocardial infarction: an early intervention randomized controlled trial, *Psychosomatic Medicine*, 64: 580–86.

Prochaska, J.O., DiClemente, C.C. and Norcross, J.C. (1992) In search of how people change: applications to addictive behaviors, *American Psychologist*, 47: 1102–14.

Prochaska, J.O. and Velicer, W.F. (1997) The transtheoretical model of health behavior change, *American Journal of Health Promotion*, 12: 38–48.

Prochaska, J.O., Redding, C.A. and Evers, K.E. (2002) The transtheoretical model and stages of change, in K. Glanz, B.K. Rimer and F.M. Lewis (eds) *Health Behavior and Health Education: Theory, Research, and Practice* (3rd edn, pp. 99–120). San Francisco: Jossey-Bass.

Prochaska, J.O., Velicer, W.F., Rossi, J.S. et al. (1994) Stages of change and decisional balance for 12 problem behaviours, *Health Psychology*, 13: 39–46.

Steed, L., Lankester, J., Barnard, M. et al. (2005) Evaluation of the UCL Diabetes Self-management Programme (UCL-DSMP): a randomized controlled trial, *Journal of Health Psychology*, 10: 261–76.

Sutton, S. (2001) Back to the drawing board? A review of applications of the transtheoretical model to substance use, *Addiction*, 96: 175–86.

Sutton, S. (2002a) Testing attitude-behaviour theories using non-experimental data: an examination of some hidden assumptions, *European Review of Social Psychology*, 13: 293–323.

Sutton, S. (2002b) Using social cognition models to develop health behaviour interventions: problems and assumptions, in D. Rutter and L. Quine (eds) *Changing Health Behaviour: Intervention and Research with Social Cognition Models* (pp. 193–208). Maidenhead: Open University Press.

Sutton, S. (2004) Determinants of health-related behaviours: theoretical and methodological issues, in S. Sutton, A. Baum and M. Johnston (eds) *The Sage Handbook of Health Psychology* (pp. 94–126). London: Sage Publications.

Sutton, S. (2005) Stage theories of health behaviour, in M. Conner and P. Norman (eds) *Predicting Health Behaviour: Research and Practice with Social Cognition Models* (2nd edn, pp. 223–75). Maidenhead: Open University Press.

Talbot, F., Nouwen, A., Gingras, J., Gosselin, M. and Audet, J. (1997) The assessment of diabetes-related cognitive and social factors: the multidimensional diabetes questionnaire, *Journal of Behavioral Medicine*, 20: 291–312.

Toobert, D.J. and Glasgow, R.E. (1994) Assessing diabetes self-management: the summary of diabetes self-care activities questionnaire, in C. Bradley (ed). *Handbook of Psychology and Diabetes: a Guide to Psychological Measurement in Diabetes Research and Practice* (pp. 351–75). Chur, Switzerland: Harwood Academic.

Toobert, D.J., Hampson, S.E. and Glasgow, R.E. (2000) The summary of diabetes self-care activities measure: results from 7 studies and a revised scale, *Diabetes Care*, 23: 943–50.

Weinman, J., Petrie, K.J., Moss-Morris, R. and Horne, R. (1996) The Illness Perception Questionnaire: a new method for assessing the cognitive representations of illness, *Psychology and Health*, 11: 431–45.

Weinstein, N.D., Rothman, A.J. and Sutton, S.R. (1998) Stage theories of health behavior: conceptual and methodological issues, *Health Psychology*, 17: 290–99.

West, R. (2005) Time for a change: putting the Transtheoretical (Stages of Change) Model to rest, *Addiction*, 100: 1036–39.

Wyer, S.J, Earll, L., Joseph, S. et al. (2001) Increasing attendance at a cardiac rehabilitation programme: an intervention study using the Theory of Planned Behaviour, *Coronary Health Care*, 5: 154–59.

4 Different types and components of self-management interventions

Kathleen Mulligan, Liz Steed and Stanton Newman

The definition of self-management given by Barlow et al. (2002) (see introduction) highlights that self-management of a chronic illness is complex, requiring the individual 'to manage the symptoms, treatment, physical and psychosocial consequences and life style changes inherent in living with a chronic condition'. The extent to which self-management interventions have addressed each of these aspects nevertheless varies a great deal. Examination of just a few interventions soon brings to light their diversity, which has arisen for a number of reasons. It is partly explained by the variety of disciplines and theoretical approaches from which they have evolved (see Chapter 3). Furthermore, most self-management interventions have been developed to deal with the demands of a single illness and, in part, the considerable variability results from differences between illnesses. Diversity has also arisen because interventions vary in which aspects of managing an illness they choose to address and they do not necessarily address all the different aspects of self-management. For example, some focus on helping people to manage their medication regimen whereas others may focus on lifestyle changes or on managing emotional aspects of living with a chronic illness.

Any single self-management task may nevertheless require many different skills and these are reflected in the reasons why performance of the tasks may break down. The example of taking medication illustrates this. Failure to adhere to recommended treatment may be simply the result of a misunderstanding about the correct number of medications to take and when to take them or it may be due to a difficulty in remembering to take medication or in organizing when and how to take it. Barriers to taking medication also potentially involve emotional, cognitive and social factors (Sherbourne et al. 1992). For example, individuals may have difficulty coming to terms with having a chronic illness and the need to take medicine for a long period. They may hold beliefs about medication that influence adherence, such as reservations about its necessity or concerns about long-term side-effects (Horne and Weinman 1999). Lack of social support may also hinder taking medication; for example, an unsupportive partner or social network may undermine factors such as confidence and mood that could affect the performance of health behaviours (DiMatteo 2004). This example is intended to highlight how a single self-management task such as taking medication may be influenced by many factors and also that there may be an overlap between the different aspects of self-management described by Barlow et al. (2002). Interventions that aim to facilitate self-management as a result may need to include several different components in order to address these tasks.

This chapter describes some of the most commonly used components of self-management interventions. It is not the intention to be prescriptive about which components should be included in an intervention, as the efficacy of different components, or combinations of components, is not considered in this chapter. The section on individual illnesses later in the book discusses the evidence for the relative efficacy of different approaches in those illnesses. Also, the descriptions given below do not comprise an exhaustive list of components that have been included in self-management interventions but rather an overview of those that have been widely used and/or which are most closely linked to particular theoretical approaches. Although the components are described individually, in practice there may be an overlap between aspects of different components and self-management interventions typically comprise a combination of components.

Information

An important distinction between traditional education programmes and self-management interventions is the way in which information about the disease and its treatment is imparted. Patient education programmes typically provide information about the disease and its treatment and advice about what participants need to do to manage their illness effectively. Reviews of patient education programmes for chronic illness have shown consistently that the provision of information alone is not usually sufficient to bring about significant benefits in terms of better self-management behaviour or health outcomes (Coates and Boore 1996; Gibson et al. 2002; Riemsma et al. 2002). This does not mean that information is not a necessary and important part of self-management. Without a clear understanding of the illness and its recommended treatment, people with chronic illness lack the appropriate foundations on which to base their self-management decisions. The limitation of traditional education programmes would appear to be that they do not take into account the barriers that may exist for participants to put the advice they are given into practice.

Barriers to following advice can arise for several reasons. People may experience difficulties in remembering the advice they have been given or in understanding how to integrate it into their daily lives. The beliefs people hold about their illness and its treatment may also act as a barrier to successful self-management. Self-management interventions provide participants with the information they need to manage their illness but, rather than simply using a didactic approach to deliver this information, they ideally use a more patient-centred approach where participants' understanding and beliefs about the illness are first elicited. This helps to identify the participants' perspectives and any barriers to putting the advice into practice. The information is then imparted using skills-based methods which are considered in more detail below.

Self-monitoring

According to Creer and Holroyd (1997) 'self-monitoring provides the foundation for self-management'. Systematic recording of information, about symptoms for example, is used to increase people's awareness of their symptoms and how they change over time. It can also be used to help people identify conditions that affect the outcome being monitored and the continual feedback can serve to encourage the change process (Bandura 1997). The self-monitoring process can also enable patients to identify whether they are reaching their goals.

Skills training

People may need to learn new illness-related skills to self-manage effectively. Testing blood glucose levels in diabetes, monitoring peak flow levels in asthma, adjusting medication in response to symptoms and incorporating dietary recommendations into one's daily life are just a few examples of new skills that may need to be learned. In illnesses where such skills are important, many self-management interventions can teach these new skills through practice during the intervention sessions.

Behaviour change

Managing a chronic illness entails adopting new behaviours and changing many pre-existing behaviours. Adopting and maintaining healthy behaviours can be very difficult and research has shown that possessing knowledge of which behaviours to perform or avoid does not guarantee that behaviour change will occur (e.g. Coates and Boore 1996; Taal et al. 1997; Gibson et al 2002). An important part of self-management interventions is therefore to employ techniques that have been shown to help promote behaviour change. These techniques have their origins in a variety of theoretical approaches (see Chapter 3). Some of the most commonly used techniques in self-management interventions are described below. This is not an exhaustive list of the constructs that could be applied to bring about behaviour change but rather a description of those that have been most widely used and/or appear to be central to a self-management approach. Further discussion of the application of psychological theory to behaviour change interventions can be found in Michie et al. (2005).

Promoting readiness to change

The transtheoretical model (Prochaska and DiClemente 1984) maintains that the likelihood of individuals adopting and maintaining self-management behaviours is influenced by their motivation, or readiness, to change (for a further discussion of this model see Chapter 3). It might be assumed that anyone who chooses to attend a self-management programme will be motivated and ready to change their behaviour but this is not necessarily the case. They may have chosen to attend for a variety of reasons and while many may be in the 'preparation' stage, others may be attending purely because they have been advised to, for example, and may be at an earlier motivational stage. For any one individual, motivation to change may differ in relation to different behaviours. Furthermore, many people are ambivalent about behaviour change and motivation to change may be more fluid than suggested by the transtheoretical model (Resnicow et al. 2002).

One method that has been used to help promote readiness to change is motivational interviewing (Miller and Rollnick 1991). This was developed for use in alcohol addiction (Miller 1983) but has since been used in a range of health care settings (Knight et al. 2006). Motivational interviewing grew from a recognition that the therapeutic style adopted by health care professionals has an important influence on the process of change.

The key clinical principles of motivational interviewing are:

- expressing empathy by using reflective listening skills – an empathic style can help establish good rapport and enable people to be more open about discussing difficulties in behaviour change;
- developing discrepancy between people's goals and their current behaviour to help them raise the case for change;
- avoiding argumentation, which is considered counterproductive and likely to generate or increase resistance to change;
- rolling with resistance by acknowledging and exploring it rather than directly confronting it;
- supporting self-efficacy (see below).

Rollnick and Miller (1995) argue that motivational interviewing should not be seen simply as a set of techniques that can be applied to patients but is an interpersonal style. As such, it may be seen to complement other components of self-management interventions.

Enhancing self-efficacy

One of the most influential psychological models in self-management research is the social cognitive model of Bandura (1977, 1986), particularly the concepts of 'self-efficacy', which refers to confidence in one's ability to perform a specific behaviour, and 'outcome expectations' which are beliefs about the consequences of performing the behaviour (see Chapter 3). These concepts are considered to play a pivotal role because, whatever a person's motivation, unless they believe that they can achieve the behaviour and that it will lead to the desired outcome, they will have little incentive to perform a behaviour or persevere to overcome difficulties. Self-efficacy is therefore considered to influence the goals people set for themselves, the outcomes they expect to achieve through their efforts and the perseverance they will show in the face of obstacles (Bandura 2000).

Bandura (2000) outlined four factors considered to influence self-efficacy that can be targeted in order to increase self-efficacy and encourage behaviour change.

One way of increasing self-efficacy proposed by Bandura is through *mastery*, which is achieved through direct experience of the behaviour. Success in performing a behaviour should enhance self-efficacy thereby increasing the likelihood that the behaviour will continue and more ambitious goals will be set. By contrast, failure is likely to undermine self-efficacy and discourage continued performance of the behaviour. An important aspect of self-management interventions based on social cognitive theory is therefore to encourage participants to gain mastery through practice of the target behaviours. According to social cognitive theory, self-efficacy beliefs can also be strengthened through *vicarious experience*. This is gained through modelling the successful behaviour of a person with whom one identifies, such as another patient living with the same illness. *Social persuasion* may also strengthen a person's sense of self-efficacy; for example, an encouraging health professional or other participants in a group intervention may help to persuade patients that they have the capability to perform a given behaviour. Finally, self-efficacy beliefs may be strengthened by reducing feelings of stress that can lead people to misinterpret their physical states and thus misjudge their capabilities.

Problem-solving

Problem-solving has been described by Lorig and Holman (2003) as a key self-management skill. Training in problem-solving skills developed from a cognitive behavioural approach, which recognized the importance of these skills in enabling people to adapt to the range of problems they may encounter through their lives (D'Zurilla and Nezu 2001). This technique does not involve trying to solve people's problems for them by advising them what to do, but entails helping people to think through the difficulties they encounter and decide on a solution that best suits them.

D'Zurilla and Goldfried (1971) set out five key components to the problem-solving process. These are:

1 *Problem orientation:* the way a problem is perceived by the individual is crucial for successful problem-solving. Facilitation of a positive problem orientation is important so that the individual can see the problem as a challenge which can be overcome in contrast to a negative problem orientation in which the problem is viewed in a pessimistic way that can inhibit problem-solving attempts.

2 *Problem definition and formulation:* this involves gaining a clear understanding of the nature of the problem and breaking it down into smaller, more manageable parts.

3 *Generation of alternative solutions:* by brainstorming several alternative possible ways of dealing with a problem, it should be possible for participants to identify the strategy which is likely to be most effective for them.

4 *Decision-making:* this involves participants weighing up the pros and cons of each alternative generated in the previous step and selecting the one which is considered the most appropriate for them. It is crucial that the participant, not the intervention facilitator, chooses which strategy will be tried.

5   *Solution implementation and verification:* the final step involves participants trying out the chosen strategy, evaluating its effectiveness and adapting the strategy or choosing a new strategy as appropriate.

Although these steps have been presented sequentially, successful problem-solving is likely to involve movement back and forth between the different stages before the process is complete.

Implementation intentions and contract setting (also referred to as 'goal-setting')

The problem-solving steps outlined above include selecting and implementing strategies for behaviour change. A further step considered important to facilitate this process is the setting of 'implementation intentions', which are plans to translate intentions into actions. Much research has highlighted the gap between what people say they intend to do and actual performance of that behaviour (Sheeran 2002). Gollwitzer's (1999) 'Model of Action Phases' differentiates between goal intentions and implementation intentions; while the former specify a desired end state, the latter specify how that state will be achieved. By breaking down when, where and how the given behaviour will be performed, the goal is more likely to be achieved (Sheeran 2002).

Goal-setting, involving the selection of strategies and formulating implementation intentions, forms part of many self-management interventions. Successful implementation of these strategies may be considered to provide *mastery experiences* as described in social cognitive theory which may help to enhance self-efficacy and encourage the continued performance of the self-management behaviours. An important role for the facilitator of a self-management intervention would be to help ensure that the goals selected are achievable, because failure to reach the selected goal is likely to undermine self-efficacy and hinder further performance of the behaviour. One simple and practical technique to assess whether the goal is appropriate is to ask participants to evaluate their confidence in achieving their goal on a scale of 1–10. If participants rate their confidence at less than 7, this suggests a high risk of failure and consequently the goal can be amended to a more achievable target. Conversely, participants may rate themselves as totally confident in achieving their goal, which could indicate that they are setting their sights too low and suggests they could increase their goal and still be successful. An important skill required of those who facilitate self-management interventions is to explore with the participants how realistic they are in evaluating their abilities. Participants' enthusiasm may lead them to be overly confident and fail to consider any barriers they could encounter in pursuing their goals. Part of the facilitator's role is to gently question participants about possible barriers to ensure that the goal remains achievable under these circumstances or to amend it accordingly. This approach is likely to lead to the participant learning not to set goals too high. The idea is for the participants of self-management interventions to learn this process as a general skill and thus allow them to generalize to other behaviours and issues that may present in the future.

Once goals and implementation intentions are chosen, participants are often encouraged to write a contract that they will carry out the goal.

Challenging unhelpful beliefs

The way people think is an important influence on their behaviour and emotions and thus can act as a barrier to effective self-management. Working with participants' beliefs is therefore important to the success of self-management interventions.

Among the beliefs people hold that could influence how they manage their illness are general beliefs about themselves, such as 'I'm too old to make changes in my life', self-efficacy beliefs, as described above, and beliefs about the illness and its treatment. Illness beliefs have been examined extensively within the framework of the self-regulatory model (Leventhal et al. 1984), described in the previous chapter. They have been found to fall into five main domains – beliefs about the cause, identity (symptoms the person perceives to be related to the illness), timeline, consequences of the illness and how amenable it is to cure or control. Beliefs about treatment that may influence self-management include the concerns people hold and how necessary they consider their medication to be (Horne and Weinman 1999).

In order to modify beliefs that are either incorrect; for example, a belief that angina is a small heart attack (Furze et al. 2003) or potentially unhelpful; for example, seeing oneself as a person who does not take medication, it is first necessary to elicit these beliefs from participants in order to understand and possibly challenge them. Beliefs that are incorrect can be discussed, enabling the correct information to be presented. Potentially unhelpful beliefs can be challenged using cognitive restructuring, a technique employed in cognitive behavioural therapy, which involves helping people to gain awareness of unhelpful ways of thinking and learning how to challenge and substitute them with more helpful beliefs. For example, people may hold 'catastrophizing' beliefs, such as 'having arthritis means I'll be in pain for ever'. The self-management intervention facilitator can try to help participants examine the consequences of this way of thinking and to consider other ways of looking at the problem, with a view to developing more helpful beliefs; for example, 'I can learn new techniques that will help me to manage the pain'.

Managing emotions

Coping skills training and stress management

The term 'coping' refers to what individuals attempt to do to limit the impact of a stress such as a chronic illness (Lazarus and Folkman 1984). Coping skills training aims to provide people with a collection of skills thereby increasing the resources they have to help them deal with the demands of the illness. It is argued that increasing these coping resources helps to reduce the perceived 'threat' posed by the illness and thus reduces stress and promotes a greater sense of control over the illness. Coping skills training often combines cognitive and behavioural strategies including relaxation exercises, activity pacing, distraction techniques to cope with symptoms such as pain, coping self-statements, cognitive restructuring to modify unhelpful beliefs and communication skills training. Stress management may be considered a more specific type of coping skills training which focuses on coping with the emotional demands of the illness.

A more recently developed intervention which could come under the general heading of coping or stress management techniques is the use of expressive writing (Pennebaker 1997). Participants write down their thoughts and feelings about stressful events following a structured procedure. This process is thought to help with cognitive restructuring and result in a greater sense of control over emotions.

Coping skills training can be seen to complement many of the other commonly used components of self-management interventions such as problem-solving in that it attempts to increase the range of strategies (or resources) that are available for participants to choose from. It also complements self-efficacy approaches by helping to reduce the feelings of stress that could undermine self-efficacy.

Managing depression and anxiety

In some cases the emotional consequences of an illness may be more serious and patients may experience high levels of depressed and/or anxious mood. For example, depressive symptoms and high anxiety levels are common following a myocardial infarction (Grace et al. 2002). Anxiety and depression are important consequences of chronic disease in their own right but they also have the potential to adversely affect patient self-management behaviour. Interventions that help to manage anxiety and depression are therefore an important part of self-management for some patients. One example is in cardiac rehabilitation (see Chapter 13) where the treatment of anxiety and depression is seen as an important independent component following myocardial infarction (e.g. Lewin et al. 1992).

Managing anxiety includes learning to recognize the symptoms of anxiety and what triggers them. The way people interpret their symptoms may serve to exacerbate them; for example, misinterpreting an increased heart rate as a sign of a heart attack. Part of anxiety management therefore involves learning to reinterpret these symptoms as feelings of anxiety that, although unpleasant, are not dangerous (Lewin et al. 1992). Relaxation techniques are also taught to help reduce feelings of anxiety.

A key feature of depression is the presence of negative ways of thinking (Beck et al. 1979). An important part of tackling depression is therefore to help patients identify and modify distorted thought patterns. This may include questioning how realistic the thoughts are and using positive self-talk to replace negative thoughts with more helpful ones (cognitive restructuring). An intervention may also include scheduling enjoyable activities into the day in order to tackle the reduction in positive experiences that are common in depression.

Enhancing communication skills and social support

Chronic illness self-management may be enhanced with receipt of appropriate social support (e.g. Delamater et al. 2001). The term social support is used in various ways but within self-management, viewing it as both practical and emotional support presents a useful way of conceptualizing it for patients and also serves to help individuals recognize the need for both these types of support. Participation in a group self-management programme may provide a supportive environment in which to share experiences with others and the introduction of topics by other participants that are sensitive often enables the more reticent to participate. In addition to this implicit support, some self-management programmes directly address support and communication by including spouses, friends or relatives in the programme and/or providing training in communication skills (e.g. Lorig 1995). This may include training in communicating with health care professionals in order to enhance participants' ability to ask about issues that concern them and elicit appropriate advice. Interventions may also include sessions which aim to help people develop a support network and utilize community resources (e.g. Glasgow et al. 2002).

Maintaining behaviour change

An important issue for self-management interventions is the duration of effects. Participants may change their behaviour in the short term following an intervention but maintaining these changes is essential if longer-term benefits are to be realized. Maintaining behaviour change can be addressed in the intervention by including it as a topic in problem-solving and coping skills training, often in the format of relapse prevention. It is important to acknowledge how difficult behaviour change can be, yet many self-management interventions expect long-term behaviour change to result from a brief intervention. One possible way of tackling this issue is to include one or more booster sessions a few months after the intervention to review and address any problems that have arisen.

Types of self-management interventions

The way in which the components described above are combined differs both within and between illnesses. One reason for this variation is that the composition of self-management interventions has been influenced by the demands of different illnesses. For example, self-monitoring is important in the self-management of chronic illnesses but its features will vary between illnesses. Regular monitoring of blood glucose levels is necessary for insulin dose adjustment in diabetes (see Chapter 10). In asthma (see Chapter 12), it is recommended that patients who experience frequent exacerbations keep a diary of their peak flow readings in order to identify when their asthma is deteriorating and help facilitate decisions about medication change. These are examples of when self-monitoring is recommended as a continuous aspect of managing the illness. But self-monitoring may be useful in other ways. For example, monitoring how one responds emotionally or behaves in response to particular demands of the illness is important in understanding one's coping skills. It may therefore form part of coping skills training in which participants monitor causes of and responses to stressors.

The self-management tasks that interventions address has also tended to vary across illnesses. For example, interventions for asthma have generally concentrated on management of medical aspects of the illness and used a fairly narrow range of components to do so. These are typically information, self-monitoring and implementation intentions in the form of action plans for adjusting medication. Managing the psychosocial consequences of living with asthma has rarely been addressed in self-management interventions and it may be the case that broader self-management interventions would provide additional benefits (see Chapter 12).

Self-management interventions for diabetes (see Chapter 10) are usually much broader than for asthma as they focus on self-monitoring and lifestyle change. To achieve this, they typically include skills training and components directed at behaviour change such as problem-solving and implementation intentions. In contrast, in a painful chronic illness such as arthritis (see Chapter 11), the focus tends to be on managing pain and reducing disability. Training in cognitive pain coping skills such as distraction techniques and imagery-guided relaxation is therefore common. Behaviour change is also important; for example, in physical activity, and many interventions in arthritis include components directed at these changes.

Use of components to manage the emotional aspects varies across chronic illnesses. These are rarely included in asthma self-management, for example, but some interventions exist which aim to improve coping with stress in diabetes. This type of intervention is also more common in arthritis (see Chapter 11) and while most arthritis interventions include some coping skills training (e.g. Lorig 1995), others make it a core component (e.g. Keefe et al. 1996).

One variant of a self-management intervention which adopts a different approach from most others is the Chronic Disease Self-Management Programme (CDSMP) (Lorig et al. 1999) (see Chapter 5). This intervention is not specific to a single illness so group participants may have a variety of different illnesses. The intervention therefore does not include any disease-specific information or skills but concentrates on generic skills such as problem-solving and enhancing self-efficacy. The rationale for this approach is that many people, particularly the elderly, have more than one chronic illness and the key to managing them is being able to apply generic problem-solving skills. Participants would nevertheless have to be able to learn illness-specific skills elsewhere.

These examples show that diversity in self-management interventions has arisen partly because of the differing demands of different illnesses. Another source of diversity is that many interventions have limited their focus so that they do not necessarily address all aspects of self-management.

Other issues

When examining self-management interventions, it is important to be aware that there may be some discrepancy between the title of an intervention and its content.

Some interventions that are described as 'self-management' may be fairly limited in content, for example, mostly giving information rather than facilitating self-management skills. Others, however, may adopt a self-management approach but call themselves 'patient education' while interventions that focus on the emotional aspects of living with the illness are often titled 'stress management' or 'coping skills interventions'.

A further important distinction is between self-management interventions, cognitive behavioural interventions and cognitive behaviour therapy (CBT). The latter is a form of psychological intervention developed by Beck (1976) as a specific form of treatment for psychological conditions such as clinical depression and anxiety. CBT aims to alter 'maladaptive' thought patterns that are said to work at a range of levels, including surface-level negative automatic thoughts, deeper false assumptions and rules for living, and more ingrained negative core beliefs. In contrast, self-management interventions in physical health conditions are generally focused around outcome and are about helping the individual to make adjustments to living with a chronic illness and adapting to the 'normal' psychological changes this entails. Cognitions and behaviours are as central to self-management interventions as they are to CBT and theories such as social cognitive theory and self-regulatory theory, which hypothesize how beliefs and behaviours specific to physical health can influence emotional and physical outcomes. An important distinction however is that while self-management interventions seek to understand and work with an individual's beliefs, particularly those focused around the illness, there is less focus on these beliefs being necessarily maladaptive or incorrect. Even where thoughts are negative within chronic illness they may reflect a true status; for example, the belief that eventually the illness will cause death or disability.

Self-management interventions may help individuals understand how thoughts influence behaviour and feelings and explore different ways of viewing situations. They also may use some of the same techniques that are applied in CBT; however, the initial beliefs are not viewed as part of a pathological system. In addition, self-management interventions rarely deal with thoughts at the level of false assumptions and core beliefs which requires a more in-depth individualistic approach than is usually presented for self-management (but see Michie 2005 for further discussion). The term 'cognitive behavioural intervention', rather than defining desired outcome like self-management interventions, or underlying theory such as CBT, is a more generic term that reflects the type of strategies used in the intervention, that is, those focused around changing both cognitions and behaviours. To this extent cognitive behavioural interventions may be synonymous with self-management interventions where improved self-management is the outcome. Alternatively, where the focus is to challenge maladaptive thoughts, they may be a component of CBT.

Conclusion

This chapter has described the main components that are usually included in self-management interventions. It has also highlighted the diversity in the application of these components both within and between chronic illnesses. When designing a self-management intervention, it is important to be clear about which tasks are to be addressed by the intervention and which skills are required to put those tasks into practice.

References

Bandura, A. (1977) *Social Learning Theory*. Englewood Cliffs, NJ: Prentice Hall.

Bandura, A. (1986) *Social Foundations of Thought and Action: A Social-cognitive Theory*. Englewood Cliffs, NJ: Prentice Hall.

Bandura, A. (1997) *Self-efficacy: The Exercise of Control*. New York: Freeman.

Bandura, A. (2000) Health promotion from the perspective of social cognitive theory, in Understanding and Changing Health Behaviour: From Health Beliefs to Self Regulation. P. Norman, C. Abraham and M. Connor (eds) Amsterdam: Harwood Academic Publishers 299–339.

Barlow, J., Wright, C., Sheasby, J., Turner, A. and Hainsworth, J. (2002) Self-management approaches for people with chronic conditions: a review, *Patient Education and Counseling*, 48: 177–87.

Beck, A. (1976) *Cognitive Therapy and the Emotional Disorders*. New York: Penguin.

Beck, A.T., Rush, A.J., Shaw, B.F., Emery, G. (1979) *Cognitive Therapy for Depression*. New York: Guilford Press.

Coates, V.E. and Boore, J.R. (1996) Knowledge and diabetes self-management, *Patient Education and Counseling*, 29(1): 99–108.

Creer, T.L. and Holroyd, K.A. (1997) Self-management, in A. Baum et al. (eds) *Cambridge Handbook of Psychology, Health and Medicine* (pp. 255–58). Cambridge: Cambridge University Press.

Delamater, A.M., Jacobson, A.M., Anderson, B., Cox, D., Fisher, L., Lustman, P., Rubin, R. and Wysocki, T. (2001) Psychosocial therapies in diabetes: report of the psychosocial therapies working group, *Diabetes Care*, 24(7): 1286–92.

DiMatteo, M.R. (2004) Social support and patient adherence to medical treatment: a meta-analysis, *Health Psychology*, 23(2): 207–18.

D'Zurilla, T.J. and Goldfried, M.R. (1971) Problem solving and behavior modification, *Journal of Abnormal Psychology*, 78: 107–26.

D'Zurilla, T.J. and Nezu, A.M. (2001) Problem-solving therapies, in K.D. Dobson (ed.) *Handbook of Cognitive-behavioral Therapies* (2nd edn, pp. 211–45).

Furze, G., Bull, P., Lewin, R. J. and Thompson, D.R. (2003) Development of the York Angina Beliefs Questionnaire, *Journal of Health Psychology*, 8(3): 307–15.

Gibson, P.G., Coughlan, J., Wilson, A.J., Abramson, M., Hensley, M.J. and Walters, E.H. (2002) Limited (information only) patient education programs for adults with asthma, *The Cochrane Database of Systematic Review* Issue 2, No. CD001005.

Glasgow, R.E., Toobert, D.J., Hampson, S.E. and Strycker, L.A. (2002) Implementation, generalization and long-term results of the 'choosing well' diabetes self-management intervention, *Patient Education and Counseling*, 48(2): 115–22.

Gollwitzer, P.M. (1999) Implementation intentions: strong effects of simple plans, *American Psychologist*, July: 493–503.

Grace, S.L., Abbey, S.E., Shnek, Z.M., Irvine, J., Franche, R.L. and Stewart, D.E. (2002) Cardiac rehabilitation I: review of psychosocial factors, *General Hospital Psychiatry*, 24(3): 121–26.

Horne, R. and Weinman, J. (1999) Patients' beliefs about prescribed medicines and their role in adherence to treatment in chronic physical illness, *Journal of Psychosomatic Research*, 47(6): 555–67; 47(6): 555–67.

Keefe, F.J., Caldwell, D.S., Baucom, D., Salley, A., Robinson, E., Timmons, K., Beaupre, P., Weisberg, J. and Helms, M. (1996) Spouse-assisted coping skills training in the management of osteoarthritic knee pain, *Arthritis Care and Research*, 9(4): 279–91.

Knight, K.M., McGowan, L., Dickens, C. and Bundy, C. (2006) A systematic review of motivational interviewing in physical health care settings, *British Journal of Health Psychology*, 11(2): 319–32.

Lazarus, R.S. and Folkman, S. (1984) *Stress, Appraisal and Coping.* New York: Springer.

Leventhal, H., Nerenz, D.R. and Steele, D.J. (1984) Illness representations and coping with health threats, in A. Baum, S.E. Taylor and J.E. Singer *Social Psychological Aspects of Health* (pp. 219–52). Mahwah, NJ: Erlbaum.

Lewin, B., Robertson, I.H., Cay, E.L., Irving, J.B. and Campbell, M. (1992) Effects of self-help post-myocardial-infarction rehabilitation on psychological adjustment and use of health services, *Lancet*, 339(8800): 1036–40.

Lorig, K. (1995) Arthritis self-help course, *HMO Practice*, 9(2): 60–61.

Lorig, K.R. and Holman, H. (2003) Self-management education: history, definition, outcomes, and mechanisms, *Annals of Behavioral Medicine*, 26(1): 1–7.

Lorig, K.R., Sobel, D.S., Stewart, A.L., Brown, B.-W.J., Bandura, A., Ritter, P., Gonzalez, V.M., Laurent, D.D. and Holman, H.R. (1999) Evidence suggesting that a chronic disease self-management program can improve health status while reducing hospitalization: a randomized trial, *Medical Care*, 37(1): 5–14.

Michie, S., Johnston, M., Abraham, C., Lawton, R., Parker, D., Walker, A. and on behalf of the Psychology Theory Group (2005) Making psychological theory useful for implementing evidence based practice: a consensus approach, *Quality and Safety in Health Care*, 14(1): 26–33.

Michie, S. (2005) Is cognitive behaviour therapy effective for changing health behaviours? Commentary on Hobbis and Sutton, *Journal of Health Psychology*, 10(1): 33–36.

Miller, W.R. and Rollnick, S. (1991) *Motivational Interviewing: Preparing People to Change Addictive Behaviors*. New York: Guildford Press.

Pennebaker, J.W. (1997) Writing about emotional experiences as a therapeutic process., *Psychological Science*, 8(3): 162–66.

Prochaska, J.O. and DiClemente, C.C. (1984) *The Transtheoretical Approach: Crossing Traditional Boundaries of Change*. Homewood, Ill: Dow-Jones/Irwin.

Resnicow, K., Dilorio, C., Soet, J.E., Ernst, D., Borrelli, B. and Hecht, J. (2002) Motivational interviewing in health promotion: it sounds like something is changing, *Health Psychology*, 21(5): 444–51.

Riemsma, R., Taal, E., Kirwan, J. and Rasker, J. (2002) Patient education programmes for adults with rheumatoid arthritis, *British Medical Journal*, 325(558): 559.

Rollnick, S. and Miller, W.R. (1995) What is motivational interviewing?, *Behavioural and Cognitive Psychotherapy*, 23(4): 325–34.

Sheeran, P. (2002) Intention-behavior relations: A conceptual and empirical review, *European Review of Social Psychology*, 12: 1–36.

Sherbourne, C.D., Hays, R.D., Ordway, L., DiMatteo, M.R. and Kravitz, R.L. (1992) Antecedents of adherence to medical recommendations: results from the Medical Outcomes Study, *Journal of Behavioral Medicine*, 15(5): 447–67.

Taal, E., Rasker, J. and Wiegman, O. (1997) Group education for rheumatoid arthritis patients, *Seminars in Arthritis and Rheumatism*, 26(6): 805–16.

5   Delivery of self-management interventions

Patrick McGowan and Kate Lorig

Introduction

It is generally acknowledged that a widening gap exists between the care that people should receive for their chronic health condition(s) and the care they do receive (Glasgow and Strycker 2000). Therefore, there is a need to develop innovative and effective approaches to ensure people receive this care, especially in hard-to-reach populations (Corkery et al. 1997; Philis-Tsimikas et al. 2004). The self-management approach can be considered as an innovative and effective approach in addressing this gap.

The basic philosophical orientation of self-management programmes represents a paradigm shift from traditional education where health professionals were perceived as experts, to a collaborative approach where expertise is shared between professional and patient. As well, this shift has encouraged interactive interventions that teach problem-solving and coping skills rather than didactic approaches that provide information. Two fundamental assumptions lie at the foundation of these self-management programmes: that individuals can learn to live and cope with their condition and solve problems when they arise; and knowledgeable individuals practising self-management will experience decreased symptoms and improved physical function, and quality of life.

Major impediments in researching and synthesizing the literature on self-management includes lack of agreement as to what constitutes self-management, lack of information on the theoretical orientation and essential components of self-management programmes for specific conditions and that self-management interventions are commonly complex with multi-components. In addition, there is a trend for meta-analyses to incorporate generous inclusion criteria. However, drawing on evaluation research, this section briefly summarizes the strengths, weaknesses and challenges of the various methods used to deliver self-management.

This chapter describes three main ways that evidence-based self-management is delivered: through specially developed self-management programmes delivered by health care professionals or lay leaders; by health professionals supporting self-management in routine clinical practice, using the '5As' approach (Glasgow et al. 2003a) as an example; and through interactive technology including the Internet and telephone. The chapter provides a brief discussion of each approach, along with a critique of their strengths, weaknesses and challenges.

Self-management programmes

The most familiar and common way that evidence-based self-management is delivered is through specially designed programmes that emerged during the last two decades. These include both disease-specific and generalized programmes that are led predominantly by health care professionals as well as programmes led by lay persons (Lorig et al. 1985; Lorig et al. 1999; Barlow et al. 2002c; Newman et al. 2004; Kennedy et al 2007). The following section discusses several aspects of how self-management programmes are delivered including: duration; setting; professional versus lay leaders; disease-specific versus generic programmes, and group versus individual programmes.

Programme composition

Programme composition includes factors such as number and length of sessions and ideal group size. There has been considerable variance in such factors. For example, the delivery of self-management programmes varies in both frequency and duration, and may range from as little as one hour weekly for four weeks (Lord et al. 1999) to extended sessions (i.e. 1½–2½ hours) over the course of a few months (Lorig et al. 1999; Brown et al. 2002). Evidence to suggest optimal number of sessions or duration is infrequently presented. Research has also not addressed the ideal group size for the delivery of self-management programmes and therefore it is difficult to ascertain this. The Centers for Medicare and Medicaid Services in the USA (Health Care Finance Administration 2000) has recommended a group size for patient education of 2–20 members with an average of 10 participants. According to Barlow et al. (2002c), self-management group size varies but is typically between 6–12 persons. Final group size is also influenced by attrition. Again attrition rates are difficult to summarize in that published reports do not consistently include this information (Newman et al. 2004). In the review conducted by Newman et al. (2004), attrition for both group or individual delivery ranged from 0 per cent to 50 per cent. In evaluations of group self-management programmes Lorig et al. (1999, 2004) reported average session attendance of 4.1 of the six sessions, which is consistent with the results of the analysis of 4000 people entering self-management programmes in British Columbia, Canada (McGowan 2006). Recommendations for optimal programme composition are therefore currently difficult to make.

Programme setting

Self-management programmes are delivered in a variety of settings and according to Barlow et al. (2002c) the most popular locations in which health professionals deliver programmes are clinical settings (e.g. hospitals). In contrast, the most popular settings for lay-led programmes are community settings such as senior centres, libraries and recreation centres (Wathen 1985). It is not clear that one setting is always better than others; however, in a meta-analysis of self-management programmes for arthritis, Warsi et al. (2003) reported that there was a lack of evidence on the effectiveness of 'settings' other than community. This is also consistent with the findings of the Task Force on Community Preventive Services (Norris et al. 2002b) that for adults with type 2 diabetes, data on glycaemic control provided sufficient evidence that self-management education is effective in community gathering places. The Task Force on Community Preventive Services (2002) recommended that self-management education delivered in a community settings should be coordinated with the participant's primary care provider but this is rarely practised. Nonetheless, according to Funnell and Anderson, a community-based approach may offer advantages.

> This approach allows health professionals to have a direct experience with the community where their patients are caring for their diabetes. Such knowledge can help diabetes educators tailor the self-management education to their patients' environment ... the message that is conveyed is that diabetes self-management is a part of everyday life as opposed to the message given when patient education classes are held in a psychologically, socially, or physically distant medical center.
>
> (Funnell and Anderson 2002: 4)

In addition, providing group programmes in community settings may be advantageous in that it provides increased access especially in geographic rural and remote areas without medical settings.

Self-management programmes have had less success in ensuring participation of specific subgroups; namely, people with limited education and low economic resources (Foster et al. 2003); and ethnic groups and males (Warsi et al. 2003; Sheikh et al. 2004). With respect to ethnic populations, these challenges are being addressed through cultural adaptation of programmes (Griffiths et al. 2005).

Professional versus lay-leaders

There is an ongoing debate regarding who should deliver self-management programmes, health professionals or lay leaders. It has been demonstrated that both professionals and lay leaders deliver effective self-management programmes (Cohen et al. 1986; Lorig et al. 1986; Barlow et al. 2002c; Fu et al. 2003), but each group may bring different strengths and assets. For example, an advantage of having health care professionals deliver self-management programmes is the opportunity for them to combine traditional medical education (i.e. information and technical skills about the disease) with self-management education (Bodenheimer et al. 2002) thus developing a linkage with the person's primary health care team. As well, professionals may have an advantage in being able to deliver self-management at the same time as the patients' regular medical appointment, whereas the patient may be reluctant to participate in an additional educational activity. Patients may also be more receptive to receive this education from a health professional due to the prestige and expertise the profession represents. Cultural factors may also be influential; for example, Fu et al. (2003) note that it is very uncommon in China to have lay leaders provide health education. Lastly, their peers in the medical community may more readily accept professionally led self-management education.

Professionals may however find delivering self-management programmes challenging because they are generally trained in the acute care model (i.e. familiar with didactic directive approaches that may focus less on process, interactive exercises and developing the patient's problem-solving skills (Heisler 2006). Physicians, nurses and dieticians have traditionally been trained to provide expert (often unsolicited) advice about the benefits of health behaviour change (Goldstein et al. 1998b), and learning self-management techniques may represent a total retooling of their orientation (Rollnick 1996; Emmons and Rollnick 2001). Newman et al. (2004) concur that training in group facilitation, problem-solving, goal-setting and cognitive behavioural techniques needs to be enhanced to increase the use of these programmes. Although lay leaders would also need to be trained they would not have to 'retool' (see also Chapter 6).

There are other advantages for having volunteer lay leaders deliver self-management programmes. An important advantage relates to the prevalence of chronic health conditions and the high costs of health care professionals. In the early stages of self-management programme development (Lorig et al. 1985), cost was one of the main incentives for involving volunteers in delivering the programme in that they were plentiful and capable. However, Griffiths et al. (2007) have recommended a cautious position on the evidence suggesting cost-effectiveness of lay-led programmes. Although outcomes such as self-efficacy have been shown to improve in some studies, this is not always associated with improvement in self-rated health or health care utilization. Similar findings have been reported in the recent Cochrane Review (Foster et al. 2007) on lay-led self-management programmes (using only levels 1 or 2 evidence criteria or effect sizes to estimate impact) although the results of this review are being challenged on the basis of the appropriateness of the outcome measures and time frames used in these recent studies (Battersby 2006).

In addition to the use of community volunteer leaders obviating the need for expensive professional personnel, they may strengthen the programme in that they serve as influential role models for promoting self-management skills and self-efficacy. However, a review of lay-led self-management of chronic illness conducted by Bury et al. (2005: 3) questioned the belief that the use of lay leaders is essential because they 'act as role models' or that 'messages transmitted by peers are more credible or otherwise have a higher possible capacity to promote a sense of mastery among course participants'. The implication may be that it is the intervention rather than the influence of group leaders that is the main source of benefit in self-management.

Finally, as volunteers are community residents, they are in a good position to encourage participation of others who normally do not participate in community programmes and they can deliver programmes outside traditional working hours. Also, acting as a group leader in the delivery of a self-management course may have several benefits for the leaders themselves, who are often drawn from older and difficult-to-reach populations (Lorig et al. 1985; McGowan and Green 1995; Barlow et al. 2005). Challenges of involving volunteers include the need for ongoing recruitment and training and providing an infrastructure to support the leaders (Eve et al. 2003). In addition, the ethics of using unpaid volunteers should be considered.

Disease-specific versus generic programmes

A frequently asked question about delivery of self-management group programmes is whether they should be disease-specific or generic programmes. As co-morbidity is common in the ageing population (Coebergh et al. 1999; Fillenbaum et al. 2000), there is growing need for interventions that can be applied across chronic diseases. Therefore, standard interventions requiring minimal adaptation to a particular disease have the potential to be more cost-effective and less complicated to translate into practice than those requiring extensive adaptation to each condition (National Institutes of Health 2000). According to Barlow et al:

> Despite the unique nature of each condition and its typical manifestation, there are many commonalities in the nature of self-management tasks ...Thus, although disease specific self-management is needed for certain aspects of chronic conditions (e.g., medication), there are opportunities for shared or generic approaches to self-management training for psychosocial, communication and lifestyle issues.
>
> (Barlow et al. 2002b: 369)

Self-management approaches could combine dedicated modules for specific tasks (e.g. blood glucose monitoring for diabetes or analgesia in arthritis) combined with a generic approach for common issues and combining these approaches could be a means of optimizing one's ability to effectively self-manage across the course of the disease duration. However, research has not addressed optimal times for each approach.

Another frequently asked question relates to whether there are differences in effectiveness between disease-specific programmes compared to more general self-management programmes for participants with specific conditions. The study conducted by Lorig et al. (2005) compared the results of the Arthritis Self-Management Program with those of the Chronic Disease Self-Management Program, a general programme, and found both had positive effects, with the disease-specific programme having advantages over the more generic programme. However, as both programmes had positive effects, the more general programme was considered a viable alternative.

Group versus individual programmes

The evidence on whether self-management is optimally delivered as group or individual intervention is currently unclear. For example, a meta-analysis of diabetes self-management interventions which considered the effectiveness of group versus individual self-management programmes found no differences between these two methods (Norris et al. 2002a). In other studies, group self-management programmes fostered greater interaction and interpersonal dynamics, social modelling and problem-solving, compared to individually delivered self-management programmes (Heller et al. 1988; Rickheim et al. 2002; Mensing and Norris 2003; Tang et al. 2006). In a study examining the preferences for different educational formats involving persons with rheumatoid arthritis, Barlow et al. (2002a) revealed that people preferred individualized delivery by health professionals for education of the disease and its treatment but preferred a group format for self-management, exercise and relation-ship issues. However, in a review of individual versus group diabetes self-management education programmes, Tang et al. (2006) found no clear and consistent differences in diabetes-related health outcomes between the two formats, but noted data that supported the notion that group-based diabetes self-management education can be more cost-effective, lead to greater treatment satisfaction and can be slightly more effective for lifestyle changes.

Although potentially more cost-effective, the disadvantages to group pro-grammes may include lack of anonymity, privacy and confidentiality. For example, disclosure of HIV status in a group setting may deter participation (US Health Resources and Services Administration HIV AIDS Bureau 2005).

Supporting self-management in clinical practice

The main job of managing one's chronic health condition lies with the patient, yet a great responsibility still remains with health care providers who can use their expertise to inform, activate and assist patients in the self-management of their condition. This activity, defined by the United States Institute of Medicine, is defined as: 'the systematic provision of education and supportive interventions by health care staff to increase patients' skills and confidence in managing their health problems, including regular assessment of progress and problems, goal setting, and problem-solving support' (Adams et al. 2004: 57).

Despite growing evidence that individual and group interventions to support self-management are effective with chronic conditions, there is a considerable misconception among health care providers as to what really constitutes self-management support. In a review of health care organizations involved in imple-menting components of the Chronic Care Model, Wagner et al. (2001: 74) found that many organizations 'believed that they had provided self-management support, assuming that it was a new jargon term for traditional, didactic classroom teaching or counselling'. Many patients received little or no self-management support. This may be due, in part, to providers' lack of training and tools in self-management or because they have little time to spend on it (Eichner and Blumenthal 2003). As well, many of the components of self-management interventions are not taught in most health science schools (Newman et al. 2004).

Currently, a greater emphasis is being focused on health care providers to deliver self-management support and use behavioural techniques during routine clinic visits to enhance patients' abilities to be effective self-managers. These provid-ers can use a variety of techniques such as: setting goals; checking the patient's readiness for self-management; breaking goals and tasks into small action plans; getting personalized feedback; self-monitoring; enlisting social support; checking patient commitment to key tasks; and importantly, following up on patient goals achievement. All these techniques may be used singly or in combination. A comprehensive approach which defines a set of activities that health care providers can use is known as the '5As'. These activities are not necessarily linear with each step following the other sequentially. The next section of this chapter briefly describes the 5As. This is not the only approach that may be useful for health care professionals; the Flinders Model (Flinders Human Behaviour Health and Research Unit 2006), developed at Flinders University in Adelaide, South Australia, is another example; however, space does not permit the description of other models.

The 5As approach

A model known as the '4As' was originally developed for the National Cancer Institute to guide physician intervention in smoking cessation (Glynn and Manley 1989). This changed over time with the addition of a fifth A and has been applied to primary care interventions for a variety of behaviours (Ockene et al. 1995; Goldstein et al. 1998a; Pinto et al. 2001). It has also been recommended for use as an underlying approach in describing counselling interventions for a variety of health-related behaviours (Whitlock et al. 2002).

The 5As are Assess, Advise, Assist, Arrange and Agree. Essentially the 5As is a model of behaviour change counselling that is evidence-based and appropriate for a broad range of different behaviours and health conditions, and is feasible to utilize in primary care settings. The goal of the 5As, in the context of self-management support, is to develop a personalized, collaborative action plan that includes specific behavioural goals and a specific plan for overcoming barriers and reaching those goals.

In the first specific activity, 'Assess', the clinician assesses the patient's level of behaviour, beliefs and motivation. Three activities can take place:

1   collaboratively establishing the agenda for the interaction;
2   gathering health behaviour information;
3   assessing the client's readiness for change.

The second activity of the 5As (Advise) involves advising patients based on their personal health risks. This is where clear, specific and personalized behaviour change advice, including information about personal health harms and benefits, is given, as well as personally relevant, specific recommendations for behaviour change.

The third activity of the 5As (Agree) involves collaboratively setting goals and making short-term action plans. Patient and health care provider select appropriate treatment goals and methods based on the patient's interest in and willingness to change a specific behaviour.

The fourth aspect of the 5As (Assist) refers to health care provider activities that address barriers to change, increase the patient's motivation and self-help skills and/or help the patient secure the needed supports for successful behaviour change (Whitlock et al. 2002). Problem-solving and motivational interviewing as described in

Chapter 4 are both important elements here. It is also during the 'Assist' phase that health care providers provide traditional patient education, including how to monitor the condition and solve problems. Health care providers can also inform patients about community self-management programmes where they would learn skills and develop confidence in managing their condition. In addition, patients can be told about existing community resources such as self-help and support groups.

The fifth 'A' (Arrange) represents follow-up contacts (in person or by telephone) to provide ongoing assistance and support and to adjust the treatment plan as needed and includes referral to more intensive or specialized treatment.

Through the 5As approach, health care providers can assist patients to become better self-managers, and Bodenheimer and Grumbach (2007) make a strong case that the provision of self-management support needs to include all or most of the 5As. In practice, however, 'Assist' and 'Arrange', two components especially critical for long-term maintenance are delivered the least often. They acknowledge that it is difficult to isolate one component of the 5As to determine individual effectiveness, but that 'the triad of goal setting, action planning, and problem-solving, while not rigorously evidence based, appear to be important techniques to improve health-related behaviours and clinical outcomes, and that regular and sustained follow-up is essential' (Bodenheimer and Grumbach 2007: 94).

Perhaps the greatest challenge that health care providers have for using the strategies contained in the 5As is the perception that self-management support is not an essential part of their role but merely an 'add-on' activity at the end of the visit if there is time (Glasgow and Eakin 2000). This perception, however, is being re-evaluated. The US Institute of Medicine's Committee on Quality of Health Care in America established an agenda to address the quality of health care with a focus on five common and high-burden chronic conditions. Patient self-management support was identified as one of the six critical cross-cutting topics applicable to these chronic conditions. A key strategy in the Summit Report (Adams et al. 2004: 58) was to 'recognize the centrality of self-management support to good patient care and incorporate this recognition into the health care culture'. The key issue is that the typical one on one 15-minute visit – developed for acute care – does not work, especially for chronic and multiple conditions.

The use of 'motivational interviewing' (a component within the 'Assist' phase of the 5As) may certainly hold great potential once implementation challenges have been addressed. Individuals have typically delivered motivational interviewing with training in psychology or counselling. Training in this technique may be challenging for health professionals as it may represent a total 'retooling of their orientation' (Miller and Rollnick 2002: 254). Health professionals have been trained to provide expert advice about the benefits of health change behaviour (Goldstein et al. 1998b). Additional challenges to using motivational interviewing in medical settings include limited amount of time, the probability of not seeing the same health care provider again and no follow-up.

A recent meta-analysis by Rubak et al. (2005) evaluated the effectiveness of using motivational interviewing in different areas of disease. They found that this technique produced significant effects in some areas (body mass index, total blood cholesterol, systolic blood pressure) but not in others (cigarettes per day and HbAlc). They also found that health care providers (ie; nurses; midwives and dieticians) obtained an effect in only 48 per cent of studies compared to psychologists and physicians in 80 per cent of studies. Sixty-four per cent of studies showed an effect in brief 15-minute visits and noted that more than one encounter ensured effectiveness. They emphasized the need for large-scale studies to investigate the implementation of motivational interviewing into the daily clinical work in primary and secondary health care. Despite the promise that the technique holds for promoting behaviour change, there are few controlled studies evaluating its efficacy with health problems (Burke et al. 2003; Britt et al. 2004). This point of view is consistent with that of Bodenheimer and Grumbach (2007) that the effectiveness of motivational interviewing in enhancing physical activity and managing chronic illness is inconclusive.

Use of interactive technology to deliver self-management

The potential for interactive health technologies and their evidence base, including Internet-based self-management interventions, is reviewed in more detail in Chapter 7. They are discussed here as one possible mode for the delivery of self-management interventions.

Internet-based self-management

There is a growing potential for provision of self-management via the Internet. This mode of delivery offers easy access, time and cost efficiency, and no need for in-person contact.

Between 1996–2003 there was a twelve-fold increase in MEDLINE citations for 'web-based therapies'. A meta-analysis of 22 studies conducted by Wantland et al. (2004) examined the effectiveness of web-based interventions versus non-web-based interventions. The analyses showed improved outcomes for knowledge and/or behavioural change in persons using web-based interventions.

McKay et al. (2001) evaluated the short-term benefits of an Internet-based supplement to usual care for sedentary patients with type 2 diabetes. This randomized controlled trial involved 78 participants who were placed either in an Internet-information-only group or in an Internet-information plus self-management group. People in the self-management intervention group learned goal-setting and received personalized feedback, learned how to identify strategies to overcome barriers and used email to communicate with an online occupational therapist coach. Also, participants could communicate with others in the intervention group. People in the information-only group could read diabetes-specific articles on the web site and were able to track their glucose level over the eight-week period. At the eight-week follow-up, both groups had improved physical activity levels. Participants in the 'active lives intervention group' who used the site more frequently derived greater benefits. While there were no between-condition differences in outcomes, the use of the Internet appeared to be effective for increasing activity levels among the patients who used the service with sufficient regularity. And there was a significant relation between the extent of web site use and level of improvement in physical activity. There was a steep decline in the use of the Internet intervention over the eight-week period, and the authors emphasized a need to investigate ways to enhance use.

Internet-based self-management support programmes using one or more elements of self-management have been used with other health conditions. The Comprehensive Health Enhancement Support System (CHESS) program, developed for persons facing life-threatening illnesses, has been implemented with health conditions such as HIV/AIDS (Gustafson et al. 1999) and breast cancer (Gustafson et al. 2001). In the breast cancer study participants accessed the CHESS web site for a period up to six months and viewed different modules. They accessed the web site an average of six times per week over a 26-week period. Participants logged on at their own pace accessing information and decision support, and could access medical experts and other persons in the intervention group. Strom et al. (2000), using a waitlist control group design, investigated the effectiveness of a six-week Internet-based program that included relaxation, problem-solving and monitoring to test the effectiveness for headache control. They found the intervention groups experienced reductions in headache severity. In addition, Nguyen et al. (2005) found that people with chronic obstructive pulmonary disease who participated in a nurse-facilitated Internet-based program that included modelling, action planning and goal-setting experienced reductions in dyspnoea.

A recent study (Lorig et al. 2006) examined the effectiveness of a web-based self-management program compared to usual care. This randomized controlled trial involved 958 subjects with either heart or lung disease or with type 2 diabetes. It compared an Internet-based self-management program (similar to the small-group Chronic Disease Self-Management Program) to usual care and to the results of the original small-group program study (Lorig 1999). The Internet-based program mirrors the original Chronic Disease Self-Management Program except it does not require real-time attendance, has no face-to-face interaction and uses email reminders. Subjects were recruited through advertisements placed on established web sites in discussion groups, and in newspapers. Group size averaged 25 subjects, and members were assigned a password to access the web site. Two trained web-based moderators led each program. Subjects also received the book *Living a Healthy Life with Chronic Conditions* through the mail. Course moderators emailed participants to remind them to log on. Participants were asked to log on to the web site at least three times for a total of 1–2 hours each week. Participants read the weeks' course content, posted their action plan on a bulletin board, did self-tests and sent emails to a friend. Throughout the program moderators modelled action-planning and problem-solving on the bulletin board, offered encouragement and monitored all the posts to the bulletin board. Outcome measures included health indicators and behaviours, utilization and self-efficacy. Measures were taken at baseline, and at six and twelve months. Compared with usual care, the Internet-based group showed improvements in health statuses, and the Internet group had similar results to the original small-group Chronic Disease Self-Management Program.

Telephone self-management

Another mode of delivering self-management interventions is via the telephone. It may involve all aspects of the intervention being delivered in this way or the telephone may be used as a route for providing 'booster sessions' following an initial intervention delivered in person. In a randomized controlled trial (Weinberger et al. 1989) trained non-medical interviewers contacted persons with osteoarthritis to review medications, symptoms and barriers to keeping scheduled visits. Study participants experienced significant decreases in physical disability and pain. A literature review on interactive voice response systems, where patients report clinical information using their keypad or voice and receive recorded messages, conducted by Piette (2000) found that patients reported in a reliable manner and were more inclined to report health problems to an interactive voice response (IVR) system than to a clinician. Two rigorous multi-site randomized trials, one with patients with depression (Simon et al. 2004), and the other with patients with heart failure (Goldberg et al. 2003), demonstrated that telephone care could improve outcomes. However, a review by Currell et al. (2004: 4) concluded that the 'evidence for the effectiveness of telephone is mixed, and that the quality of most telephone care studies makes it difficult to discern consistent findings'. There is also some evidence that telephone care improves clinical outcomes, but little evidence that it decreases the overall cost of health care, particularly in the short term (Piette 2005).

Although the picture is not complete, there is some evidence that telephone-based self-management support can improve chronic disease outcomes and help patients become more effective advocates for their own care. One could make a logical assumption that several activities included in the 5As approach could be conducted by telephone. For example, it may be possible for a clinician to complete a health risk assessment questionnaire by telephone, and apply the communication techniques used in 'Advise'. The telephone may be an easy way to give patients health information and access information to other programs and services available in the community. Telephone access is important to homebound patients and to patients who may be intimidated by a busy medical office environment (Fries et al. 2000). Importantly, the telephone may be an effective method to get feedback on action plans and to engage the patient in problem-solving, especially when this activity is linked with outpatient care and clinician follow-up (Piette 2005). In addition, there is some preliminary evidence on the effectiveness of using motivational interviewing over the telephone. By allowing clinicians and patients to communicate without the formal office visit, telephone communication can address disease management problems in a more timely way.

Conclusion

This chapter described several methods used in the delivery of self-management to persons experiencing chronic health conditions and has cited evidence relating to the effectiveness of each method in bringing about the desired outcomes and effectiveness of delivery methods in reaching target populations. When considering the way that knowledge is developed, the process usually begins with basic biomedical or social sciences to clinical trials or other experimental studies to test the efficacy and effectiveness of interventions. The techniques found effective are then submitted to applied research on their management and dissemination. Much of the work that has been done at the levels of basic science and controlled trials remains to be applied and disseminated widely, especially to marginalized populations. The basic efficacy and effectiveness questions have been answered for more innovations than have been effectively implemented by practitioners or applied to or by populations needing a program (Leeman 2006). Therefore, the research most needed in the area of implementing interventions is at the demonstration and dissemination end of the spectrum. Here the research questions have more to do with delivery, adaptation, implementation, sustainability and diffusion of innovations.

A comprehensive framework that may be able to help plan and evaluate the potential public health impact of an intervention and consider several stages of knowledge development and dissemination is the Reach, Effectiveness, Adoption, Implementation and Maintenance (RE-AIM) framework (Glasgow et al. 1999; Glasgow et al. 2003b). The five dimensions of RE-AIM build on conceptual work by Rogers (2003) and Green and Kreuter (2005) and are discussed in detail in Chapter 8.

Traditional evaluations have mainly focused on only one or two dimensions from knowledge development to dissemination. Examining all five dimensions may yield a more thorough evaluation, thus giving decision-makers more information on which to base their decision to adopt or discontinue a program. The model is still evolving (Glasgow et al. 2006).

Meanwhile, it would appear that the lay-led self-management program model developed by the Stanford Patient Education Research Center has satisfactorily addressed the RE-AIM factors in that these programs have been around since the mid-1980s and are currently being delivered in approximately 20 countries. These self-management programs have undergone randomized controlled trials (Lorig et al. 1985; Lorig et al. 1999; Gifford et al. 1998), dissemination studies (Sobel et al. 2002), follow-up and cost analysis studies (Lorig et al. 2001), and have demonstrated external validity through successful implementation and producing similar results in different countries and with different populations (McGowan and Green 1995; Fu et al. 2003; Griffiths et al. 2005; Fu et al. 2006; Swerissen et al. 2006; Nolte et al. forthcoming).

The provision of self-management by health care providers, however, faces many challenges that may take years to resolve. In many ways, self-management support techniques do not coincide with the prevalent way that professionals deliver care and may require mandated macro-level changes to resolve both legislative and administrative supports. At the micro level, accruing skills to change one's orientation to that of partnership may be achieved through formal and continuing education if willingness, recognition and support are provided. And importantly, the involvement of all staff is required. According to Best (2006: ii), 'the greatest challenge for the delivery of self-management interventions is not at the individual level – where there are effective, evidence-based strategies – but at the systems level, where the optimal mix of clinical, community, and informal/personal strategies is difficult to manage'.

Self-management delivery methods using interactive technologies including the Internet and telephone have a promising potential and can look forward to addressing implementation, feasibility and viability issues. In addition, there may be an exciting opportunity and potential for combining the different approaches and evaluations of cost, and cost-effectiveness will be needed. Certainly, there is no 'one best way' for the delivery of self-management as each method has its unique strengths and limitations. An effective delivery approach:

> must include a population-based strategy that includes a menu of patient-centred options that can be tailored to the capacities and circumstances of the clinical or community setting where they are offered, as well as to the individual's and family's capacities, circumstances and preferences.
>
> (Best 2006: i)

All in all, delivery of self-management is still a work in progress.

References

Adams, K., Greiner, A.C. and Corrigan, J.M. (eds) (2004) *Report of a Summit. The 1st Annual Crossing the Quality Chasm summit – a Focus on Communities.* Washington, DC: National Academies Press.

Barlow, J.H., Bancroft, G.V. and Turner, A.P. (2005) Volunteer, lay tutors' experiences of the Chronic Disease Self-Management Course: being valued and adding value, *Health Education Research*, 20(2): 128–36.

Barlow, J.H., Cullen, L.A. and Rowe, I.F. (2002a) Educational preferences, psychological well-being and self-efficacy among people with rheumatoid arthritis, *Patient Education and Counseling*, 46(1): 11–19.

Barlow, J.H., Sturt, J. and Hearnshaw, H. (2002b) Self-management interventions for people with chronic conditions in primary care: examples from arthritis, asthma and diabetes, *Health Education Journal*, 61(4): 365–78.

Barlow, J., Wright, C., Sheasby, J., Turner, A. and Hainsworth, J. (2002c) Self-management approaches for people with chronic conditions: a review, *Patient Education and Counseling*, 48: 177–87.

Battersby, M. (2006) A risk worth taking, *Chronic Illness*, 2: 265–69.

Best, A. et al. (2006) *A population-based Framework for Chronic Disease Self-management.* Vancouver, BC: Vancouver Coastal Health Research Institute.

Bodenheimer, T. and Grumbach, K. (2007) *Improving Primary Care: Strategies and Tools for a Better Practice.* New York: Lange Medical Books/McGraw-Hill.

Bodenheimer, T., Lorig, K., Holman, H. and Grumbach, K. (2002) Patient self-management of chronic disease in primary care, *JAMA*, 288(19): 2469–75.

Britt, E., Hudson, S.M. and Blampied, M. (2004) Motivational interviewing in health settings: a review. *Patient Education and Counseling*, 53: 147–55.

Brown, S.A., Garcia, A.A., Kouzekanani, K. and Hanis, C.L. (2002) Culturally competent diabetes self-management education for Mexican Americans: the Starr County border health initiative, *Diabetes Care*, 25: 259–68.

Burke, B.L., Arkowitz, H. and Menchola, M. (2003) Motivational interviewing is equivalent to more intensive treatment, superior to placebo, and will be tested more widely, *Journal of Consulting Clinical Psychology*, 71: 843–61.

Bury, M., Newbould, J. and Taylor, D. (2005) *A Rapid Review of the Current State of Knowledge Regarding Lay-led Self-management of Chronic Illness: Evidence Review* (www.nice.org.uk/page.aspx?o=526636: accessed 23 January 2007).

Coebergh, J.W.W., Janssen-Heijnen, M.L.G., Post, P.N. and Razenberg, P.P.A. (1999) Serious co-morbidity among unselected cancer patients newly diagnosed in the Southeastern part of the Netherlands in 1993–1996, *Journal of Clinical Epidemiology*, 52: 1131–36.

Cohen, J.L., Sauter, S.V., deVellis, R.F. and deVellis, B.M. (1986) Evaluation of arthritis self-management courses led by laypersons and by professionals, *Arthritis and Rheumatism*, 29(3): 399–93.

Corkery, E., Palmer, C., Foley, M.E. et al. (1997) Effect of a bicultural community health worker on completion of diabetes education in a Hispanic population, *Diabetes Care*, 20(3): 254–57.

Currell, R., Urquhart, C., Wainwright P. and Lewis, R. (2004) Telemedicine versus face to face patient care: effects on professional practice and health care outcomes. Cochrane Database of Systematic Reviews 2000, Issue 2. Art. No.: CD002098. DOI: 10. 1002/ 14651858. CD002098.

Eichner, J. and Blumenthal, D. (eds) (2003) *Medicare in the 21st Century: Building a Better Chronic Care System*. Washington, DC: National Academy of Social Insurance.

Emmons, K.M. and Rollnick, S. (2001) Motivational interviewing in health care settings: opportunities and limitations, *American Journal of Preventive Medicine*, 20(1): 68–74.

Eve, R., Mares, P. and Munro, J. (2003) *The Future of Self-management Education for People with Chronic Conditions: An Aid for PCTs and Other Commissioners* (www.innovate.org.uk/Library/SME%20Briefing.pdf: accessed 23 January 2007).

Fillenbaum, G.G., Pieper, C.F., Cohen, H.J., Cornoni-Huntley, J.C. and Guralnik, J.M. (2000) Co-morbidity of five chronic health conditions in elderly community residents: determinants and impact on mortality, *Journal of Gerontology and Medical Science*, 55A: M84–9.

Flinders Human Behaviour and Health Research Unit (2006) *Flinders Model* (www.som.flinders.edu.au/FUSA/CCTU/Self-Management.htm: accessed 2 November 2006).

Foster, G., Taylor, S.J.C., Eldridge, S.E., Ramsay, J. and Griffiths, C.J. (2007) Self-management education programmes by lay leaders for people with chronic conditions. *Cochrane Database of Systematic Reviews*, Issue 4, No. CD005108. DOI: 10.1002/14651858.CD005108.pub2.

Foster, M., Kendall, E., Dickson, P. et al. (2003) Participation and chronic disease self-management: are we risking inequitable resource allocation? *Australian Journal of Primary Health*, 9: 132–40.

Fries, J.F., Weinberger, M. and Lorig, K.R. (2000) Behavioral interventions, in D.T. Felson (conference chair) Osteoarthritis: new insights. Part 2: treatment approaches, *Annals of Internal Medicine*, 133: 730–32.

Fu, D., Fu, H., McGowan, P. et al. (2003) Implementation and quantitative evaluation of chronic disease self-management programme in Shanghai, China: randomized controlled trial, *Bull World Health Organ*, 81(3): 174–82.

Fu, D., Ding, Y., McGowan, P. and Fu, H. (2006) Qualitative evaluation of Chronic Disease Self-Management Program (CDSMP) in Shanghai, *Patient Education and Counseling*, 61: 389–96.

Funnell, M.N. and Anderson, R.M. (2002) Working toward the next generation of diabetes self-management education, *Journal of Preventive Medicine*, 22(4S): 3–5.

Gifford, A.L., Laurent, D.D., Gonzalez, V.M., Chesney, M.A. and Lorig, K.R. (1998) Pilot randomized trial of education to improve self-management skills of men with symptomatic HIV/AIDS, *Journal of Acquired Immune Deficiency Syndromes and Retrovirol Sequences*, 18(2): 136–44.

Glasgow, R.E. and Eakin, E.G. (2000) Medical office-based interventions, in F.J. Snock and C.S. Skinner (eds) *Psychological Aspects of Diabetes Care*. London: John Wiley & Sons Ltd.

Glasgow, R.E. and Strycker, L.A. (2000) Preventive care practices for diabetes management in two primary care samples, *American Journal of Preventive Medicine*, 19: 9–14.

Glasgow, R.E., Vogt, T.M. and Boles, S.M. (1999) Evaluating the public health impact of health promotion interventions: the RE-AIM framework, *American Journal of Public Health*, 89: 1322–27.

Glasgow, R.E., Davis, C.L., Funnell, M.M. and Beck, A. (2003a) Implementing practical interventions to support chronic illness self-management, *Joint Commission Journal on Quality and Safety*, 29(11): 563–74.

Glasgow, R.E., Boles, S.M., McKay, H.G., Feil, E.G. and Barrera Jr., M. (2003b) The D-Net diabetes self-management program: long term implementation, outcomes, and generalization results, *Preventive Medicine*, 36: 410–19.

Glasgow, R.E., Klesges, L.M., Dzewaltowski, D.A. et al. (2006) Evaluating the impact of health promotion programs: using the RE-AIM framework to form summary measures for decision making involving complex issues, *Health Education Research*, 21(5): 688–94.

Glynn, T.J. and Manley, M.W. (1989) *How to Help Your Patients Stop Smoking. A Manual for Physicians*. Bethesda, MD: National Cancer Institute.

Goldstein, M.G., DePue, J. and Kazuira, A. (1998a) Models for provider-patient interaction: applications to health behavior change, in S.A. Shumaker, E.B. Schon, J.K. Ockene and W.L. McBeem (eds) *The Handbook of Health Behavior Change* (2nd edn). New York: Springer Publishing.

Goldstein, M., DePue, J., Monroe, A. et al. (1998b) A population-based survey of physician smoking cessation counseling practices, *Preventive Medicine*, 27: 720–29.

Green, L.W. and Kreuter, M.W. (2005) *Health Promotion Planning: An Educational and Ecological Approach*. New York: Mayfield Publishing.

Griffiths, C., Motlib, J., Azab, A. et al. (2005) Randomised controlled trial of a lay-led self-management programme for Bangladeshi patients with chronic disease, *British Journal of General Practice*, 55(520): 831–37.

Griffiths, C., Foster, G., Ramsay, J., Eldridge, S. and Taylor, S. (2007) How effective are expert patient (lay led) education programmes for chronic disease? *British Medical Journal*, 334: 1254–56.

Gustafson, D.H., Hawkins, R., Boberg, E. et al. (1999) Impact of a patient-centred, computer-based health information/support system, *American Journal of Preventive Medicine*, 16(1): 1–9.

Health Care Finance Administration (2000) Rules and regulations, *Fed Regist*, 65: 83129–54.

Heisler, M. (2006) *Building Peer Support Programs to Manage Chronic Disease: Seven Models for Success*. Oakland, CA: California Healthcare Foundation.

Heller, S.R., Clarke, P., Daly, H. et al. (1988) Group education for obese patients with type 2 diabetes: greater success at less cost, *Diabetes Medicine*, 5: 552–56.

Kennedy A., Reeves D., Bower, P., Lee, V., Middleton, E., Richardson, G., Gardner, C., Gately, C. and Rogers, A. (2007) The effectiveness and cost effectiveness of a national lay-led self care support programme for patients with long-term conditions: a pragmatic randomised controlled trial, Journal of Epidemiology and Community Health, 61(3): 254–61.

Leeman, J. (2006) Interventions to improve diabetes self-management: utility and relevance for practice, *The Diabetes Educator*, 32(4): 571–83.

Lord, J., Victor, C., Littlejohns, P., Ross, F.M. and Axford, J.S. (1999) Economic evaluation of a primary care-based education programme for patients with osteoarthritis of the knee, *Health Technology Assessment*, 3: 1–55.

Lorig, K. (2006) Action planning: a call to action. *Journal of the American Board of Family Medicine*, 19(3): 324–25.

Lorig, K., Holman, H., Sobel, D. Laurent, D., Gonzales, V., & Minor, M. (1003). Living a healthy life with chronic conditions. Palo Alto. CA:Bull Publishing Company. 1993

Lorig, K., Lubeck, D., Kraines, R.G., Seleznick, M. and Holman, H.R. (1985) Outcomes of self-help education for patients with arthritis, *Arthritis & Rheumatism*, 36(4): 439–46.

Lorig, K., Feigenbaum, P., Regan, C., Ung, E. and Holman, H.R. (1986) A comparison of lay-taught and professional-taught arthritis self-management courses, *Journal of Rheumatology*, 13(4): 763–67.

Lorig, K., Ritter, P., Stewart, A. et al. (2001) Chronic disease self-management program: two-year health status and health care utilization, *Medical Care*, 39(11): 1217–23.

Lorig, K., Ritter, P.L., Laurent, D.D. and Fries, J. (2004) Long-term randomized controlled trials of tailored-print and small-group arthritis self-management interventions, *Medical Care*, 42(4): 346–54.

Lorig, K., Ritter, P.L., Laurent, D.D. and Plant, K. (2006) Internet-based chronic disease self-management: a randomized trial. *Medical Care*, 44(11): 964–71.

Lorig, K., Ritter, P. L. and Plant, K. (2005) A disease-specific self-help program compared with a generalized chronic disease self-help program for arthritis patients, *Arthritis & Rheumatism*, 53(6): 950–57.

Lorig, K.R., Sobel, D.S., Stewart, A.L. et al. (1999) Evidence suggesting that a chronic disease self-management program can improve health status while reducing hospitalization: a randomized trial, *Medical Care*, 37(1): 5–14.

McGowan, P. (2006) *The Chronic Disease Self-Management Program – Program Evaluation British Columbia 2003–2006* (www.coag.uvic.ca/cdsmp/cdsmp_research.htm: accessed 10 April 2007).

McGowan, P. and Green, L.W. (1995) Arthritis self-management in native populations of BC: an application of health promotion and participatory research principles in chronic disease control, *Canadian Journal on Aging*, 14(1): 201–12.

McKay, H.G., King, D., Eakin, E.G., Seeley, J.R. and Glasgow, R.E. (2001) The diabetes network internet-based physical activity intervention: a randomized pilot study, *Diabetes Care*, 24(18): 1328–34.

Mensing, C.R. and Norris, S.L. (2003) Group education in diabetes: effectiveness and implementation, *Diabetes Spectrum*, 16: 96–103.

Miller, W.R and Rollnick, S. (2002) *Motivational Interviewing: Preparing People for Change* (2nd edn.). New York, NY: Guilford Press.

National Institutes of Health (2000) *Self-management Strategies Across Chronic Diseases, PA-00–109* (www.grants.nih.gov/grants/guide/pa-files/PA-00–109.html: accessed 23 January 2007).

Newman, S., Steed, L. and Mulligan, K. (2004) Self-management for chronic illness, *Lancet*, 364: 1523–37.

Nguyen, H.Q., Carrieri-Kohlman, V., Rankin, S.H., Slaughter, R. and Stulbarg, M.S. (2005) Is Internet-based support for dyspnea self-management in patients with chronic obstructive pulmonary disease possible? Results of a pilot study, *Heart & Lung*, 34(1): 51–62.

Nolte, S., Elsworth, G., Sinclair, A. and Osborne, R.H. (forthcoming) The extent and breadth of benefits from participating in chronic disease self-management courses: a national patient-reported outcomes survey, *Patient Education and Counseling*, doi: 10.1016/j.pec.2006.08.016.

Norris, S.L., Lau, J., Smith, S.J., Schmid, C.H. and Engelgau, M.M. (2002a) Self-management education for adults with type 2 diabetes: a meta-analysis of the effect on glycemic control, *Diabetes Care*, 25: 1159–71.

Norris, S.L., Nichols, P.J., Caspersen, C.J. et al. (2002b) Increasing diabetes self-management education in community settings: a systematic review, *American Journal of Preventive Medicine*, 22(4S): 39–66.

Ockene, J.K., Ockene, I.S., Quirk, M.E. et al. (1995) Physician training for patient-centered nutrition counseling in a lipid intervention trial, *Preventive Medicine*, 24(6): 563–70.

Philis-Tsimikas, A., Walker, C., Rivard, L., Talavera, G., Reimann, J.O., Salmon, M. et al. (2004) Improvement in diabetes care of underinsured patients enrolled in project dulce: a community-based, culturally appropriate, nurse case management and peer education diabetes care model, *Diabetes Care*, 27(1): 110–15.

Piette, J.D. (2000) Interactive voice response systems in the diagnosis and management of chronic disease, *American Journal of Managed Care*, 6: 817–27.

Piette, J.D. (2005) *Using Telephone Support to Manage Chronic Disease*. Oakland, CA: California Health Care Foundation.

Pinto, B.M., Lynn, H., Marcus, B.H., DePue, J. and Goldstein, M.G. (2001) Physician-based activity counseling: intervention effects on mediators of motivational readiness for physical activity, *Annals of Behavioral Medicine*, 23(1): 2–10.

Rickheim, P.L., Weaver, T.W., Flader, J.L. and Kendall, D.M. (2002) Assessment of group versus individual diabetes education, *Diabetes Care*, 25: 269–74.

Rogers, E.M. (2003) *Diffusion of Innovations* (5th edn). New York: Free Press.

Rollnick, S. (1996) Behaviour change in practice: targeting individuals, *International Journal of Obesity & Related Metabolic*, 20(Suppl. 1): S22–S26.

Rubak, S., Sandboek, A., Lauritzen, T. and Christensen, B. (2005) Motivational interviewing: a systematic review and meta-analysis, *British Journal of General Practice*, 55(513): 305–12.

Sheikh, A., Netuveli, G., Kai, J. and Panesar, S.S. (2004) Comparison of reporting of ethnicity in US and European randomized controlled trials, *British Medical Journal*, 329: 87–8.

Simon, G.E., Ludman, E.J., Tutty, S., Operskalski, B. and Von Korff, M. (2004) Telephone psychotherapy and telephone care management for primary care patients starting antidepressant treatment, *Journal of the American Medical Association*, 292(8): 935–42.

Sobel, D.S., Lorig, K.R. and Hobbs, M. (2002) Chronic Disease Self-Management Program: from Development to Dissemination. *Permanente Journal*, Spring 2002, 6(2) (www.xnet.kp.org/permanentejournal/spring02/selfmanage.html: accessed 2 November 2006).

Strom, L., Pettersson, R. and Andersson, G. (2000) A controlled trial of self-help treatment of recurrent headache conducted via the Internet, *Journal of Consultative Clinical Psychology*, 68(4): 722–27.

Swerissen, H., Belfrage, J., Weeks, A. et al (2006) A randomized control trial of a self-management program for people with a chronic illness from Vietnamese, Chinese, Italian and Greek backgrounds, *Patient Education and Counseling*, 64: 360–68.

Tang, T.S., Funnell, M.M. and Anderson, R.M. (2006) Group education strategies for diabetes self-management, *Diabetes Spectrum*, 19(2): 99–105.

Task Force on Community Preventive Services (2002) Recommendations for health-care system and self-management education interventions to reduce mortality and morbidity from diabetes, *American Journal of Preventive Medicine*, 22(4S): 10–14.

US Health Resources and Services Administration HIV AIDS Bureau (2005) *Applying Elements of the Chronic Care Model to HIV/AIDS Clinical Care: Moving CARE Act Clients from Intensive Case Management Toward Self Management* (www.hab.hrsa.gov/special/ccm/ccm.htm: accessed 8 April 2007).

Wagner, E.H., Austin, B.T., Davis, C. et al. (2001) Improving chronic illness care: translating evidence into action, *Health Affairs (Millwood)*, 20(6): 64–78.

Wantland, D.J., Portillo, C.J., Holzemer, W.L., Slaughter, R. and McGhee, E. (2004) The effectiveness of web-based vs. non-web-based interventions: a meta-analysis of behavioral change outcomes, *Journal of Medical Internet Research*, Article e40 (www.jmir.org/2004/4/e40/: accessed 2 November 2006).

Warsi, A., LaValley, M.P. Wang, P.S. et al. (2003) Arthritis self-management education programs: a meta-analysis of the effect on pain and disability, *Arthritis and Rheumatism*, 48(8): 2207–13.

Wathen, G. (1985) Arthritis self-management: American style, *British Journal of Occupational Therapy*, 48(5): 129–30.

Weinberger, M., Tierney, W.M., Booher, P. and Katz, B.P. (1989) Can the provision of information to patients with osteoarthritis improve functional status? A randomized controlled trial, *Arthritis and Rheumatism*, 32: 1577–83.

Whitlock, E.P., Orleans, C.T., Pender, N. and Allan, J. (2002) Evaluating primary care behavioral counseling interventions: an evidence-based approach, *American Journal of Preventive Medicine*, 22(4): 267–84.

6 Training and quality assurance of self-management interventions

Wendy Hardeman and Susan Michie

Self-management interventions aim to equip people with the means to manage (or regulate) their own behaviour, thinking and emotions in order to reach their own (or others') goals.[1] Following an introduction to the area (section 1), this chapter addresses two relatively neglected areas in research and clinical practice: training practitioners in the knowledge and skills to deliver self-management interventions (section 2), and assuring the quality of design, delivery and receipt of these interventions (section 3). In section 2 we discuss the training of practitioners in the skills required to facilitate self-management interventions, and the personal and situational characteristics that lead to effective training. In section 3 the focus is on quality assurance of the delivery and receipt of interventions. We make a distinction between the *promotion* of faithful delivery and receipt of interventions and methods to *assess* delivery and receipt. Section 4 contains some concluding remarks and directions for future research.

1 Introduction

In this section we define some key concepts in relation to quality assurance, and explain why quality assurance is important during the development, implementation and evaluation of self-management interventions.

What is quality assurance?

In the literature quality assurance in interventions or treatments is often referred to as *treatment fidelity*. Treatment fidelity includes methodological strategies used to monitor and enhance the reliability and validity of interventions (Bellg et al. 2004). These strategies comprise, for instance, observation of intervention sessions or consultations in clinical practice, and assessment of practitioners' skills in intervention delivery during training.

Originally, treatment fidelity focused on whether the treatment or intervention was delivered as intended (treatment integrity). Moncher and Prinz (1991) added the concept of treatment differentiation: the extent to which various treatments or interventions differ from each other in the intended manner. This is particularly important when the same practitioner delivers more than one type of intervention. For instance, in randomized controlled trials practitioners may deliver a theory-based intervention to patients in the experimental group and usual care to patients in the control group. Lichstein et al. (1994) added the concepts of treatment receipt and enactment. Receipt involves optimizing and assessing the degree to which the client or participant understands and demonstrates knowledge of and ability to use skills learned during the intervention. Enactment refers to assessing and optimizing the degree to which the participant applies the skills learned in their everyday life. The Behavior Change Consortium added study design and training of practitioners to the framework of treatment fidelity (Bellg et al. 2004). By design they mean that the intervention is specified in sufficient detail so that the active ingredients are delivered, and that the extent to which practitioners adhere to the protocol is assessed. Training was added to the framework because the competence of the practitioner influences to what extent contextual and interpersonal variables affect delivery of the intervention (Moncher and Prinz 1991).

In sum, treatment fidelity now encompasses five aspects (Bellg et al. 2004):

1   *Design*: Is the intervention developed in congruence with relevant theory and clinical experience?
2   *Training of practitioners*: Are the practitioners adequately trained to deliver the intervention as intended, and to maintain standardization of delivery over time?
3   *Intervention delivery*: Is the intervention delivered in practice as intended, for instance as specified in a manual or in protocols?
4   *Reach*: Does the target group understand and demonstrate knowledge of, and the ability to use the skills learned during the delivery of the intervention?
5   *Enactment*: To what extent does the target group implement the skills learned in relevant real life settings?

Thus, quality assurance needs our attention during the *development* of self-management interventions, before they are implemented in research studies or clinical practice. First, the self-management intervention needs to be described clearly, so that the practitioners understand what they are expected to deliver (*design*). Manuals or protocols should describe the intervention techniques used by the practitioners in specific terms; for example 'ask the participant to set a SMART goal to become more active: Specific, Measurable, Attainable, Realistic, and Timely', rather than 'help the participant set a goal'. Second, we need to assess whether practitioners show competence in the knowledge and skills required to deliver the intervention (*training*). After training, quality assurance involves gathering evidence about the extent to which the intervention is delivered as planned (*delivery*). Finally, it is important to know to which degree participants show an understanding of what they are asked to do in the intervention (*reach*), and whether they are able to use self-management skills in their everyday life (*enactment*). Goals for each of the five aspects of treatment fidelity are outlined by Bellg et al. (2004).

Why does quality assurance matter?

The promotion of faithful intervention delivery and assessment of fidelity in behavioural interventions can be time-intensive, and is thus costly. One may wonder whether this is worth the resources. Several reasons have been provided for the importance of quality assurance (Moncher and Prinz 1991; Bellg et al. 2004; Woolf and Johnson 2005):

- *Internal validity*: without insight into fidelity, it would be difficult to interpret data on the efficacy of interventions, to compare interventions fairly, or to replicate interventions. Without this knowledge, practitioners may omit important intervention components, or add components to the intervention.
- *External validity*: without evidence of fidelity we may reject effective interventions, or accept ineffective interventions for implementation in clinical practice.
- *Theory development*: if we have evidence that theories informing our interventions have been applied, we are able to test the theories more rigorously. This would aid theory development and improve the design of future interventions.
- *Understanding mechanisms underlying behaviour change*: measures of fidelity can be used to test causal pathways between intervention delivery and process and outcome measures. This increases our confidence that changes in cognitions and behaviour are attributable to changes in the variables targeted in the intervention (e.g. increases in physical activity are mediated by increased self-efficacy about being more physically active).
- *Costs*: instead of investing heavily in technological innovations that only moderately improve efficacy of treatments, we could use our resources for improving the delivery of existing care packages.

The emphasis on treatment fidelity may vary according to whether self-management interventions are delivered in the context of research or clinical practice. When testing the efficacy of an intervention, in other words whether the intervention works under ideal conditions, it is important to ensure as much as possible that the intervention is delivered according to protocol. When more than one practitioner is involved, consistency in intervention delivery across practitioners is important. In pragmatic studies and clinical practice it would still be helpful to assess intervention delivery, as this information can be used to support and supervise practitioners. However, the emphasis on protocol adherence may be less stringent.

2 Training in self-management interventions

To determine the skills necessary for effective training in self-management interventions, it is necessary to know what such interventions consist of. Self-management has been defined variously (Boekaerts et al. 2000; Maes and Karoly 2005) but tends to incorporate problem-solving, goal-setting, self-monitoring and action-planning, and may involve managing emotions (see also Chapter 4).

An example of a national public health self-management intervention is the 'health trainer' (Department of Health 2004). Recruited from their local communities, health trainers work in a variety of health care and other settings across England to teach people skills to manage behaviours that impact on their health. As stated in the White Paper:

"Providing information and persuasive messages can increase people's knowledge of health risks and what action to take to deal with them. This is an essential framework for changing our way of life, but it is rarely enough on its own. There is good evidence that a range of approaches grounded in psychological science can help people in changing habits and behaviour ... These sorts of approaches help people:

- Learn how to watch for things around them that can trigger or reinforce the behaviour they want to change.
- Set goals and plan how to achieve them.
- Build confidence to make the changes that they want to ... These important skills and techniques in supporting behavioural change will be a key element of health trainers' work."

The requisite competences, understanding and knowledge for health trainers to deliver their self-management training are shown in Box 6.1.

Box 6.1

Case example: health trainers

The competences required for the health trainer role were developed by Skills for Health as part of the National Occupational Standards for the Practice of Public Health. One of the competences, 'Enable individuals to change their behaviour to improve their own health and well-being' was based on self-management principles, and developed by consultant health psychologists working with the Department of Health. The performance criteria for these competences include:

1   encourage individuals to
    (a)   assess how their behaviour is affecting their health and well-being;
    (b)   identify the changes that might benefit their health and well-being;
    (c)   identify their motivation to change their behaviour;
    (d)   identify the situations that will help them change;
    (e)   identify barriers to change and ways of managing them;

2   assist individuals to
  (a)   identify specific, measurable, achievable, realistic and timely goals for changing their behaviour;
  (b)   identify one easily achievable goal to start working on;
  (c)   identify any skills that need to be learned to achieve this goal;
  (d)   develop a personal action plan that will help them achieve their goals;
  (e)   identify who and what will help them achieve their plan;
  (f)   make sure they get the support they need in achieving their plan;
  (g)   record their progress in achieving their plan;
  (h)   identify when and how their plan will be reviewed.

These are active, practical skills that can be best trained by an active, practical approach. In many ways, training can, itself, be thought of as a self-management intervention. Those being trained need to learn skills of imparting skills, of how to enact them appropriately, how to monitor their effectiveness, how to make adjustments in response to the feedback they get, how to make goals for their training and how to plan to achieve those goals.

Personal and situational characteristics that lead to effective training

In the absence of training, health care professionals do not usually possess the knowledge and skills needed to deliver self-management interventions (Whitehead 2001; Rubak et al. 2005). Knowledge is required of models and theories of behaviour change and self-management, and of group processes, and how these relate to behaviour change techniques and their application either one-to-one or in groups. Skills required include those of communication, facilitating groups, monitoring of group processes, eliciting thoughts and beliefs to change behaviour and adherence to manuals and protocols.

Knowledge

Knowledge is essential but not sufficient for training. Trainers need to know about theories and techniques of behaviour change, both in terms of imparting that knowledge and in terms of using it in their training. Imparting knowledge effectively requires giving the necessary information in an appropriate format, in appropriate quantities (not too much at a time) and at appropriate times. There should be a variety of practical tasks (e.g. discussion, quizzes, demonstrations) to ensure that the knowledge has been understood and can be recalled when needed. Links between this knowledge and practitioners' behaviour should be clear and well rehearsed.

The limitations of relying on knowledge to change behaviour have been demonstrated in many areas; for example, health promotion, education and therapeutic clinical interventions. For example, strategies to improve adherence to clinical interventions achieved a 64 per cent success rate by changing knowledge alone, but an 85 per cent success rate by using behavioural strategies, rising to 88 per cent if combined with educational strategies (Haynes 1976).

Skills

There are three sets of skills essential for those training self-management. The first are general skills of good communication and building relationships with practitioners that encourage learning. Training usually occurs in groups, so skills of managing groups are also essential for successful training. Third, specific behaviour-change skills (e.g. goal-setting, self-monitoring, action-planning). These skills are best taught by active, participatory methods (e.g. role-play and video feedback) rather than the didactic methods of instruction and advice commonly used to train health practitioners.

Communication and relationship-building skills

Good communication depends on what is said, how it is said, what is heard and the development of positive interaction. Trainers should use simple, non-technical language and be specific and concrete about what they are asking practitioners to learn and do (Michie and Johnston 2004; Michie and Lester 2005). They should use active listening skills, such as asking for clarification, paraphrasing, reflecting and summarizing what was said. To encourage interaction, open-ended questions and responses are helpful, as well as facilitating practitioners to ask questions and communicate their views even if those views are different than those of others. Taking a person-centred/active participation/collaborative approach is more effective than taking a 'mastery' role in training (Michie et al. 2003).

Developing a safe and comfortable atmosphere helps practitioners to express any uncertainty, anxiety or confusion they may feel, and raise problems and barriers as they arise. Trainers should regularly check for comprehension and acceptance of the goals and processes of the training as a whole, and of each part of the training as it proceeds.

In developing a trusting relationship with practitioners, it is necessary to express positive feelings through behaviour (expressions, gestures, language) to promote a sense of worth and security. Relationships with practitioners can be enhanced by the trainer getting to know their individual characteristics, tailoring their messages and activities accordingly and giving praise and encouragement appropriate to each individual. Blanket or undifferentiated praise is much less effective than that targeted appropriately to specific individuals and specific behaviours. Trainers should be aware of their non-verbal as well as their verbal behaviour; if body language and voice quality is not consistent with what is being said, the training value of the message is undermined.

Skills of managing groups

Groups provide a potentially powerful laboratory for training skills of self-management. Individuals bring different experiences, strengths and contributions to the learning experience and can provide effective support and encouragement to other group members. There is considerable flexibility for using a variety of training approaches with groups. For example, practitioners can work in pairs or small groups and feedback to the larger group to observe similarities and differences of approach and think about the reasons for this. They can role-play and observe each other, and learn how to give feedback in a skilled fashion; for example, start with praise and be specific and constructive. Pairing people is also a very good way of doing homework tasks, since practitioners can serve a reminder and motivational function for each other. Skilled trainers can harness the energy, motivation and confidence of the more able group members to provide positive leadership for the whole group. Humour can play an important role in maintaining a positive atmosphere and deflecting potential problems. When groups work well, the whole is much greater than the sum of its parts.

Managing groups requires not just being able to target training and several individuals simultaneously, but understanding and working with the relationships between group members. Individuals' strengths and weaknesses are likely to be very different, as are their styles of behaviour; for example, loud and dominating versus quiet and submissive, judgemental and intolerant versus open and accepting, rigid versus flexible. Skills for dealing with these differences within the same room and at the same time are required, in order to bring out the best in each individual and for the group as a whole. For example, using attention selectively and reinforcement contingently can both reduce contributions from domineering practitioners and increase involvement of retiring practitioners. Highly skilled trainers can assess the reason for behaviours that are problematic for the group, for example, if someone is attention-seeking, this may be because of insecurity or a more general cultural style. The use of praise for appropriate behaviours may help in both cases, but especially so in the former.

Conflicts may arise between group members over style of behaviour, expressed values or insensitive comments. It is up to the trainer to watch for this and intervene early on rather than let negative feelings and behaviour build up. An effective method is to work with such differences and conflicts as part of the training. The first step is to reflect to the group any difficulties observed and get the views of the individuals concerned and group. Once there is a shared understanding of the situation, it can be worked with as an example of the kind of situation practitioners are likely to encounter when they run self-management groups. A problem-solving approach can be taken: define the problem, generate a range of solutions, evaluate the strengths and weaknesses of each, select one that appears feasible and likely to have short-term success, and develop an action plan for it. Conducting this in small groups with the relevant individuals in separate groups helps to depersonalize and generalize the issue as a learning point for the whole group.

Specific behaviour-change skills

More specific skills include facilitation and encouraging responsibility and goal-setting as well as exploring beliefs, confidence and barriers/enablers. The methods required to teach such skills are well covered by Bandura's social cognitive theory (Bandura 1969). This states the following as necessary for successful behaviour change (training):

1   having clear goals for the outcome of the training;
2   having a conducive environment; for example, audio-visual facilities, a quiet training room, access to 'on-the-job' training;
3   having helpful beliefs – that the training will be effective and that you (the trainer) have the competence to impart the necessary skills. One of the barriers identified by nurses delivering preventive interventions is their lack of confidence in their skills and knowledge, and the belief that they are ill prepared for this role (see Burke and Fair 2003).
4   being competent in training skills, for example:
    (a)   modelling skills (e.g. role-playing), and setting up effective role-plays for practitioners;
    (b)   breaking tasks down into graded hierarchies, starting with the easiest task;
    (c)   giving encouragement to increase motivation and confidence;
    (d)   minimizing performance anxiety.

Carver and Scheier's self-regulation model complements the above by emphasizing methods of monitoring current behaviour so that discrepancies between current and desired behaviour can be easily detected and appropriate strategies put into place to reduce those discrepancies (Carver and Scheier 1999). Targets need to be negotiated, ideally with each practitioner, and small, specific goals for incremental change identified. There is evidence that involvement of people in setting their own goals leads to greater goal achievement than when goals are imposed (see Locke and Latham 2002). A plan for ongoing assessment and evaluation of progress needs to be jointly agreed.

Having agreed the goals of training, priorities and specific plans about how to achieve the goals need to be set. There is evidence that specifying and writing down who will do what, when, where and how is conducive to goal achievement (Gollwitzer and Sheeran 2006). Formulating effective plans depends on identifying enablers and barriers to the required change and harnessing enablers in the plan and developing 'mini action plans' to avoid or overcome the barriers.

Self-monitoring is a useful skill for changing behaviour and is useful for trainer and practitioner alike (also see Chapter 4). Reviewing self-monitoring records provides an opportunity for practitioners to identify problem areas, think about how they might be addressed, what are the specific behaviours they consider need to be changed, and develop an action plan to achieve this. Self-monitoring should be used not just to identify the need for action plans but also to evaluate the extent to which the action plan was successful. A problem-solving approach helps to learn from the experience: if the plan was not successful, what were the reasons, what is learned about the individual and the situation that can be used to adapt the plan in the future?

Relapse prevention is key to long-term maintenance of change, whether that is of training or self-management skills. It is important for practitioners to be aware from the beginning that learning is never straightforward, but proceeds in ups and downs depending on the interaction of individual and situation at any time. Lapses should be introduced as events that provide useful material to learn from and something to be valued. Such preparation reduces the likelihood that people will experience lapses as failure and a sign of inadequacy. Methods to identify and learn from lapses can also help to prevent one-off lapses becoming long-term relapse.

The impact of training on treatment fidelity

Training and supervision may increase practitioners' preparedness and comfort, and convince them of the utility and effectiveness of the intervention (Dane and Schneider 1998). Consistent supervision may also increase their feelings of account-ability. However, the evidence on the impact of training on treatment fidelity is limited (Dusenbury et al. 2003). For example, it is unclear whether video or live training is better in terms of increasing fidelity, and only few studies have compared training methods. Indirect, didactic training (verbal information about the treatment, no direct contact with trainer) of four teachers who dealt with students' problem behaviours was associated with lower fidelity of treatment delivery than direct training using rehearsal (modelling, role-play) and feedback (positive reinforcement and corrective feedback) (Sterling-Turner et al. 2002). In a study of 64 students three types of training were compared: didactic training, modelling training (videotape), and rehearsal and feedback training (training with experimenter and confederate, verbal prompts, being corrected while implementing the protocol, and contingent praise). Rehearsal and feedback training resulted in the highest levels of fidelity of delivery, followed by modelling and didactic training, respectively (Sterling-Turner et al. 2001). The use of pilot participants, role-playing, and booster sessions is also recommended (Lichstein et al. 1994).

3 Quality assurance in self-management interventions

In this section we present an overview of evidence for the use of self-management skills in research studies and clinical practice. We then introduce various strategies to promote faithful delivery of self-management interventions and their receipt by participants, and discuss methods to assess fidelity.

Fidelity of delivery: how are we doing?

Evidence for practitioners' use of self-management skills

Once training in self-management skills is completed, we often expect that health practitioners will consistently apply these skills in clinical practice and intervention studies. However, the available evidence suggests that the use of new skills decreases over time if they are not reinforced. For instance, in a study in which general practitioners and practice nurses were trained in a patient-centred method for the management of type 2 diabetes, only one-fifth of the practitioners reported that they still consistently used the method by the end of the three-year study period (Pill et al. 1999). In a randomized controlled trial evaluating an intervention to increase physical activity in individuals at risk of type 2 diabetes, practitioners delivered about half of the specified behaviour change techniques (e.g. goal-setting), and adherence decreased in later sessions (Hardeman et al. 2008). Adherence in a cardiovascular prevention counselling programme was 66 per cent (Harting et al. 2004). In a school intervention to increase fruit and vegetable consumption, teachers delivered 50 per cent of the intervention package (Davis et al. 2000), and teachers delivered 58 per cent of a Life Skills Training curriculum (Dusenbury et al. 2005). Higher levels of adherence (over 80 per cent) were found in a study of family, peer and school interventions to promote competence and reduce risk for conduct disorder, substance abuse and school failure (Dumas et al. 2001). The different methods used to assess adherence to skills across studies may partly explain the variations in levels of reported adherence.

The intervention studies above are examples of only a minority of studies that assess intervention delivery. Most of these studies report whether the sessions took place or their duration, but not what happened *during* the sessions. Several literature reviews of mainly psychotherapy interventions illustrate the absence of evidence about intervention delivery. Only 16 per cent of 539 applied behavioural analysis interventions published in the *Journal of Applied Behavioral Analysis* between 1968–1980 performed some check of the accuracy of the implementation of the independent variable (e.g. the cognitions and behaviours targeted in the intervention) (Peterson et al. 1982). An extension of this review to eight journals in clinical psychology, behaviour therapy, psychiatry and marital and family therapy found that 55 per cent of 359 intervention studies published between 1980–1988 ignored assessment of intervention delivery altogether (Moncher and Prinz 1991). Of 158 applied behavioural analysis studies among children, published in the *Journal of Applied Behavioral Analysis* between 1980–1990, only 16 per cent systematically measured and reported levels of implementation for all the independent variables (Gresham et al. 1993). Dane and Schneider reviewed interventions of primary and secondary prevention of behavioural, social and academic problems published between 1980–1994 (Dane and Schneider 1998). Only 39 out of 162 studies (24 per cent) featured specific procedures for the documentation of intervention delivery. Finally, a recent review by Borrelli et al. showed that only 27 per cent of psychosocial interventions reported checking adherence to protocol (Borrelli et al. 2005). In sum, the evidence on the extent of practitioner adherence to self-management skills is sparse, but suggests that we cannot assume that practitioners use these skills consistently over time. Continuous efforts are required to promote their use in research and clinical practice.

Reasons for low adherence to self-management skills

Various factors may explain the decrease in use of self-management skills over time. Self-management interventions tend to be complex (see Campbell et al. 2000). They consist of various components that require special skills on behalf of practitioners, and may involve multidisciplinary teamworking (Dusenbury et al. 2003). Other explanations for low adherence include a perceived lack of time by practitioners, lack of confidence in the use of self-management skills, pessimism about the patient's ability to change, lack of organizational support, limited availability of materials, and no reimbursement for the use of preventative skills (see Orleans et al. 1985; Pinto et al 1998). Pill et al. (1999) found that the failure to implement patient-centred diabetes care over time was related to a basic tension in the relationship between nurses and patients: the nurses' definition of their responsibility to the patients, and patients' perception of their responsibility for their own health. When biochemical measures showed suboptimal control of diabetes, nurses were less willing to allow the patient freedom to decide what to do in order to manage their diabetes, and used a more didactic approach.

Promotion of fidelity of intervention delivery, receipt and enactment

To promote the use of newly learned self-management skills, practitioners need to know precisely which skills they are expected to deliver in practice. The impact of training method on fidelity has been covered in section 2. In this section we introduce strategies to promote faithful intervention delivery by practitioners, and to promote the receipt of the intervention by participants. We then discuss what constitutes an optimal level of fidelity in interventions.

Manuals and protocols

Reported use of manuals in interventions and treatments is low. A meta-analysis of treatment outcome studies by Shapiro and Shapiro (Moncher and Prinz 1991) showed that less than 20 per cent of studies reported using a manual. A recent review of psychosocial interventions showed that 35 per cent reported manual use (Borrelli et al. 2005). There is some evidence that manual-based training promotes adherence among practitioners (Miller and Binder 2002). However, the relationship between manual-based training and treatment or intervention outcomes remains unclear (see also Lichstein et al. 1994), due to methodological limitations of the studies. Some studies found negative side-effects of manual-based training: embedded criticism in interactions with participants, increased hostility, and decreased warmth and affect (Miller and Binder 2002).

Ideally, a manual or protocol should include an explicit description of techniques and strategies that comprise acceptable implementation of the intervention (Moncher and Prinz 1991). In other words, general descriptions such as 'help the participant set a goal to eat healthier' are insufficient. Instead, the manual should provide details about what goal-setting involves; for example, the steps involved in helping the participant to identify an achievable goal, and making a specific plan of where, when and how the participant will implement their goal (see Box 6.2).

Box 6.2

Case example: promotion of fidelity in the *ProActive* programme

The *ProActive* programme is aimed at promoting increased physical activity among people at risk of developing type 2 diabetes, due to a family history of the disease and a sedentary lifestyle. The programme was evaluated in a randomized controlled trial among 365 participants between 30–50 years old (Williams et al. 2004; Hardeman et al. 2005). The programme was theory-based, informed by the theory of planned behaviour, self-regulation theory, operant theory and relapse prevention theory. Practitioners with experience of working in primary or community care delivered the programme at the homes of the participants or by telephone. The training of practitioners included a didactic part in which the theories were explained, including the behaviour change techniques informed by them, and role-play to practise the techniques. The practitioners also received an extensive training manual with the programme's theoretical basis, overview of relevant empirical evidence, case-based examples and exercises. They worked with several pilot participants under supervision before taking on participants in the trial. During intervention delivery monthly supervision sessions were held in which individual cases were discussed. The practitioners recorded the use of specified techniques after each intervention session, and tape-recorded sessions for feedback.

Other factors impacting on promotion of fidelity

Dusenbury et al. (2003) report several factors that are key to successful implementation: adaptive planning that is responsive to the needs of practitioners, tailoring the training to local sites, a critical mass of practitioners to provide support and prevent isolation, and local development of materials for the intervention. Additional factors that may impact on fidelity are characteristics of the programme (e.g. complexity), practitioners (e.g. their attitudes and confidence towards intervention delivery) and the organizations involved (e.g. receptivity to the intervention, culture) (Dusenbury et al. 2003).

Box 6.3

Case example: promotion of fidelity in the Diabetes Educational Programme (DEP)

DEP is an educational programme for people with newly diagnosed type 2 diabetes, delivered by the Cambridgeshire Primary Care Trust. The programme is a collaboration between the Intermediate Care Diabetes Service and the University of Cambridge General Practice and Primary Care Research Unit. The theoretical base of the programme is the self-regulation model (Leventhal et al. 1997), which provides a framework that aids understanding of how people cope after a diagnosis with diabetes, and how they think about their illness. DEP targets five dimensions of illness beliefs: cause, identity, consequences, timeline and cure/control. The programme consists of five hours of education in two sessions held a week apart, with 6–12 people in each group (with or without their partners). Session 1 is run by a diabetes specialist nurse (DSN) with a supporting community based nurse, and session 2 by a dietitian.

Quality assurance mechanisms were introduced for training, delivery and audit. Training for DEP educators includes an introduction to the psychological approach, and training in and practising adult and group education principles. The sessions have clear aims and learning objectives, which are defined in a manual. Quality assurance criteria along NICE guidelines were put in place. They include regular training for educators, formal administrative features (such as referral and attendance logs), educator experience logs, regular team meetings, annual internal and external assessment, patient questionnaires and regular audit (Holmes et al. 2006).

Promotion of participant receipt and enactment

If the receipt of the intervention by participants is suboptimal, the efficacy or effectiveness of the intervention may be confounded by the communication between practitioner and participant (Lichstein et al. 1994). Few studies have paid attention to the promotion of receipt and enactment. Lichstein et al. report the following strategies to promote *receipt* of the intervention: use of slides during the intervention, role-playing with participant including feedback, verbal cues, instructions, reminders, and questioning the participant's understanding of material. To promote the use of self-management skills by participants in everyday life, Lichtstein et al. recommend the use of concrete prompts, reminders or motivational cards, forms for recording home practice, and handing out tapes or materials (*enactment*).

How much fidelity is needed?

An important issue is what levels of fidelity one should be aiming for in self-management interventions. Some authors defined high treatment fidelity as at least 80 per cent adherence to protocol (Borrelli et al. 2005), but the evidence base for this cut-off point seems unclear. Several concerns have been aired against a too rigid implementation of the treatment fidelity guidelines as recommended by Bellg et al. (2004). Leventhal and Friedman (2004) argue that rigid implementation of all the goals of treatment fidelity will hinder the science and practice of behavioural interventions, particularly when interventions are implemented in clinical practice. In particular, they criticize 'forcing the delivery procedure in a rigid, manualized treatment'. Miller and Binder argue that fidelity does not capture the fluid nature of competent performance of practitioners.

Leventhal and Friedman (2004) also argue that systematic implementation of an intervention is difficult because there is no empirically based set of theoretical concepts and procedures for understanding the processes between the steps beginning with the design of the intervention through to final behavioural adherence. However, in the absence of evidence about whether the intervention delivered is the one planned, one can make no claims about the theoretical basis of effective interventions (Michie 2005).

The degree of emphasis on treatment fidelity in self-management interventions is a topic of ongoing debate. An ideal balance may be achieved when practitioners deliver the active ingredients of the intervention while they engage the participant by adapting delivery to the participant's personal and contextual characteristics. Adaptations to the protocol; for example, tailoring the training and adapting the intervention to various cultural backgrounds, may be inevitable for the successful implementation of an intervention (Perrin et al. 2006). Finding the optimal balance is challenging; it may vary according to whether the intervention is tested in research, where consistent delivery is important, or implemented in clinical practice, where more variation in delivery may be allowed.

Assessment of intervention fidelity

Few studies have assessed fidelity of intervention delivery. Consequently, we have little insight into *why* interventions are effective or not, and we may be reinventing the wheel (Michie and Abraham 2004). We discuss which components of self-management interventions could be assessed, and introduce various strategies to the assessment of intervention delivery.

Which components of interventions to assess?

Self-management interventions usually consist of several components, for example, general communication skills (e.g. summarizing), behaviour change techniques (e.g.

goal-setting, action-planning), modes of delivery (e.g. face-to-face, group versus individual, printed material), and providers (e.g. teachers, health practitioners) (see also Chapter 4). It can be challenging to decide which components to assess when there are limited resources. Many studies record the proportion of participants who attended sessions, or the duration of the intervention sessions. However valuable this information might be (e.g. knowing whether we are reaching our intended target group), it does not provide an insight into what happened during the sessions. We need to assess 'the black box' of intervention delivery if the aim is to understand how interventions work or not, to support practitioners in delivery of the intervention, and to test the theories which informed the intervention. This type of assessment is time-intensive and costly, and it requires protocols describing the intervention or treatment. On the other hand, lack of evidence about the extent of intervention delivery can be costly in the long run, particularly if ineffective interventions are disseminated into clinical practice.

Assessing protocol adherence involves gathering evidence about whether the practitioner performed the major operations prescribed by the intervention, and did not engage in unprescribed procedures (Moncher and Prinz 1991). Waltz et al. make an important distinction between assessing adherence and competence. They define *adherence* as 'the extent to which practitioners used interventions and approaches prescribed by the treatment manual and avoided the use of proscribed intervention procedures' (Waltz et al. 1993). *Adherence measures*, they argue, should include four types of techniques used by practitioners:

1   techniques that are essential to the intervention and unique to it;
2   techniques that are essential to the intervention but not unique to it;
3   techniques that are compatible with the intervention, but neither necessary nor unique;
4   techniques that are proscribed.

Competence refers to the level of skill shown by the practitioner in delivering the treatment. It presupposes adherence, but adherence does not necessarily imply competence (see also Miller and Binder 2002). *Competence measures* are used to determine whether an intervention has been adequately delivered in relation to the stage of the intervention, client difficulty and client presenting problems (Waltz et al. 1993).

The decision as to which aspects of the intervention to assess depends on the research question: it may be adherence, treatment dose, quality of delivery, participant responsiveness or programme differentiation (Dusenbury et al. 2003). In terms of practitioner behaviour, the assessment may focus on their use of patient-centred skills (e.g. paraphrasing, proportion of practitioner versus participant talk), empathy or use of behaviour change techniques (e.g. goal-setting). Ideally an assessment should not only focus on whether the protocol was adhered to, but also on what else was delivered, as this might have an equally important impact on effectiveness.

Sampling of intervention sessions

Gresham et al (1993) mention two practical considerations that need to be addressed when assessing intervention delivery: the number of observation sessions, and reactivity of practitioners to observation. There is plenty of evidence that practitioners may change their behaviour when they are aware that they are being assessed. Typically, this leads to higher levels of adherence. Strategies to reduce reactivity include spot-checks, being as unobtrusive as possible, and not revealing the aim of the observation (Gresham et al. 1993). For instance, pseudo-patients were used to assess whether pharmacists enquired about patients' medication use when selling nonprescription analgesic products (De Almeida Neto et al. 2000).

There is an absence of evidence on how many sessions should be sampled to gain a representative sample of sessions. Schlosser (2002) states that ideally 20–40 per cent of sessions should be assessed, or they should be equally balanced across study phases. Waltz et al. recommend that for the assessment of adherence one randomly selects interactions across participants, whereas for competence one rates all the sessions for randomly selected participants (Waltz et al. 1993). However, in practice the decision will often be guided by available resources, time and finances.

Calculation of adherence to protocols or manuals

Gresham et al. (1993) suggest recording the occurrence and non-occurrence of the implementation of each intervention component, and calculating the percentage of components implemented. This could be done for each component within and across sessions (component integrity), and for all components within each session (session integrity). This approach was adopted in the *ProActive* trial, where proportions were used to calculate adherence to behaviour-change techniques specified in protocols: the number of component behaviours in a given technique that practitioners applied in practice, divided by the number of protocol-specified component behaviours for that technique (Hardeman et al. 2008).

Box 6.4

Case example: assessment of fidelity in the ProActive programme

Adherence to specified behaviour change techniques was assessed in a theory-based intervention to increase physical activity (*ProActive*; N = 365). The intervention was delivered by four facilitators. Coding frames were developed from the intervention protocol for the four key sessions in order to assess component behaviours of the techniques. For instance, 'elicit perceived advantages of becoming more active' as part of the technique 'increasing motivation to become more active'. Facilitator behaviours were scored either as 'applied' or 'not applied'. Four raters reliably classified facilitator behaviours under 14 techniques (e.g. goal-setting, use of rewards) to calculate adherence to techniques. An independent assessor coded transcripts of 108 sessions with a sub-sample of 27 participants, using the coding frames. A second assessor coded half of the transcripts to assess inter-rater reliability. This was high with an intra-class correlation of .96 for all behaviours across the four sessions. The median observed adherence to techniques across participants was 44 per cent (*IQR* 35–62%). Adherence differed between the four facilitators and decreased across the four sessions (Hardeman et al. 2008).

Tools for the assessment of intervention delivery

Tools to measure fidelity are available, but they are weak. There is no widely accepted standardized methodology to assess intervention delivery (Dusenbury et al. 2003). Three main methods can be used to assess fidelity: external observers or interviewers; self-report by practitioners; and participant report (Bellg et al. 2004).

External sources include independent observers, fake patients or participants, and audio- and video-taped sessions. Self-report consists of ratings or checklists that practitioners or participants complete after the session. The gold standard is the coding of intervention sessions, either observed, tape- or video-recorded or transcripts, using a priori criteria of what constitutes adequate intervention delivery.

The three methods may yield different estimates of fidelity of intervention delivery. Self-report measures usually show higher levels of intervention delivery than observed measures (Resnicow et al. 1998; Davis et al. 2000; Sterling-Turner et al. 2002; Hardeman et al. 2008). Resnicow et al. (1998) compared three fidelity measures in a school-based intervention to increase fruit and vegetable intake: interviews with teachers; teacher self-report; and observation.

They found non-significant correlations between observed fidelity and the self-report measures. The three measures also showed different patterns of associations with study outcomes (e.g. cognitions and behaviour). Adjusting for pre-intervention values, interview scores and observed fidelity were associated with change in knowledge, but none of the fidelity scores was associated with changes in fruit and vegetable intake. In other words, each measure seemed to tap into a different aspect of intervention delivery.

This illustrates that fidelity assessment should not rely exclusively on practitioner-reported adherence, which is susceptible to bias (Peterson et al. 1982). Practitioners' self-report may be more suitable as a method to promote fidelity than as an accurate assessment of intervention delivery.

4 Conclusions

The preceding sections illustrate that training and quality assurance of self-management interventions is a significant undertaking. Quality assurance starts at the early stages of developing the intervention and requires attention during the entire period of implementing the intervention. Quality assurance mechanisms need adequate resources, and research funders of self-management interventions and health care commissioners should recognize this.

We finish this chapter with some recommendations for future research. First, more research is needed to establish which training methods are most effective, both for teaching self-management skills and for maximizing protocol adherence and competence. Such research should evaluate individual and combined training methods, and measure mediating processes so that knowledge about mechanisms of change can be accumulated. Second, research may focus on what constitutes optimal fidelity of delivery of self-management interventions. Faithful delivery of intervention is important in order to understand why self-management interventions work (or do not), and to test the theories that inform interventions. However, adaptations to the protocol may be necessary to keep the participant engaged, and to take individual and contextual circumstances into account. Ideally, protocols or manuals should describe where and how intervention delivery can be adapted, without compromising the core elements of the intervention and its effectiveness (Dusenbury et al. 2003). Third, more research is needed to establish which aspects of intervention delivery to assess, and how this could be done cost-effectively. Reliable and less time-intensive tools to assess fidelity are needed so that a representative sample of intervention sessions can be coded. Fourth, causal pathways between indicators of intervention fidelity and process and outcome measures need further investigation. The current evidence is mainly based on small samples, so that causal pathway analyses have been underpowered. Further work may involve both conceptual modelling and testing causal pathways in trial datasets. It is clear that causal pathways are complex, involving practitioners' delivery, participants' receipt of the intervention and enactment of its principles, through to cognitions and behaviour change.

Note

1   In this chapter we generally use the words 'practitioner' and 'participant', but one could also use 'therapist', 'provider' or 'professional', and 'patient' or 'client', respectively.

References

Bandura, A. (1969) *Principles of Behavior Modification*. New York: Holt, Rinehart & Winston.

Bellg, A.J., Borrelli, B., Resnick, B., Hecht, J., Minicucci, D.S., Ory, M. et al. (2004) Enhancing treatment fidelity in health behavior change studies: best practices and recommendations from the Behavior Change Consortium, *Health Psychology*, 23: 443–51.

Boekaerts, M., Pintrich, P.R. and Zeidner, M. (2000) Self-regulation: an introductory overview, in M. Boekaerts, P.R. Pintrich and M. Zeidner (eds) *Handbook of Self-regulation*. San Diego, CA: Academic Press.

Borrelli, B., Sepinwall, D., Ernst, D., Bellg, A.J., Czajkowski, S.M.E., Breger, R. et al. (2005) A new tool to assess treatment fidelity and evaluation of treatment fidelity across ten years of health behavior research, *Journal of Consulting and Clinical Psychology*, 73: 852–60.

Burke, L.E. and Fair, J. (2003) Promoting prevention: skills sets and attributes of health care providers who deliver behavioral interventions, *Journal of Cardiovascular Nursing*, 18: 256–66.

Campbell, M., Fitzpatrick, R., Haines, A., Kinmonth, A.L., Sandercock, P., Spiegelhalter, D. et al. (2000) Framework for design and evaluation of complex interventions to improve health, *British Medical Journal*, 321: 694–96.

Carver, C.S. and Scheier, M.F. (1999) Themes and issues in the self-regulation of behavior, in R.S.Wyer (ed.) *Perspectives on Behavioral Self-regulation: Advances in Social Cognition*, Vol. XII (pp. 1–105). London: Lawrence Erlbaum Associates.

Dane, A.V. and Schneider, B.H. (1998) Program integrity in primary and early secondary prevention: are implementation effects out of control? *Clinical Psychology Review*, 18: 23–45.

Davis, M., Baranowski, T., Resnicow, K., Baranowski, J., Doyle, C., Smith, M. et al. (2000) Gimme 5 fruit and vegetables for fun and health: process evaluation, *Health Education and Behavior*, 27: 167–76.

De Almeida Neto, A.C., Benrimoj, S.I., Kavanagh, D.J. and Boakes, R.A. (2000) Novel educational training program for community pharmacists, *American Journal of Pharmaceutical Education*, 64: 307.

Department of Health (2004) *Choosing Health: Making Healthier Choices Easier*. London: Her Majesty's Stationery Office.

Dumas, J.E., Lynch, A.M., Laughlin, J.E., Smoth, E.P. and Printz, R.J. (2001) Promoting intervention fidelity: conceptual issues, methods and preliminary results from the EARLY ALLIANCE Prevention Trial, *American Journal of Preventive Medicine*, 20: 38–47.

Dusenbury, L., Brannigan, R., Falco, M. and Hansen, W.B. (2003) A review of research on fidelity in implementation: implications for drug abuse prevention in school settings, *Health Education Research*, 18: 237–56.

Dusenbury, L., Brannigan, R., Hansen, W.B., Walsh, J. and Falco, M. (2005) Quality of implementation: developing measures crucial to understanding the diffusion of preventive interventions, *Health Education Research*, 20: 308–13.

Gollwitzer, P.M. and Sheeran, P. (2006) Implementation intentions and goal achievement: a meta-analysis of effects and processes, *Advances in Experimental Psychology*, 38: 249–68.

Gresham, F.M., Gansle, K.A. and Noell, G.H. (1993) Treatment integrity in applied behavior analysis with children, *Journal of Applied Behavior Analysis*, 26: 257–63.

Hardeman, W., Sutton, S., Griffin, S., Johnston, M., White, A., Wareham, N. et al. (2005) A causal modelling approach to the development of theory-based behaviour change programmes for trial evaluation, *Health Education Research*, 20: 676–87.

Hardeman, W., Michie, S., Fanshawe, T., Prevost, A.T., McLoughlin, K. and Kinmonth, A.L. (2008) Fidelity of delivery of a physical activity intervention: Predictors and consequences. *Psychology & Health*, 23, 1: 11–24.

Harting, J., van Assema, P., Van der Molen, H.T., Ambergen, T. and de Vries, N.K. (2004) Quality assessment of health counseling: performance of health advisors in cardiovascular prevention, *Patient Education and Counseling*, 54: 107–18.

Haynes, R.B. (1976) Introduction, in D.I. Sackett and B.R. Haynes (eds) *Compliance with Therapeutic Regimens* (pp. 1–8). Baltimore, MD: John Hopkins University Press.

Holmes, S., Barnes, R., Benson, J., Dinneen, S., Hardeman, W. and Reynolds, J. (2006) 'Small is beautiful': the development and delivery of structured group education for type 2 diabetes. Poster presentation at the 12th Regional Conference WONCA Europe, Florence, Italy, 27–30 August.

Leventhal, H., Benyamini, Y.B.S., Diefenbach, M., Leventhal, E.A., Patrick-Miller, L. and Robitaille, C. (1997) Illness representations: theoretical foundations, in D.J. Petrie and J.A. Weinman (eds) *Perceptions of Health and Illness: Current Research and Applications* (pp. 19–45). Singapore: Harwood Academic Publisher.

Leventhal, H. and Friedman, M.A. (2004) Does establishing fidelity of treatment help in understanding treatment efficacy? Comment on Bellg et al. (2004), *Health Psychology*, 23: 452–56.

Lichstein, K.L., Riedel, B.W. and Grieve, R. (1994) Fair test of clinical trials: a treatment implementation model, *Advances in Behavior Research and Therapy*, 16: 1–29.

Locke, E.A. and Latham, G.P. (2002) Building a practically useful theory of goal setting and task motivation: a 35-year odessey, *American Psychologist*, 57: 705–17.

Maes, S. and Karoly, P. (2005) Self-regulation assessment and intervention in physical health and illness: a review, *Applied Psychology: An International Review*, 54: 267–99.

Michie, S. (2005) Changing behavior: theoretical development needs protocol adherence, *Health Psychology*, 24: 439.

Michie, S. and Abraham, C. (2004) Interventions to change health behaviours: evidence-based or evidence-inspired? *Psychology and Health*, 19: 29–49.

Michie, S. and Johnston, M. (2004) Changing clinical behaviour by making guidelines specific, *British Medical Journal*, 328: 343–45.

Michie, S. and Lester, K. (2005) Words matter: increasing the implementation of clinical guidelines, *Quality and Safety in Health Care*, 14: 367–70.

Michie, S., Miles, J. and Weinman, J. (2003) Patient-centredness in chronic illness: what is it and does it matter? *Patient Education and Counseling*, 51: 197–206.

Miller, S.J. and Binder, J.L. (2002) The effects of manual-based training on treatment fidelity and outcome: a review of the literature on adult individual psychotherapy, *Psychotherapy: Theory, Research, Practice, Training*, 39: 184–98.

Moncher, F.J. and Prinz, F.J. (1991) Treatment fidelity in outcome studies, *Clinical Psychology Review*, 11: 247–66.

Orleans, C.T., George, L.K., Houpt, J.L. and Brodie, K.H. (1985) Health promotion in primary care: a survey of U.S. family practitioners, *Preventive Medicine*, 14: 636–47.

Perrin, K.M., Burke, S.G., O'Connor, D., Walby, G., Pitt, C.S.S., McDermott, R.J. et al. (2006) Factors contributing to intervention fidelity in a multi-site chronic disease self-management program, *Implementation Science*, 1: 26.

Peterson, L., Homer, A.L. and Wonderlich, S.A. (1982) The integrity of independent variables in behavior analysis, *Journal of Applied Behavior Analysis*, 15: 477–92.

Pill, R., Rees, M.E., Stott, N.C.H. and Rollnick, S.R. (1999) Can nurses learn to let go? Issues arising from an intervention designed to improve patients' involvement in their own care, *Journal of Advanced Nursing*, 29: 1492–99.

Pinto, B.M., Goldstein, M.G., DePue, J.D. and Milan, F.B. (1998) Acceptability and feasibility of physician-based activity counseling: the PAL Project, *American Journal of Preventive Medicine*, 15: 95–102.

Resnicow, K., Davis, M., Smith, M., Lazarus-Yaroch, A., Baranowski, T., Baranowski, J. et al. (1998) How best to measure implementation of school health curricula: a comparison of three measures, *Health Education Research*, 13: 239–50.

Rubak, S., Sandbaek, A., Lauritzen, T. and Christensen, B. (2005) Motivational interviewing: a systematic review and meta-analysis, *British Journal of General Practice*, 55: 305–12.

Schlosser, R.W. (2002) On the importance of being earnest about treatment integrity, *Augmentative and Alternative Communication*, 18: 36–44.

Sterling-Turner, H.E., Watson, T.S. and Moore, J.W. (2002) The effects of direct training and treatment integrity on treatment outcomes in school consultation, *School Psychology Quarterly*, 17: 47–77.

Sterling-Turner, H.E., Watson, T.S., Wildmon, M., Watkins, C. and Little, E. (2001) Investigating the relationship between training type and treatment integrity, *School Psychology Quarterly*, 16: 56–67.

Waltz, J., Addis, M.E., Koerner, K. and Jacobson, N.S. (1993) Testing the integrity of a psychotherapy protocol: assessment of adherence and competence, *Journal of Consulting and Clinical Psychology*, 61: 620–30.

Whitehead, D. (2001) Health education, behavioural change and social psychology: nursing's contribution to health promotion? *Journal of Advanced Nursing*, 34: 822–32.

Williams, K., Prevost, A.T., Griffin, S., Hardeman, W., Hollingworth, W., Spiegelhalter, D. et al. (2004) The *ProActive* trial protocol – a randomised controlled trial of the efficacy of a family-based, domiciliary intervention programme to increase physical activity among individuals at high risk of diabetes [ISRCTN61323766], *BMC Public Health*, 4: 48.

Woolf, S.H. and Johnson, R.E. (2005) The break-even point: when medical advances are less important than improving the fidelity with which they are delivered, *Annals of Family Medicine*, 3: 545–52.

7 Facilitating self-management through telemedicine and interactive health communication applications

Debbie Cooke, Sheetal Patel and Stanton Newman

Background

Telemedicine, or interactive health communication applications (IHCAs) as this is sometimes referred to, are significant technological advances which may have a role to play in facilitating the implementation and delivery of self-management within health care.

Telemedicine is the delivery of health care at a distance (Sood et al. 2007). It has been defined as:

> ... the use of telecommunications for medical diagnosis and patient care. It involves the use of telecommunications technology as a medium for the provision of medical services to sites that are a distance from the provider.
>
> The concept encompasses everything from the use of standard telephone services through high speed, wide band width transmission of digitised signals in conjunction with computers, fibre optics, satellites and other sophisticated peripheral equipment and software.
>
> (Scannell et al. 1995)

Interactive Health Communication has been defined in a recent *Cochrane Review* based upon work carried out in the USA (Science Panel on Interactive Communication and Health 1999) as: 'the interaction of an individual – consumer, patient, caregiver, or professional – with or through an electronic device or communication technology to access or transmit health information or receive guidance and support on a health-related issue' (Murray et al. 2005: 2).

In absentia health care or the provision of health care without personal contact has been in existence probably for as long as the practice of medicine. Many well-known physicians have practised medicine remotely; for example, Galen was apparently so skilled in understanding symptomatology that there were times when he preferred to diagnose without questioning the patient. He would then prescribe, with confidence, by post (Porter and Porter 1989). Modern health care technology has meant that in absentia care has evolved into what is now known as telemedicine.

The development of telemedicine needs to be viewed within the wider context of the huge advances in telecommunications technologies that have been made over the last couple of decades and with the result that these now pervade much of everyday life. This particularly applies to the Internet and mobile phone technologies. Society has witnessed the evolution of e-banking and e-learning. People now book holidays online and can get sacked by a text message. In many ways these technological advances can be perceived as liberating because they are enabling easy communication. However, in other ways their influence may be seen as more menacing, representing a method of control and surveillance.

The advances in the technologies underlying the Internet revolution show no sign of slowing down. According to Moore's Law, the power of a computer chip will double about every 18 months (Manasian 2003). Many experts believe that this law will continue to apply for the next 50 years. There are also dramatic advances in the storage and transmission technologies. The power of these computing and communication technologies continues to grow and their price to fall at a fairly steady rate. With reference to the Internet's role in health, Rainie (2006) argues that we are at the beginning of the second stage of a four-stage process (see Table 7.1). Eighty-five per cent of adults in the UK now use a mobile phone and 63 per cent have access to the Internet. A digital divide exists; that is, the ability to disseminate health information and deliver health care digitally is limited by disparities in access to and ability to use technology (see Chapter 2). In the UK, at least, mobile phone use is evenly distributed across social groups while Internet use is lower among the lower income groups and people over 65 years of age (Ipsos MORI 2006). Based on previous trends, the proportions of people using these technologies will increase which may narrow the digital divide. Coupled with this is the increasing challenge that health care systems are faced with in managing chronic disease (see Chapter 1). Telemedicine may, therefore, begin to be used more frequently in the provision or support of aspects of health care for chronic disease management, particularly if its clinical and cost-effectiveness can be demonstrated.

Table 7.1 The role of the Internet in the provision of health care

	Phase	
1	Informational	Internet viewed as source of medical information
2	Interactive	Use of email to communicate with health care providers
3	Instrumental	Health care users and providers will share information (telemonitoring)
4	Interventional	Medical treatment occurs online

There are many different applications of telemedicine used in a wide variety of medical specialities. Pathology, radiology, psychiatry and dermatology have particularly focused on diagnostic accuracy. One application of telemedicine is telemonitoring which involves the remote monitoring of health status or vital signs monitoring. This, in particular, has the potential to assist the patient with self-monitoring by allowing transmission of information on health status back to the health care professional and thereby enabling remote consultation. Self-monitoring has been described as the cornerstone of self-management (Creer and Holroyd 1997). In diseases such as diabetes and asthma, there is evidence that close monitoring of symptoms or clinical indicators of disease severity (e.g. glucose levels in diabetes) can lead to better health outcomes (Diabetes Control and Complications Trial Research Group 1993; Expert Panel Report 2 1997). It is therefore not surprising to find that asthma and diabetes are two of the disease areas in which telemonitoring interventions are commonly applied. Figure 7.1 outlines an example of a telemonitoring system that is used in diabetes (e.g. Ferrer-Roca et al. 2004; Farmer et al. 2005a). Rieckmann and colleagues discuss telemonitoring systems that have been used to facilitate self-management in hypertension (see Chapter 16).

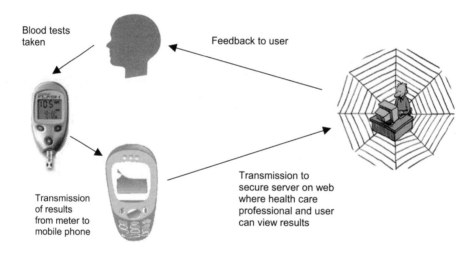

Blood tests taken

Feedback to user

Transmission of results from meter to mobile phone

Transmission to secure server on web where health care professional and user can view results

Figure 7.1 Example of a telemonitoring system for people with diabetes

Potentially, the remote delivery of health care is easier for the patient as it may reduce the need for travel and hence waiting times. It may provide reassurance for the user and allow communication at times that are more convenient to them; for example, when they are on holiday. Murray and colleagues propose that IHCAs lead to changes in health behaviours and, in turn, clinical outcomes by increasing knowledge and self-efficacy and also providing motivation for behaviour change.

Other telemedicine interventions also incorporate several components traditionally viewed as enabling self-management. An example is the Watch, Discover, Think and Act computer-assisted program for asthma self-management in children (Shegog et al. 2001). This uses three types of computer-based strategy to provide asthma self-management skills training: a simulation of real-world activities so the child can learn and practise self-regulation; tutorials for the child to practise asthma-specific skills; and a game which involves the child successfully managing a character's asthma in order to progress from one scenario to the next. There are many other examples of IHCAs.

Franklin and colleagues have developed a system called 'Sweet Talk' based on social cognition theory, the Health Belief Model and goal-setting (Franklin et al. 2003). They sent teenagers with diabetes personalized text messages reminding them of their treatment goals and allowing them to send questions to the diabetes team. This intervention significantly increased self-efficacy and reduced HbA1c when compared to a conventional treatment group. In another intervention, Internet software provided individually tailored dietary information, menu suggestions, help with meal composition and evaluation of calorific requirements that reduced the intake of calories among obese adults after 12 months in comparison to a group receiving normal care (Turnin et al. 2001).

The Stanford Chronic Disease Self-Management Program (CDSMP) was adapted to be delivered via the Internet. An evaluation of this program showed equivalent results in terms of health outcomes to the original CDSMP that was delivered face-to-face in a group setting (Lorig et al. 2006). An online version of the Expert Patient Program, based upon the CDSMP, is currently being evaluated in the UK. More detail on the web-based CDSMP and other examples of online self-management interventions are provided in Chapter 5.

It is important to acknowledge the tensions present between the potential for such interventions to promote autonomy and independence and foster new dependencies (i.e. on the technology itself). In the same way that interventions are often labelled as self-management when they do not contain any components that are traditionally defined as self-management, IHCAs or telemedicine applications per se do not automatically meet definitions of self-management (see also Chapter 4). Used within a traditional biomedical model of illness, telemedicine may enforce a didactic approach to chronic disease management rather than moving towards a more collaborative, self-management approach to health care delivery.

Challenges in implementation of telemedicine systems

Table 7.2 summarizes the challenges faced in implementing telemedicine systems to support the management of chronic disease. Each of these issues is considered.

Table 7.2 Challenges in the implementation of telemedicine systems

Type of challenge	Factors to be addressed
Providing an evidence-base	Demonstrating clinical effectiveness
	Demonstrating cost-effectiveness
Need for evaluation frameworks	Development of frameworks for evaluation that are specific to this area and take account of the factors outlined here

Type of challenge	Factors to be addressed
Acceptability	To users, carers, health care professionals and health care systems
Change in clinical practice	Redefining role and skills required of health care professionals
Ethical Issues	Confidentiality
	Data security
	Malpractice liability

Several reviews of the clinical efficacy of telemedicine are available both within specific disease areas (Wainwright and Wootton 2003; Farmer et al. 2005b; Martinez et al. 2006) and more broadly across different areas (Currell et al. 2000; Hailey et al. 2002). There is an emerging evidence base for the clinical effectiveness of telemedicine technologies (Barlow et al. 2007), although the evidence is suggestive, and the majority of studies do not meet robust evaluation standards (Bensink et al. 2006; Barlow et al. 2007; Whitten et al. 2007). Much of the available literature refers to pilot projects and short-term outcomes. Very few of the studies reviewed have assessed the long-term or routine use of telemedicine. One of the most relevant systematic reviews for the purpose of this chapter included 24 RCTs of IHCAs (Murray et al. 2005). The IHCAs had a significant positive effect on knowledge, social support, behavioural outcomes (e.g. calorific intake, exercise and medication-taking) as well as clinical outcomes (e.g. asthma symptoms, HbA1c levels among people with diabetes and body mass index). The evidence also suggested a positive effect on self-efficacy. It was not possible to determine whether they had an effect on emotional outcomes or overall health care resource use.

Glasgow and Bull (2001) provide a discussion of the strengths and limitations of IHCAs as an adjunct to self-management education in the field of diabetes. They apply the Reach, Efficacy, Action, Implementation and Maintenance (RE-AIM) framework (see Chapter 8) to their critique of these interventions that include the use of the Internet, CD-ROMs, automated phone disease management systems and hand-held, portable or mobile devices. These technologies offer wide availability, speed, consistent and individually tailored techniques for carrying out routine tasks and behaviours, and good follow-up support. However, they are limited in their ability to deal with novel, unanticipated situations.

Little is known about the psychological, behavioural and emotional consequences of using telemedicine systems. Certainly, research in this area would benefit from greater use of theoretical models (Mackert 2006). Mackert argues that models used in Information Systems research could be applied; for example, the Theory of Planned Behaviour (Ajzen 1991) and the Technology Acceptance Model (Davis 1989) which states that perceptions of value and ease of use of a new technology explain intentions to use it.

An important issue is how people with chronic disease, their families and informal carers respond to using such technologies. How acceptable are these interventions to users, their health care professionals and carers/family? Understanding the factors that lead to the successful adoption and integration of these technologies into routine practice is critical. Applications of individual behaviour change domains (e.g. knowledge, motivation and goal-setting) identified by Michie and colleagues will aid this understanding (Michie et al. 2005). Similarly, application of the Normalization Process Model (May 2006; May et al. 2007) and WISE (Whole System Informing Self-Management Engagement) Model (Kennedy and Rogers 2001) are likely to assist in understanding the process of integration into routine practice. These offer theoretical frameworks for the evaluation of new interventions within broad social and organizational contexts. The Normalization Process Model takes a bottom-up approach to understanding normalization and looks at four domains: 1) interaction between professionals and patients within a consultation and its temporal order; 2) embeddedness of trust in professional knowledge and practice; 3) distribution of work, knowledge and practice across divisions of labour or within an organization; and 4) organizational capacity. The WISE model has a wider conceptual approach to diffusion of innovation, focusing on appropriate information and improved access to services for patients, and training for health care professionals in patient-centred consultation skills.

The resistance of health care professionals to using these technologies has been identified as one of the main barriers preventing their successful implementation (Debnath 2004). Use of these technologies may require different clinical skills; for example, different approaches to information-giving that may significantly alter the nature of the clinical encounter and the relationship between the professional and the patient (Currell et al. 2000). As with the delivery of self-management interventions without IHCAs, this would result in fundamental changes in clinical interactions. Professional roles and ways of working would need to be redefined including the delegation of particular tasks to patients and carers (Nicolini 2006). This may result in loss of interpersonal cues (May et al. 2001). Development of new telemedicine applications, especially those providing information or decision support, is also likely to change the role and skills required of health care professionals and thus affect the form and content of education programmes (Alpay and Heathfield 1997). Awareness of potential cultural differences in attitudes to technology or barriers to use will be essential in introducing any of these technologies into everyday clinical practice.

There is evidence that the communication and collaboration aspects of implementing telemedicine systems are more challenging than the technical or policy aspects (Alpay and Murray 1998): 'Thus far, most telemedicine research has a technological focus. We know a great deal about bandwidths and resolution, but little about the human dimensions that make the practice possible' (Mair and Whitten 2000: 1519).

To examine the acceptability of telemedicine interventions, Mair and Whitten (2000) reviewed 32 studies of patient satisfaction with telemedicine across a range of disciplines. Patient satisfaction is commonly defined as when an individual's expectations of treatment and care are met. Generally, patient's reported satisfaction with telemedicine. Definite advantages were increased accessibility of specialist expertise, less travel required and reduced waiting times. Some reservations were expressed mainly relating to communication between provider and client. It is likely that in most studies there was a selection bias favouring those who were more likely to be positive about the interventions. As these were research studies, they were subject to the requirements of informed consent and this meant that it was unlikely that any patients with a marked aversion to a new technology or who disliked the idea of the technology would have volunteered for these studies (Currell et al. 2000). The samples therefore represent self-selected groups of those people who are at least willing to try the new technology. Accurate assessments of satisfaction and acceptability will only be possible when the technologies are in more widespread use. The methodologies in these studies for assessing satisfaction were not always specified. Most sought to measure whether patients would use the telemedicine system again or were 'satisfied' with the service. Very few actually defined what they meant by satisfaction. The currently available evidence does not provide an understanding of the reasons underlying the satisfaction or dissatisfaction that was found. Most of the studies only presented initial impressions and did not consider patient satisfaction over time. The restriction to an early assessment makes it possible that the novelty value of the technology resulted in a positive bias. A more recent review identified similar methodological problems in the area but also found higher levels of concern regarding delivery of telemedicine and more barriers to implementation among health care providers than consumers (Whitten and Love 2005).

There are cost implications to the roll-out of these devices but economic evaluations in the area are scarce. The telemedicine literature in general has been criticized by several commentators for its lack of evidence on cost-effectiveness (Whitten et al. 2002). Is telemedicine just a way of saving money by obviating the need for clinic visits? Is it a threat to community or to traditional methods of health care delivery? Telemedicine's role in the delivery of health care remains ambiguous because of uncertain impact on cost savings and benefits (Reardon 2005). These points relate to the role of patient-reported outcomes in planning and evaluating services as well. A systematic review of cost-effectiveness studies of telemedicine found that of 600 cost-related articles identified only 9 per cent contained any cost–benefit data (Whitten et al. 2002). Only 4 per cent of those articles met quality criteria justifying inclusion in their formalized systematic review. They concluded that there was little published evidence to confirm whether or not telemedicine is a cost-effective alternative to standard health care delivery.

There is an assumption that people with chronic illness who are successfully managing their condition will make less demand of health care services. However, it is of course possible that they will place a greater demand on health care services and so increase costs. Research in this area is needed if the implications on service use are to be understood. Telemedicine interventions are advocated as they may help to increase access for geographically isolated populations (Mair and Whitten 2000). The net result will be increased usage if groups currently unable to access health care are brought into the system. In this way the issue of equity of access to health care will be improved but costs may increase. There is concern regarding the social implications of remote access, in that telemedicine has the potential to create a second tier of care for those remote and isolated populations (Bashshur 1997) as well as vulnerable populations (Cashen et al. 2004).

In relation to clinical efficacy and effectiveness and cost-effectiveness, there is a need for evaluation frameworks (Sisk and Sanders 1998). In the UK, the Department of Health have recognized this need and are in the process of developing an evaluation framework for technologies that assist self-care and self-management (Barlow 2006).

Concern regarding the security of personal information in electronic form is another potential obstacle that the widespread introduction of telemedicine raises. There are many views on this. Some believe that electronic patient records are more susceptible to unauthorized access and dissemination than are paper charts on hospital wards. Others believe that proper safeguards make electronic information more secure than paper records. There are several ethical issues to consider: confidentiality, data security, consent, competence, interprofessional and professional-patient relationships, and organization of medical services (Ashcroft and Goddard 2000). Patients wary of electronic data may be reluctant to use telemedicine systems that result in the creation or transmission of confidential information. Similarly, if health care providers believe that electronic systems may increase the risk of breaching patient confidentiality, they may also be reluctant to use these. Other barriers to implementation include concerns about malpractice liability, quality of service, technical issues and, in the USA at least, public and private reimbursement policies that do not compensate for telemedicine services (Angood 2001).

Conclusion

It has been argued that discourses on patient empowerment and technological advances lead both to a consumerist approach to health care that may reinforce existing medical models of illness. In many cases, 'empowerment' and self-management are achieved through the adoption of dominant thought systems based upon the medical model (Fox et al. 2005). Fox et al. illustrate this using qualitative work with an Internet support group for users of Xenical, a drug treatment for obesity. They argue that this online environment resulted in informed consumers who simply adopted conventional thinking about weight, body shape, size and health. This tension between promotion of autonomy and dependence has already been highlighted but will need to be foremost in thinking about what technological applications in chronic disease management are attempting to achieve.

As the concept of self-management begins to help shape service provision for people with chronic illness, so telemedicine, telemonitoring and IHCAs are increasingly likely to be used to facilitate this process. The evidence base is continually being added to but more work needs to be done to establish both their clinical and cost-effectiveness and whether they enhance self-management or foster greater dependency on health care providers and possibly the technology. Careful consideration of the barriers to implementation of telemedicine systems in routine clinical practice is also required. Many of these individual, organizational, financial and ethical barriers are mirrored in the consideration of the adoption and successful integration of self-management interventions into routine health care (see Chapter 17).

References

Ajzen, I. (1991) The theory of planned behavior. *Organizational behavior and human decision processes*, 50(2): 179–211.

Alpay, L. and Heathfield, H. (1997) A review of telematics in healthcare: evolution, challenges and caveats, *Health Informatics Journal*, 3(2): 81–92.

Alpay, L. and Murray, P. (1998) Challenges for delivering healthcare education through telematics, *International Journal of Medical Informatics*, 50(1–3): 267–71.

Angood, P.B. (2001) Telemedicine, the Internet, and world wide web: overview, current status, and relevance to surgeons, *World Journal of Surgery*, 25(11): 1449–57.

Ashcroft, R.E. and Goddard, P.R. (2000) Ethical issues in teleradiology, *The British Journal of Radiology*, 73(870): 578–82.

Barlow, J. (2006) Building an evidence base for successful telecare implementation. Updated report of the Evidence Working Group of the Telecare Policy Collaborative. Department of Health/CSIP.

Barlow, J., Sing, D., Bayer, S. and Curry, R. (2007) A systematic review of the benefits of home telecare for frail elderly people and those with long-term conditions, *Journal of Telemedicine and Telecare*, 13: 172–79.

Bashshur, R. (1997) Telemedicine and the health care system, in R. Bashshur, J.H. Sanders and G. Shannon (eds) *Telemedicine: Theory and Practice* (pp. 5–36). Springfield, IL: Charles C. Thomas.

Bensink, M., Hailey, D. and Wootton, R. (2006) A systematic review of successes and failures in home telehealth: preliminary results, *Journal of Telemedicine and Telecare* 12(S3): 8–16.

Cashen, M.S., Dykes, P. and Gerber, B. (2004) eHealth technology and Internet resources: barriers for vulnerable populations, *Journal of Cardiovascular Nursing*, 19(3): 209–14.

Creer, T. L. and Holroyd, K.A. (1997) Self-Management, in A. Baum et al. (eds) *Cambridge Handbook of Psychology, Health and Medicine* (pp. 255–58). Cambridge: Cambridge University Press.

Currell, R., Urquhart, C., Wainwright, P. and Lewis, R. (2000) Telemedicine versus face to face patient care: effects on professional practice and health care outcomes (Cochrane Review), *Cochrane Database of Systematic Reviews*, Issue 2, No. CD002098.

Davis, F.D. (1989) Perceived usefulness, perceived ease of use, and user acceptance of information technology, *MIS Quarterly*, 13(3): 319–40.

Debnath, D. (2004) Activity analysis of telemedicine in the UK, *Postgraduate Medical Journal*, 80(944): 335–38.

Diabetes Control and Complications Trial Research Group (1993) The effect of intensive treatment of diabetes on the development and progression of long-term complications in insulin-dependent diabetes-mellitus, *New England Journal of Medicine*, 329(14): 977–86.

Expert Panel Report 2 (1997) Guidelines for the diagnosis and management of asthma, National Institutes of Health. National Heart, Lung and Blood Institute, NIH publication, no. 97–4051.

Farmer, A., Gibson, O.J., Tarassenko, L. and Neil, A. (2005a) A systematic review of telemedicine interventions to support blood glucose self-monitoring in diabetes, *Diabetic Medicine*, 22(10): 1372–78.

Farmer, A.J., Gibson, O.J., Dudley, C., Bryden, K., Hayton, P.M., Tarassenko, L. and Neil, A. (2005b) A randomized controlled trial of the effect of real-time telemedicine support on glycemic control in young adults with type 1 diabetes, *Diabetes Care*, 28(11): 2697–702.

Ferrer-Roca, O., Burbano, K.F., Cardenas, A., Pulido, P. and Diaz-Cardama, A. (2004) Web-based diabetes control, *Journal of Telemedicine and Telecare*, 10(5): 277–81.

Fox, N.J., Ward, K.J. and O'Rourke, A.J. (2005) The 'expert patient': empowerment or medical dominance? The case of weight loss, pharmaceutical drugs and the Internet, *Social Science and Medicine*, 60(6): 1299–309.

Franklin, V., Waller, A., Pagliari, C. and Greene, S. (2003) 'Sweet Talk': text messaging support for intensive insulin therapy for young people with diabetes, *Diabetes Technology and Therapeutics*, 5(6): 991–96.

Hailey, D., Roine, R. and Ohinmaa, A. (2002) Systematic review of evidence for the benefits of telemedicine, *Journal of Telemedicine and Telecare*, 8: 1–30.

Glasgow R. E. and Bull S. S. (2001) Making a difference with interactive technology: considerations in using and evaluating computerized aids for diabetes self-management education. *Diabetes Spectrum* 14:99–106.

Ipsos MORI (2006) Technology tracker. Technology Research at IPSOS-MORI (www.ipsos-mori-com/technology/usage.shtml: accessed 27 February 2008).

Kennedy, A. and Rogers, A. (2001) Improving self-management skills: a whole systems approach, *British Journal of Nursing*, 10(11): 734–37.

Lorig, K.R., Ritter, P.L., Laurent, D.D. and Plant, K. (2006) Internet-based chronic disease self-management: a randomized trial, *Medical Care*, 44(11): 964–71.

Mackert, M. (2006) Expanding the theoretical foundations of telemedicine, *Journal of Telemedicine and Telecare*, 12(1): 49–50.

Mair, F. and Whitten, P. (2000) Systematic review of studies of patient satisfaction with telemedicine, *British Medical Journal*, 320(7248): 1517–20.

Manasian, D. (2003) Digital dilemmas, *The Economist*, 25 January.

Martinez, A., Everss, E., Rojo-Alvarez, J.L., Figal, D.P. and Garcia-Alberola, A. (2006) A systematic review of the literature on home monitoring for patients with heart failure, *Journal of Telemedicine and Telecare*, 12(5): 234–41.

May, C. (2006) A rational model for assessing and evaluating complex interventions in health care, *BMC Health Services Research*, 6: doi:10.1186/1472-6963-6-86.

May, C., Gask, L., Atkinson, T., Ellis, N., Mair, F. and Esmail, A. (2001) Resisting and promoting new technologies in clinical practice: the case of telepsychiatry, *Social Science and Medicine*, 52: 1889–901.

May, C., Finch, T., Mair, F. et al. (2007) Understanding the implementation of complex interventions in health care: the normalization process model, *BMC Health Services Research*, 7: doi:10.1186/1472-6963-7-148.

Michie, S., Johnston, M., Abraham, C. et al. on behalf of the Psychological Theory Group (2005) Making psychological theory useful for implementing evidence based practice: a consensus approach, *Quality and Safety in Health Care*, 14(1): 26–33.

Murray, E., Burns, J., Tai, S. S., Lai, R. and Nazareth, I. (2005) Interactive health communication applications for people with chronic disease, *Cochrane Database of Systematic Reviews*, Issue no. 4. CD004274. DOI 10.1002/14651858.

Nicolini, D. (2006) The work to make telemedicine work: a social and articulative view, *Social Science and Medicine*, 62(11): 2754–67.

Porter, R. and Porter, D. (1989) *In Sickness and In Health: The British Experience*. New York: Blackwell.

Rainie, L. (2006) Foreword: E-Health Research, in M. Murero and R.E. Rice (eds) *The Internet and Health Care: Theory, Research and Practice* (pp. xxi–xxiv). London: Lawrence Erlbaum Associates.

Reardon, T. (2005) Research findings and strategies for assessing telemedicine costs, *Telemedicine Journal and e-Health*, 11(3): 348–69.

Scannell, K., Perednia, D.A. and Kissman, H. (1995) *Telemedicine: Past, Present, Future: Current Bibliographies in Medicine*. Maryland: National Library of Medicine.

Science Panel on Interactive Communication and Health (1999) *Wired for Health and Well-Being: The Emergence of Interactive Health Communication*. Washington, DC: US Department of Health and Human Services.

Shegog, R., Bartholomew, L.K., Parcel, G.S. et al. (2001) Impact of a computer-assisted education program on factors related to asthma self-management behavior, *Journal of the American Medical Informatics Association*, 8(1): 49–61.

Sisk, J.E. and Sanders, J.H. (1998) A proposed framework for economic evaluation of telemedicine, *Telemedicine Journal*, 4(1): 31–37.

Sood, S., Mbarika, V., Jugoo, S. et al. (2007) What is telemedicine? A collection of 104 peer-reviewed perspectives and theoretical underpinnings, *Telemedicine and e-Health*, 13: 573–90.

Turnin, M.C., Bourgeois, O., Cathelineau, G. et al. (2001) Multicenter randomized evaluation of a nutritional education software in obese patients, *Diabetes and Metabolism*, 27(2): 139–47.

Wainwright, C. and Wootton, R. (2003) A review of telemedicine and asthma, *Disease Management and Health Outcomes*, 11(9): 557–63.

Whitten, P. and Love, B. (2005) Patient and provider satisfaction with the use of telemedicine: overview and rationale for cautious enthusiasm, *Journal of Postgraduate Medicine*, 51(4): 294–300.

Whitten, P., Johannessen, L.K., Soerensen, T., Gammon, D. and Mackert, M. (2007) A systematic review of research methodology in telemedicine studies, *Journal of Telemedicine and Telecare*, 13(5): 230–35.

Whitten, P.S., Mair, F.S., Haycox, A. et al. (2002) Systematic review of cost effectiveness studies of telemedicine interventions, *British Medical Journal*, 324(7351): 1434–37.

Part III

Evaluation

8 Development and evaluation of self-management interventions

Liz Steed, Kathleen Mulligan and Stanton Newman

Self-management interventions are complex interventions in that they are generally made up of multiple components with multiple mechanisms through which change can occur. This makes both the development and evaluation of such interventions a challenge. This has been recognized in the UK by the recent publication of a framework for design and evaluation of complex interventions by the Medical Research Council (MRC) (Campbell et al. 2000). This framework aims to be a guide to researchers to ensure improved quality of such interventions and as such is a helpful basis from which to evaluate self-management interventions. Figure 8.1 shows the various stages depicted in the MRC framework. Although presented as a staged approach, it should be considered that both development and evaluation can be iterative processes; cycling between stages may occur, for example, when an exploratory trial highlights that more work needs to be done at earlier developmental stages (Campbell et al. 2000).

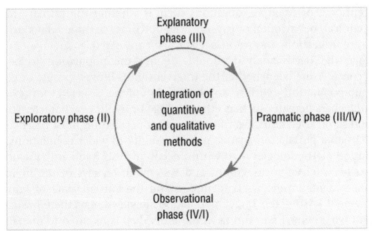

Source: Reproduced with permission from the *British Medical Journal* (BMJ) Publishing Group.

Figure 8.1 Iterative view of development or randomized controlled trials of complex interventions

This chapter uses the MRC model, together with other literature, particularly from the fields of public health evaluations, to discuss issues pertinent to developing and evaluating self-management interventions.

Needs analysis

The identification of need for development of a self-management intervention may be in response to a variety of factors. This may include a requirement for self-management within national or international disease management recommendations; for example, the American Diabetes Association, in response to recognized deficits within clinical practice or progression from research findings. It may also come from a range of sources such as patients, clinicians, managers or policy-makers. Importantly, these different groups of individuals may have different needs from the intervention, such as improving quality of life versus economic outcomes or reduction in health care utilization. For these reasons, together with the complexity and initial costs of developing and evaluating self-management interventions, any new project should be instigated only following a formal process to evaluate necessity and objectives of such an intervention (Lorig 1996). This can be conceived as a preliminary step to even that of the preclinical stage of the MRC framework.

An initial aim of the needs assessment is to address whether there is in fact a requirement for a new intervention, or whether other previously developed work may adequately address the need. If room for a new intervention is identified, then the perceived needs of all interested parties, for example, patients, clinicians, policy-makers should be identified. Competing needs may be apparent and negotiation of priorities will be required to ensure clear specification of the objectives in developing the intervention. For example, questions such as whether the primary objective is change in clinical, behavioural or psychosocial outcomes or more related to reduction of health care utilization, and so on needs to be considered.

Further, the needs analysis should identify the population to be targeted. Factors to consider include whether the intervention is illness-specific or generic and whether sub-populations within an illness should be selected, for example, by demographic characteristics such as ethnicity, age or by illness characteristics such as severity, and so on. Decisions regarding the target population must balance demands for specificity to a population against generalizability to wider populations.

Common methodologies used within needs analysis frequently include qualitative approaches such as focus groups and systematic reviews of the literature. The objective of systematic reviews is to understand the current state of knowledge of self-management within the target population. Reviews may therefore include descriptions of what behaviours and tasks the individual is required to manage and the psychological and social impact of the illness on the individual including any particular difficulties that arise in self-managing in this population. Additionally, review of interventions that have previously been conducted within the field may be presented. It has been suggested that using consistent descriptors of interventions and then looking for associations between characteristics of interventions and outcomes may be helpful in developing future interventions (Elasy et al. 2001). Previous research will also often make recommendations and, where the study of self-management is an evolved concept within an illness (e.g. diabetes or arthritis), future studies should benefit from building on prior work (Griffin et al. 1998). For a significant number of chronic illnesses, however, there may have been few studies of self-management and in these cases a review of work conducted in other illness areas will be invaluable in providing a platform for development.

In conducting systematic reviews, methodological guidelines have been developed (Sutton et al. 1998). The type of interventions included within systematic reviews of self-management interventions has been a topic of debate (Newman et al. 2004). Some reviews focus only on randomized controlled trials and or meta-analysis. However, it has been argued that this may lead to a limited understanding of self-management interventions, and it may be preferable to include other designs; for example, pre-post assessment, providing assessment of study quality is taken into account within the review.

Focus groups have also often been used in assessing the need for self-management interventions, commonly targeting health care professionals as well as the target populations (Lorig 1996). This methodology can explore in depth the perceived needs and understanding of the client and health care groups which the intervention will target. Evaluation with client groups can focus upon what they perceive as central components to their self-management regimen and specifically things they find difficult within this. It can be useful to get a sense of participants' likely openness to the concept of self-management and an initial feeling for the type of format and delivery that may be suitable for the group in question.

Focus groups with health care professionals should follow similar ground, but additionally should explore the practicality of implementing a self-management intervention in a clinical context. The success of any intervention is ultimately in its translation to clinical practice and a programme which while efficacious in a research setting cannot be used efficiently within the realities of a health care setting is likely to be of limited benefit.

Identifying theoretical basis of self-management interventions

The use of theory in the development of self-management interventions has been variable and in some illnesses infrequent (see Chapters 10–16). Interventions have often been developed on a more pragmatic basis where concepts have been taken from different theories, or developed out of, for example, disease management programmes. There is some evidence to suggest, however, that interventions based on theory have greater efficacy than those without a clear theoretical framework (Griffin et al. 1998). The role of theory within self-management interventions is discussed in Chapter 3.

The choice of theory, however, may be complex when multiple theories with often overlapping constructs are available. To aid this process Hardeman et al. (2005) have set out a causal modelling approach to developing theory-based interventions, particularly those targeted at behaviour change. Within this five criteria are defined for theory selection: A theory may be appropriate if it has:

1 been used in interventions aimed at similar target behaviours;
2 applicability to the target group;
3 clear definition of causal testable pathways between outcome determinants and outcome;
4 strength of evidence about predictive validity;
5 clear guidelines for measurement.

Choice of theory then may be based on both knowledge of the broad application of theories within the field of self-management, and within the specific target areas.

Translation of theory to intervention development

Having selected the theoretical basis of the intervention, its translation into intervention components and hence specific strategies to facilitate change can be defined. Chapter 4 describes components of self-management interventions that have been used most frequently.

Other design issues that may be considered at this stage are mode and format of delivery of the intervention. Self-management interventions have been delivered in a range of formats; for example, individual, group or combined approaches. However, evidence to suggest that one format is better than another is unclear (see Chapter 5 for further discussion). Decisions may therefore be guided by characteristics of the illness, practicalities and economics. In certain illnesses (e.g. cystic fibrosis or other lung diseases) it may not be possible to hold group interventions for risk of cross-infection. Similarly, where individuals are physically extremely limited a group may be inappropriate as members may not be able to reliably commit to attendance. The mode of delivery of self-management interventions has also varied with many programmes using direct person-to-person delivery, while others use work-books (e.g. The Heart Manual, Lewin et al. 1992), telephone interventions (Piette 2005) or Internet-based programmes (e.g. McKay et al. 2001). Further, interventions may be delivered in a variety of ways; for example, by lay leaders, health care professionals or via emerging technologies. Chapter 5 discusses the efficacy of these different approaches in more detail.

Intervention modelling

Having designed the core intervention, it has been proposed that modelling of the key mechanisms of action is a helpful step and has been used effectively in a range of complex interventions (Eldridge et al. 2005; Rowlands et al. 2005). Modelling can take different formats such as simple paper and pen mapping exercises, to complex computer modelling. The purpose is to detail both the key hypothesis within the intervention and the social context within which it is acting, hence explicating any assumptions made and the implications of these. This process aims to elucidate potential problems within the intervention design as well as pointing to important factors other than primary outcomes that may need to be measured to gain full understanding of the mechanisms through which change may occur. Although this approach has been applied to public health interventions, it is unclear the extent to which it has been used explicitly with self-management interventions. As discussed later, explicating the processes through which interventions act is relatively novel and hence greater use of modelling may be helpful.

Exploratory phase

It is recommended within MRC guidelines that for complex interventions, it is appropriate to implement an exploratory stage with possible feasibility trial prior to a full randomized controlled trial or other formal evaluation design. Such a phase is said to serve a number of purposes. For example, it can allow for implementation of the intervention while at a stage where there is still room for further development. It can answer questions such as whether the intensity of the programme is appropriate, whether there should be more/fewer sessions, whether the length of sessions are appropriate, and so on. Aspects of content or mode of delivery can be addressed, perhaps with comparison of two slightly different forms of the intervention compared. Qualitative assessment of participants at this stage may also prove useful in defining whether any critical aspects of the intervention need to be changed to ensure optimum effectiveness. Other issues such as standardization versus flexibility, documentation and training of facilitators can also usefully be addressed during the exploratory phase.

Standardization versus flexibility

The extent to which the content and delivery of complex interventions can or should be standardized has been discussed (Hawe et al. 2004) and may be usefully explored for self-management interventions at the exploratory stage of development. Traditionally within medicine, where randomized controlled trials are perceived as the gold standard of intervention evaluation, it is specified that interventions should be as consistent as possible, with standard content and delivery (Campbell et al. 2000). It has been argued by others, however, that such stringent standardization may be inappropriate for complex interventions and such stringency may in itself lead to less efficacious interventions (Hawe et al. 2004). The important point is not whether standardization occurs but 'what' of the intervention is standardized. Recommendations are that, rather than specific content be standardized, the process through which change is said to occur should be standard. For example, in self-management this may mean that rather than pre-specifying which beliefs an individual will or should hold, the process for eliciting and evaluating them, that is, in a facilitatory rather than didactic manner, should be standard.

Documentation

A criticism of some self-management interventions has been their poor documentation of what the intervention actually involves and how it has been implemented. This makes it difficult to replicate or to clearly understand the intervention in order to further develop it. A recent call has therefore been made for all self-management interventions to be formally documented and published alongside the report on efficacy (Newman et al. 2004), although as highlighted in Chapter 6 this is still a topic for debate.

Training of facilitators

Chapter 6 discusses the process of training facilitators. This, together with examination as to the ease of following implementation guidelines, can also occur during the exploratory phase. The importance of facilitators learning any new skills required is highlighted within MRC guidelines and is particularly pertinent to self-management interventions where facilitators are frequently required to learn new skills and different approaches in interventions. Although it will, in most cases, be necessary to offer training programmes for facilitators, sufficient practice within the exploratory stage of interventions will also be essential to ensure consistency once the formal trial is under way. Evaluation of intervention fidelity (i.e. the intervention is delivered as meant) is also discussed in Chapter 6. Techniques for ensuring intervention fidelity are currently not well evolved in self-management but processes such as video-taping delivery or having an external observer in sessions may be a helpful way of observing this in the initial stage where contamination of outcomes is not of primary concern.

Feasibility Trial

In addition to finalizing the development of the intervention, the exploratory phase can address issues pertinent to the formal analysis, particularly if a feasibility trial is conducted. A feasibility trial can be considered as a small-scale version of the formal design where issues around recruitment, for example, how this will be conducted and whether the targeted population have sufficient interest in such an intervention, can be explored. MRC guidelines suggest that if randomization is a component of the feasibility trial, this can lead to estimates of potential effect sizes from which power analyses can be formulated. This may be particularly important where a novel outcome is to be evaluated or the intervention is in a previously unexplored field. While a feasibility trial may be helpful for this purpose, it should be noted that this can only occur once there is relative consistency in the delivery and content of the programme as changes could have implications for power analysis.

Piloting of outcome measures is also a useful component of a feasibility trial with issues such as acceptability, time requirements, and so on, able to be estimated and hence incorporated in further interventions.

Standard care

As many studies involve comparisons between the self-management intervention and standard care, and standard care is highly variable in many chronic conditions, the need to be clear as to what standard care includes is crucial. Standard care can itself be complex; for example, incorporating regular contact with health care professionals, some form of education and pharmacological intervention. It is therefore important within the exploratory phase to define the characteristics of standard care and the parameters within which variations within this care will adhere to the definition of standard care.

Formal evaluation

Trial design

Following the exploratory phase and possible feasibility trial, incorporation of information into a final intervention design for formal evaluation of the self-managment intervention can occur. Within the medical arena randomized controlled trials (RCTs) have long been considered as the most robust form of evaluation for clinical interventions and this model has often been translated into other forms of interventions including those of self-management interventions. Within an RCT, the intervention(s) is compared to a control group and allocation to intervention or control is made through a process of randomization. The central aim of the RCT is to increase internal validity by minimizing the likelihood that differences between the control and intervention group are due to bias rather than real effects. Methods of randomization vary but should adhere to allocation concealment so that the sequence of randomization is not predictable (Altman and Schulz 2001). Blinding of treatment allocation is a further recommendation for RCTs. However, this is commonly not feasible within self-management interventions where participants within an intervention group will be quite aware of the differences between allocations and particularly whether they are receiving standard care. Clinicians who are providing routine care to study participants should, however, be kept blind to study group allocation.

Although RCTs are commonly used within the field of self-management, debate about their appropriateness for evaluation of complex interventions has been presented (McKee et al. 1999; Walach et al. 2006). A key concern is that of equipoise or the assumption of RCTs that participants and providers do not have a preference for a specific form of treatment. It is known that individuals frequently do have a preference for one or other trial group (Bradley et al. 1993). This may particularly be the case where the only way of getting a 'new' treatment is by participation in the trial. If a preference is present but unfulfilled by randomization to the participant's less preferred group, then the participant may be disappointed, or experience what has been termed 'resentful demoralization' (Cook and Campbell 1979). Individuals allocated to the control group are hence more likely to be disappointed than those

allocated to the intervention group. This sense of disappointment itself leads to a difference between groups and a potential bias in the study.

Attempts to overcome this apparent state of non-equipoise may be to offer a waiting list control group which offers all participants the opportunity to receive the intervention at some point, or alternatively to implement a patient preference design. Within a patient preference design, the difference between interventions is explicit and individuals are asked which arm of a trial they would prefer to participate in and are allocated as appropriate. Where an individual reports no preference for either arm of the trial, then randomization between groups can occur. Hence, within a trial comparing a self-management intervention to control four possible groups become apparent – prefer A, prefer B, no preference randomized A, no preference randomized B.

It is self-evident that analysis of preference trials will be more complex than routine RCTs. However, such designs provide an important opportunity to explore issues such as the characteristics of individuals with different preferences. This may provide useful information for future self-management interventions. Further, a preference trial may increase recruitment into a trial. This is based on the rationale that some individuals may refuse participation into a research trial due to the possibility of being allocated to a new treatment. If they are happy with their current treatment and have no wish to change, there is little incentive to risk this by participating within a trial. Where their preference is assured, this becomes less of a concern. A preference design may therefore include a more motivated sample of the population under investigation. One difficulty may, however, be that if one arm of the trial is more attractive than another, there may be unbalanced recruitment to this arm, leading to the potential need to recruit higher numbers to maintain power.

Due to the complexity of Self-Managmment Interventions, techniques such as cluster randomization or block randomization may also be useful. Cluster randomization typically involves recruitment from a number of health care sites and uses the sites; for example, different hospital clinics or GP surgeries, as the method of randomization. This approach has the advantage of minimizing contamination effects between intervention and control participants. However, it usually requires greater sample sizes than non-clustered randomization, due to potential variation between the cluster sites. Block randomization may also be used for practical reasons, particularly where evaluation is of a group intervention and sufficient participants must be recruited into the intervention group within a small time frame.

Recruitment

Regardless of trial design, explicit definition of inclusion and exclusion criteria and method of recruitment are essential issues within formal evaluation. Decisions with regard to inclusion/exclusion criteria must balance a desire for specificity within a trial to generalizability to the wider population. In some situations it may be preferable to institute very broad inclusion/exclusion criteria with secondary subgroup analysis conducted if information is wanted on efficacy for different groups; for example, by demographic or clinical variables.

Method of recruitment is also important. In some self-management interventions, there has been a tendency to recruit participants through general advertisements in newspapers, clinics, and so on. Although this approach may be appropriate or necessary in some studies, it is likely to attract only those individuals most motivated and interested in self-management. The likelihood of the trial being efficacious will be increased in this situation but the findings may not be generalizable to the broader population.

Outcome assessment

Chapter 9 discusses evaluation of self-management interventions. It is important within the formal evaluation that any choice of outcome follows the hypothesized changes that the intervention is intended to effect. This is important so as to avoid a conclusion being drawn that the self-management intervention has little or no effect on an outcome which the intervention was not designed to target. An example of this is within the diabetes literature and the outcomes of anxiety and depression. A systematic review reported that although few interventions had a positive effect on these outcomes, the content of the majority of these interventions did not target the mood of participants (Steed et al. 2003). These findings also highlight the importance of targeting interventions appropriately in that if participants report low levels of anxiety and depression on recruitment into the study, improvements in these variables would not be expected.

Process assessment

In addition to outcome assessment, an analysis of process is an important component of formal evaluation (Bradieu et al. 1999). This can be conceived as taking two forms. First, formal analysis of the process variables identified at the theoretical stage of intervention development. This means measuring key theoretical constructs such as change in beliefs or self-efficacy, and so on. For the intervention to act as hypothesized, a change in the specified process variables must occur. Further analysis exploring the extent that process variables mediate change in outcomes will be key to informing the mechanisms through which the intervention is working.

A second form of process evaluation is related to the implementation of self-management interventions and considers whether this is as intended; that is, the fidelity of the intervention (see Chapter 6 for further discussion). Factors that might be explored are delivery of intervention, contextual factors, recipient responses, and so on. Examination of such factors may be particularly important in multi-site trials as this allows for exploration of differences between sites (Oakley et al. 2006). Methods for evaluating these processes can be through either qualitative or quantitative methodologies and may involve techniques such as focus groups of participants, interviews, observation, analysis of video-tapes, questionnaire surveys, and so on. Often there is a benefit to integrating both types of methodologies (Bradieu et al. 1999). Although process evaluation is as central to self-management interventions as any other form of complex intervention, it is infrequently reported and hence techniques for this form of assessment are not well developed or standardized.

Predictor analysis

Process evaluation aims to determine the mechanisms through which change is occurring, either via mediating or moderating variables (Baron and Kenny 1986). It is also important to assess whether certain characteristics of participants can be identified at baseline that predict efficacy of the intervention. For example, in a study with patients with type 2 diabetes, it was shown that the intervention was not differentially effective for different demographic characteristics such as age and gender but individuals with higher levels of depression made fewer changes in dietary self-management following the intervention (Steed et al. 2005). Such predictor analysis is an important tool for developing and targeting future populations for self-management interventions. For example, one potential consequence of the predictors identified in the study above is that the intervention may be less appropriate in its current form for those with high levels of depressed mood.

Long-term implementation

Although an intervention may be shown to be efficacious within a research context, its value will only be realized if it can successfully be translated into the clinical context. The final stage of the MRC model therefore refers to long-term implementation. The challenge in translating research from self-management interventions into clinical practice is discussed in the concluding chapter of this book. A model to aid long-term implementation has been recommended (Glasgow 2003). This model is termed RE-AIM, which is an acronym of the terms reach, efficacy, adoption, implementation and maintenance.

'Reach' is the extent to which a programme penetrates the population that is targeted. It includes the participation rate and representativeness of participants versus study decliners, the reporting of which can reflect a study's reach. For interventions to have maximum reach, they need to target as broad a range of individuals as possible, including those from minority or traditionally disadvantaged groups. Traditionally, research designs tend to exclude individuals with co-morbidities or complex circumstances. However, by doing so the reach of the intervention may be reduced.

Efficacy is the effect of the intervention if implemented as described in the protocol, and it is recommended that it should include a range of outcomes including quality of life, behaviour change, and so on. In evaluating efficacy only individuals who receive the intervention as prescribed are included. It is common, however, that for a range of reasons not all participants will adhere to intervention protocols, for example, through not attending all the intervention sessions. Inclusion of these individuals is a further important component in intervention analysis as it provides a real-life reflection of the impact of the intervention. Such an analysis often using intention to treat models dictates the programme's effectiveness rather than efficacy and should additionally be evaluated for any intervention.

Adoption is the extent to which health care settings will participate in and deliver the intervention once shown to be effective. Conceptually, this is similar to reach, with the distinction that adoption refers to uptake by health care settings, while reach refers to uptake by individual participants. Traditionally, this is a neglected area of self-management intervention research but is essential to consider for successful clinical practice. A key consideration needs to be how programmes may be implemented within the community where resources may differ markedly from within secondary or tertiary care. Qualitative research looking at barriers to adoption of interventions within different spheres of the health care system may be a useful basis from which to learn more about successful adoption across the system.

Implementation relates to the extent to which the intervention is delivered as intended once in clinical practice. Implementation of a complex intervention is often more difficult than implementing simple interventions and highlights the need for any intervention to be well documented and the training needs of those who are to deliver the intervention to be specified a priori.

Maintenance occurs both at the individual level; that is, the long-term effects of the intervention and the health care setting level; that is, the extent to which the programme is sustained. At the individual level this can be addressed through teaching techniques such as relapse prevention and perhaps having booster sessions to maintain effects. At the health care setting more broad-ranging issues such as funding resources and political importance given to approaches such as self-management are key. In some states within the USA diabetes self-management programmes are now covered by medical insurance, and within the UK the Expert Patient Programme is delivered as a NHS service. Support such as this is fundamental to maintaining effects within the health care setting.

Attention to these different dimensions should be taken into account when designing and evaluating any self-management intervention. Depending on the primary goals the intervention might be designed quite differently. For example, mailed information addressing self-management behaviours may have high reach, adoption and implementation characteristics but low efficacy and maintenance. In contrast, individual counselling may be high on efficacy and implementation but have relatively limited reach and adoption (Glasgow et al. 2001). To address such concerns a stepped care approach, as used within smoking, may be a helpful model within self-management. Within this context relatively low-cost, high-reach interventions are delivered in the first instance but with the opportunity of increasingly more complex interventions offered to those who do not manage to achieve change at earlier stages (Glasgow 2003).

Conclusions

This chapter considered the process of developing and evaluating self-management interventions. To date few self-management interventions would appear to have gone through all steps recommended by the MRC model. However, this serves as a useful guideline for the development of future interventions.

References

Altman, D.G., Schulz, K.F. (2001) Concealing treatment allocation in randomised trials, *British Medical Journal*, 323: 446–47.

Baron, R.M. and Kenny, D.A. (1986) The moderator mediator variable distinction in social psychological-research: conceptual, strategic, and statistical considerations, *Journal of Personality and Social Psychology*, 51: 1173–82.

Bradieu, F., Wiles, R., Kinmonth, A-L., Mant, D., Gantley, M. for the SHIP Collaborative Group (1999) Development and evaluation of complex interventions in health services research: case study of the Southampton Heart Integrated Care Project (SHIP), *British Medical Journal*, 318: 711–15.

Bradley, C. (1993) Designing medical and educational intervention studies: a review of some alternatives to conventional randomized controlled trials, *Diabetes Care*, 16: 509–18.

Campbell, M., Fitzpatrick, R., Haines, A., Kinmonth, A.L., Sandercock, P., Spiegelhalter, D. and Tyrer, P. (2000) Framework for design and evaluation of complex interventions to improve health, *British Medical Journal*, 321: 694–96.

Cook, T.D. and Campbell, D.T. (1979) *Quasi-experimentation: Design and Analysis Issues for Field Settings*. Boston, MA: Houghton Mifflin.

Elasy, T.A., Ellis, S.E. and Brown, A. (2001) A taxonomy for diabetes educational interventions, *Patient Education and Counselling*, 43: 121–27.

Eldridge, S., Spencer, A., Cryer, C., Parsons, S., Underwood, M. and Feder, G. (2005) Why modelling a complex intervention is an important precursor to trial design: lessons from studying an intervention to reduce falls-related injuries in older people, *Journal of Health Services Research & Policy*, 10: 133–42.

Glasgow, R.E. (2003) Translating research to practice: lessons learned, areas for improvement and future directions, *Diabetes Care*, 26: 2451–56.

Glasgow, R.E., McKay, H.G., Piette, J.D. and Reynolds, K.D. (2001) The RE-AIM framework for evaluating interventions: what can it tell us about approaches to chronic illness management? *Patient Education and Counselling*, 44: 119–27.

Griffin, S., Kinmouth, A.L., Skinner, C. and Kelly, J. (1998) *Educational and Psychosocial Intervention for Adults with Diabetes*. London: British Diabetic Association.

Hardeman, W., Sutton, S., Griffin, S., Johnston, M., White, A., Wareham, N.J. and Kinmonth, A.L. (2005) A causal modelling approach to the development of theory-based behaviour change programmes for trial evaluation, *Health Education Research*, 20: 676–87.

Hawe, P., Shiell, A. and Riley, (2004) Complex interventions: how 'out of control' can a randomised controlled trial be? *British Medical Journal*, 328: 1561–63.

Lewin, B., Robertson, I.H., Cay, E.L., Irving, J.B. and Campbell, M. (1992) Effects of self-help post-myocardial-infarction rehabilitation on psychological adjustment and use of the health services. *The Lancet*, 339: 1036–40.

Lorig, K. (1996) *Patient Education: A Practical Approach*. Thousand Oaks, CA: Sage Publications.

McKay, H.G., King, D., Eakin, E.G., Seeley, J.R. and Glasgow, R.E. (2001) The diabetes network internet-based physical activity intervention: a randomized pilot study, *Diabetes Care*, 24: 1328–34.

McKee, M., Britton, A., Black, N., McPherson, K., Sanderson, C. and Bain, C. (1999) Interpreting the evidence: choosing between randomised and non-randomised studies, *British Medical Journal*, 319: 312–15.

Newman, S., Steed, L. and Mulligan, K. (2004) Self-management for chronic illness, *The Lancet*, 364: 1523–37.

Oakley, A., Strange, V., Bonell, C., Allen, E., Stephenson, J. and RIPPLE Study Team (2006) Process evaluation in randomised controlled trials of complex interventions, *British Medical Journal*, 332: 413–16.

Piette, J.D. (2005) *Using Telephone Support to Manage Chronic Disease*. Oakland, CA: California Health Care Foundation.

Rowlands, G., Sims, J. and Kerry, S. (2005) A lesson learnt: the importance of modelling in randomized controlled trials for complex interventions in primary care, *Family Practice*, 22: 132–39.

Steed, L., Cooke, D. and Newman, S. (2003) A systematic review of psychosocial outcomes following education, self-management and psychological interventions in diabetes mellitus, *Patient Education and Counselling*, 51: 5–15.

Steed, L., Lankester, J., Barnard, M. et al. (2005) Evaluation of the UCL Diabetes Self-management Programme (UCL-DSMP): a randomized controlled trial, *Journal of Health Psychology*, 10: 261–76.

Sutton, A.J., Abrams, K.R., Jones, D.R., Sheldon, T.A. and Song, F. (1998) Systematic reviews of trials and other studies, *Health Technology Assessment*, 2(19).

Walach, H., Falkenberg, T., Fonnebo, V., Lewith, G. and Jonas, W. (2006) Circular instead of hierarchical: methodological principles for the evaluation of complex interventions, *BMC Medical Research Methodology*, 6: 29.

Wolff, N. (2001) Randomised trials of socially complex interventions: promise or peril? *Journal of Health Services Research & Policy*, 6: 123–26.

9 Outcomes of self-management interventions

Robert F. DeVellis and Susan J. Blalock

As described in previous chapters, self-management interventions are designed to enable people with chronic illnesses to manage their condition more effectively. Achieving the desired changes may involve multiple variables operating at various ecological levels (e.g. Fisher et al. 2005). Interveners may choose to examine at least two types of 'outcome': proximal and distal. The long-term goal of most such interventions is to foster optimal physical, psychological and social well-being. However, more proximal outcomes, such as changes in targeted behaviours, are usually of interest as well. Thus, to assess intervention effectiveness thoroughly, the developers of an intervention must: 1) identify the outcomes of interest; 2) specify the presumed causal pathway that links proximal outcomes (e.g. targeted behaviours) to more distal outcomes (e.g. health status); and 3) devise a strategy to measure the outcomes specified in a meaningful way. In this chapter, we discuss issues that intervention developers must address to accomplish these three overarching tasks.

Identifying the outcomes of interest

The topic of this chapter begs the question, 'What is an outcome in the context of self-management interventions?' The answer to this question is perhaps more complex than it first seems. Two common but not entirely consistent meanings of the term are (a) a consequence of some process or event and (b) an endpoint. The difference between these two definitions is important. The ultimate end-point of interest within the context of self-management interventions usually relates to health status. That is, interveners usually hope to minimize disability and distress and optimize physical, psychological and social well-being. Clearly, such end-points are intervention outcomes. As an ultimate end-point, however, changes in health status do not result directly from implementation of intervention procedures. Rather, they result from a complex chain of events initiated by the intervention. For example, an intervention may lead to changes in knowledge and beliefs (e.g. belief in one's ability to reduce caloric intake), followed by changes in behaviour (e.g. reduction of caloric intake), followed by changes in physiological parameters (e.g. weight loss), and culminating in changes in health status (e.g. reduced risk of cardiovascular disease, improved sense of wellness). Thus, using the broader definition of an outcome as being a consequence of a process, each of these intervening variables can be viewed as an outcome because each results from a process initiated by the self-management intervention. This broader definition suggests that intervention developers should not only consider the ultimate end-points they hope to achieve; they should also identify each element in the chain of events initiated by the intervention that leads to those end-points.

In keeping with this point of view, we distinguish in this chapter between proximal and distal outcomes. Distal outcomes reflect the ultimate goals of a self-management intervention, whereas proximal outcomes reflect intervention effects that must occur for the distal outcomes to be achieved. Thus, as shown in Figure 9.1, proximal outcomes mediate effects of the intervention on distal outcomes.

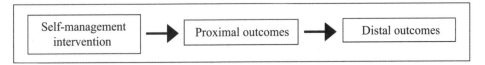

Figure 9.1 Assessing intervention effects

Distal outcomes

We use the term '*distal outcomes*' to refer to those intervention effects that would be of value even if they led to no other outcomes. Within the context of self-management interventions, the distal outcomes of interest often concern effects on symptom experience and functioning. Functioning is a broad, multidimensional construct. Dimensions of functioning include physical, psychological, social, cognitive, sexual and spiritual (e.g. Cella and Tulsky 1990). Specific self-management interventions may focus on a single dimension or a combination of dimensions. Self-management interventions may also be designed (e.g. Curtin et al. 2005) to alleviate symptoms (e.g. pain, fatigue, depression) or other negative consequences of illness (e.g. disability, missed work). In general, improvements in functioning and alleviation of symptoms are of inherent value and, consequently, fulfil our definition of distal variables. Thus, although they may lead to even more distal outcomes (e.g. lifetime earnings), intervention developers are rarely asked to establish such linkages.

Proximal outcomes

We use the term '*proximal outcomes*' to identify a wide variety of possible intervention effects. We limit the term, however, to those intervention effects that are of value primarily because they are thought to lead to distal outcomes. If one envisions a causal chain beginning with intervention delivery, the most proximal outcomes relate to participation in the intervention. Did participants attend group sessions? Did they read the self-management materials provided? Did they complete homework assignments? Clearly, these are desired effects of self-management interventions. However, their primary value lies in our belief that people who participate fully in a self-management intervention (e.g. by attending group sessions, reading provided materials, and completing homework assignments) will be more likely than others to derive maximal benefit from the intervention.

Assuming that individuals actively participate in a self-management intervention, the question becomes, 'What are the immediate effects expected from programme participation?' In answering this question, we would be likely to consider possible changes in knowledge, beliefs, attitudes, intrapsychic processes (i.e. thought patterns) and overt behaviour. For example, intervention participants may acquire knowledge required to make recommended lifestyle changes (e.g. foods that are low in fat or calories, exercises designed to strengthen specific muscle groups) and gain confidence in their ability to make such changes (e.g. Koenigsberg et al. 2004). Participation in a self-management intervention may also stimulate change in individual values. For example, individuals who are reluctant to ask for assistance with difficult tasks may come to accept that it is better to ask for assistance than to risk an illness exacerbation. Similarly, many self-management interventions target intrapsychic processes (e.g. catastrophizing, cognitive restructuring) that may either support or undermine self-management efforts (e.g. Ersek et al. 2004). Finally, many self-management interventions (e.g. Glasgow et al. 2007) attempt to change overt behaviours (e.g. eating habits, participation in regular physical activities).

The distinction between distal and proximal outcomes is especially relevant within the context of self-management interventions where behaviour change is a primary focus. In such programmes, is it sufficient to demonstrate that the targeted behaviour changed in the direction desired (e.g. caloric intake decreased, exercise activity increased)? Or, is it necessary to demonstrate change in a more distal outcome? On the one hand, it would seem appropriate to conclude that a behaviour change intervention was successful if the targeted behaviour was, in fact, changed in the intended direction. But, this assumes that behaviour change has inherent value. If a weight reduction programme demonstrated statistically significant reductions in caloric intake and increases in physical activity level, but failed to demonstrate any changes in weight or stabilization in blood glucose levels, it would seem difficult to declare the intervention a success. In that situation, it would be important to understand where the breakdown occurred. Were the findings due to (1) misspecification of the presumed causal pathway linking proximal outcomes to more distal ones or (2) measurement issues (e.g. using measures that were not valid, reliable, or sensitive to change; not allowing sufficient time for more distal outcomes to be achieved)? In the next section, we discuss how misspecification problems can be minimized by careful attention to the development of an explicit conceptual model that identifies each element in the expected chain of events initiated by the intervention, beginning with the most proximal outcomes and ending with the most distal ones. We then discuss measurement issues that are of particular relevance in relation to the many different types of outcome associated with self-management interventions.

Specifying causal pathways

An effective strategy for ensuring that potential misspecification problems can be identified is to develop an explicit representation of how the intervention is believed to work, based on previous empirical evidence and extant theory. This essentially forces the investigator to explicate assumptions and proposed causal mechanisms that link intervention components to both proximal and distal outcomes. With this type of model in hand, the investigator can design an evaluation plan that includes all relevant outcomes. Consequently, if the intervention fails to have the desired effect on the ultimate outcomes of interest, the investigator is well positioned to identify the point in the model at which the presumed causal chain was broken. On the other hand, if the ultimate outcomes of interest were achieved, but these effects were not mediated by the proximal outcomes identified by the model, the intervention developer will be forced to reconsider the presumed causal pathways articulated in the model. Improved understanding of the mechanism of action underlying intervention effects may suggest ways in which the intervention can be revised to improve effectiveness and efficiency.

A diagram is an especially useful way to model presumed mechanisms because it allows one more easily to consider multiple relationships among various elements of the model. If A leads to B and B leads to C, might there also be a direct impact of A on C not involving B? Questions such as this come readily to mind when inspecting a diagram whereas they may not when reading a verbal description of how an intervention plays out. Such a diagram can progress from a general to a more specific form through successive iterations. In its initial stages, categories of variables may suffice. For example, an early version of a model might specify that interacting with other people who have succeeded in the face of the same challenges that intervention participants are confronting will enhance their confidence. As the model evolves, the concept of 'confidence' can be further elaborated and specified (e.g. as self-efficacy for achieving particular objectives). In its final form, the model should describe a set of variables and how they are believed to relate to one another. If the model is developed with sufficient precision, it can then serve as a guide for selecting outcomes and determining how those outcomes can be operationalized.

In the process of developing this type of model, the investigator will be forced to consider explicitly several conceptual issues that too often receive scant attention. First, the anticipated strength of each hypothesized relationship should be considered. For example, the relationship between behaviour change (e.g. reduction in caloric intake) and change in physiological parameters (e.g. weight) is often taken for granted. Similarly, it is frequently assumed that changes in beliefs will lead to changes in behaviour. However, behaviour is likely to be influenced by multiple beliefs. Further, in a particular setting, behaviour may be constrained by environmental factors beyond individual control (Ajzen 1985; Ajzen 1991). Thus, the relationship between changes in a few targeted beliefs and subsequent behaviour change may be quite modest. Second, investigators should consider the normal latency required for different types of outcome to become apparent. For example, changes in knowledge and beliefs may occur immediately following intervention exposure. However, changes in physiological parameters may require weeks or months to become evident. Third, investigators should consider factors that may moderate hypothesized relationships. For example, do intervention components require a minimal level of health literacy for participants to be able to obtain maximal benefit? By grappling with these types of issue in the design stage, investigators can help ensure that their intervention rests on a firm theoretical foundation and that all relevant outcomes have been identified. It then becomes necessary to devise a measurement strategy that operationalizes these outcomes.

Measurement issues

Whether one is focusing on a distal or a proximal outcome, in order to determine whether the outcome has been achieved, we need to define the outcome of interest and then devise a means of assessing it. Moreover, both the definition and the assessment procedure have to be credible and conform to generally accepted standards. These fundamental conditions are overlooked or given inadequate attention with surprising frequency. For an investigator whose primary interest is assessing self-management outcomes, careful consideration of measurement issues may seem like an unwarranted distraction from the primary task. We believe, however, that it is of the utmost importance. Accordingly, we begin by taking a closer look at the nature of measurement and how it relates to assessing outcomes in self-management.

Accurate conceptualization of variable

The care with which we assess outcomes is critical to any evaluation of self-management in chronic illness. Although few would argue with the preceding statement in principle, it may be honoured less consistently in practice. As we suggested earlier, assessment is not typically the phase of research or evaluation that most intrigues investigators, and sometimes the most expedient measurement option is pursued with little regard for how well it might actually work. Careful measurement is critical to research because *the validity of our indicators literally determines whether we know what we are talking about.* Why is this so? Although we are generally interested in the relationships among variables or processes (e.g. between intention to exercise and sense of general well-being), what we actually assess are typically overt indicators of some sort that we hope capture the variables of interest (DeVellis 2003: 14–15). Stated differently, our empirical results most often describe the relationship between *indicators*, not the actual *variables of interest*. Only if we can have a very high degree of confidence that those indicators accurately reflect the intended variables can we use our results to make inferences about the relationship we really care about – the one between the variables themselves. Having confidence in the correspondence of our measurement operations to our concepts requires that we have a clear understanding and working definition of the latter.

Validity has a great deal to do with the quality of the observations we make, but it also has to do with the way that we define our variables of interest. Good observation does not guarantee validity if the correspondence between the observation and the variable definition is wanting. Thus, part of making sure that our indicators accurately reflect our variable of interest is choosing appropriate definitions for those variables. Sometimes, this means recognizing that the variable of interest in a specific analysis is different from some broader variable of more general interest to a larger set of research questions. For example, if a researcher's general interest is in the relationship of personality traits to self-management outcomes but the indicators available represent a specific personality trait (e.g. conscientiousness) and achievement of a specific self-management goal (e.g. improved medication adherence), it is important to recognize that the data do not address the broader concepts of interest but only those that are actually measured and analysed. Thus, the definition of 'variable of interest' and the indicator reflecting it need to correspond to a very high degree if we are to avoid confusion. Too commonly, the relationship between the construct of interest and the indicator is modest.

Ensuring variable-measure correspondence is equally important when selecting an existing instrument as a means of operationalizing a concept. It is important to establish that the way the variable has been conceptualized in the present instance is consistent with the conceptualization that underlies the existing measure. A seemingly apt name attached to an instrument is not sufficient evidence of its appropriateness. How and under what circumstances the assessment tool has actually performed are far better indicators of what it actually measures.

Consider an easily observable event: walking a specified distance. It would not be difficult to obtain a credible observation of how long it takes for someone to walk a specified distance; however, what inference would that observation support? Stated differently, what variables would those observations reflect? If the variable of interest is defined more broadly than the indicator warrants, the observed event may be an *instance* of that variable but may not accurately represent the concept as it is usually understood. For example, walking time is not the same as 'mobility', although it may be a part of it. Equating walking time with mobility does a poor job of matching the concept as it is generally understood with the observation used to assess it. More generally, observed phenomena are direct indicators only of the specific phenomenon observed under the particular conditions of the observation. An effective solution is to match the definition of constructs more closely to the actual observations used to assess them. In this case, either the 'variable of interest' could be redefined as *walking time*, or the observations could be expanded to represent the wider range of behaviours implied by the term '*mobility*'.

Slippage between a definition and an indicator can take on forms other than trying to instantiate a broad concept with a narrower indicator. Some terms can mean more than one thing and one meaning may be assumed at the conceptual level while another is applicable at the operational level. Consider the term 'desire for control'. Among the many interpretations of this term are the following two: (a) a desire to exert a strong influence over outcomes affecting oneself; and (b) a desire to exert strong influence over outcomes affecting others. In health research, the former definition is customary. We would not be surprised, however, to find the second definition more common in some disciplines, such as political theory. The potential confusion that might arise from a mismatch between conceptualizing 'desire for control' one way and operationalizing it the other way are obvious.

Important characteristics of variables

Even when we have carefully defined our variables of interest and are mindful of the need for definitions and indicators to correspond, characteristics of those variables and indicators can impact our assessment strategies. How easy or hard it is to have a high degree of confidence in our indicators is at least partially a function of the variables in which we are interested. As described earlier in this chapter, there is potentially a wide array of variables that can inform an assessment of a self-management intervention. For some of these, credible, valid assessment is straightforward while for others, it requires far more ingenuity. Different types of variable pose different assessment challenges. Some variable characteristics support more direct ascertainment while others require that we make inferences based on indirect evidence. Having to rely on less direct evidence may introduce error into our measurements of outcomes. Below, we discuss some of these features of different variables that may influence the types of indicator that we can confidently use to reflect them.

Observable versus unobservable

One fundamental difference among variables is whether they are observable or unobservable. That is, can the value of the variable be directly ascertained or must it be inferred by some indirect means? Variables of the former type that are likely to be of interest to self-management researchers and theorists are fairly few in number – perhaps fewer than is first apparent. Whether Person A or Person B is the first to complete walking a distance of 20 metres or whether someone can lift a 20-pound weight off the ground are events we can observe directly. There are other variables that we may think we observe directly when, in fact, we assess them indirectly through a proxy variable. In some cases, as when we have great confidence in the validity of the proxy variable, we may treat observation of the proxy as equivalent to observing the event of interest itself. For example, if we have a reliable timepiece, we may rely on the information it provides as equivalent to the actual passage of time and, in fact, may have no better or more direct way to measure time itself. (If we are using an hour glass rather than a precision timepiece, we may have somewhat less confidence that observing the sand pass through it amounts to observing 'time' directly.) Similarly, when we use a sphygmomanometer to assess blood pressure, we are quantifying a proxy variable (i.e. the height of a column of mercury) rather than directly observing pressure in the blood vessels. Thus, it is worth remembering that even things we may routinely regard as directly observable may not really be directly observed.

Observed versus reported

Even when a variable really is directly observable, we may assess it by some means other than direct observation. Very commonly, we rely on self-report to assess variables. That is, although an event like ability to lift 20 pounds may be observable, we often rely on someone telling us whether they can do it, rather than actually watching their performance. The extent to which reliance on self-reports represents a leap of faith depends in part on other variable characteristics such as the degree of subjectivity and social desirability.

Reports of 'judgements' versus 'sentiments'

In some cases, self-reports are about factual information, such as how many hours the respondent slept on the previous night. Although the person completing the item may not be able to provide an accurate answer, there presumably *is* a factually correct answer to a question of this sort. Nunnally (1978) applied the term 'judgements' to the process of responding to such queries. Judgements, then, are reports of objective events or states (even though the response provided may not be purely objective in practice). Other examples of judgements are reports of one's height, the number of medications taken, the presence of co-morbid conditions, ability to walk 20 metres without assistance, and the amount of time spent exercising in the past week.

In contrast, some variables concern purely subjective states or events, such as feelings of sadness, perceived competency of one's physician, belief in one's own ability to lose weight and expectations for recovery from an illness or injury. In each of these latter cases, the state, process or event about which the respondent is asked to report is inherently subjective. Nunnally referred to reports of this type as *sentiments*. Although it is easy to identify responses that are clearly of one type or the other (e.g. age v. sense of self-worth), other types of report may be more difficult to classify. For example, if an arthritis patient is asked if she can lift a two-pound package off of a high shelf, it is hard to know whether the response represents an objective (i.e. report of behaviour actually performed) or subjective (i.e. report of her belief about a hypothetical situation) appraisal, and thus whether it is a judgement or sentiment.

Cognitive accessibility of information

In the preceding discussion of judgements, we noted that even though the event being described *can* be assessed objectively, there is no guarantee that the respondent is actually reporting accurately. This brings us to another dimension along which self-reports can be classified: the cognitive accessibility of the information we request from the respondent. The information requested may be something that the respondent can readily bring to mind (e.g. age or gender) or it may entail somewhat more demanding cognitive processing in order to formulate an accurate response (e.g. Wyer 1980). Examples of the latter include *remembering* information about patterns of medication-taking, *interpreting* whether certain signs or symptoms are due to a health problem or are normal manifestations of ageing, and *comparing* whether one's strength has changed or remained the same over some period of time. When the information to be gathered is more complex and poses greater cognitive demands, there may be more opportunities for incorrect reporting (Tourangeau et al. 2000).

Thus, for less accessible information, accepting the veracity of a self-report may entail a greater leap of faith. For example, an individual may recall events incorrectly, may misinterpret an event in a way that influences whether or not it is reported, or may make a faulty comparison between events or processes.

Conflicting motivations

A factor that may render both judgements and sentiments inaccurate is conflicting motivations, or a desire to misrepresent the information for some reason (e.g. Gramzow and Willard 2006). *Social desirability* (Crowne and Marlowe 1960, 1964) is the motivation to present oneself in a favourable light. Certain indicators may tap into respondents' social desirability motivations and thus be influenced by something other than the variable they purport to measure. For example, respondents might be reluctant to answer a question about jealousy accurately because they do not want to reveal that they possess an undesirable personal attribute. In essence, the question fails to be about jealousy *per se* in such a case and becomes an indicator of a different attribute – social desirability. The opposite can also occur. An individual may be motivated to appear less desirable than he or she actually is. For example, an insurance claimant may misrepresent his or her ability to perform certain tasks in the hope that some financial benefit will result. While the presence of conflicting motivations may not be common, it is worth considering in judging whether an indicator is a credible reflection of the intended variable in a given situation.

When single items suffice

When an outcome variable possesses characteristics that support more direct ascertainment, relatively simple measurement methods may work well. Indicators that are highly representative of the variable they purport to assess and that can be observed directly or by means of a highly credible indirect means make for simple assessment. An example of such a variable is body mass index (BMI) which can be assessed indirectly by highly credible indicators (ruler and weight scale). Self-reports may be highly credible for certain types of variable, such as those that are highly accessible to the respondent and that the respondent is not motivated to distort or misrepresent. Gender, marital status and address are examples of these, although some desire to misrepresent these data may exist in some unusual circumstances. For variables such as these, a single item may be all that is necessary to assure good correspondence between the variable and the indicator.

Multi-item assessment as a means of improving accuracy

When variables require indirect assessment by means of self-report and when the information sought requires recollection, comparison, introspection or other relatively demanding cognitive processes, any single indicator may be prone to errors. For example, reporting compliance may involve trying to remember multiple behaviours over a period of days, comparing one's health status to others of the same age may entail making judgements about like-aged individuals and one's status relative to that referent, and assessing general well-being may require that a respondent dig down into her or his thoughts and feelings to formulate answers. Each of these tasks is more demanding than simply repeating over-learned information and the opportunities for error abound. One means of reducing the likelihood of such errors is to use multiple probes to assess the information (DeVellis 2003). Thus, whereas single-item measures may work well for assessing gender, marital status, address or other readily accessible information, capturing more elusive or complex information, such as mood states or compliance with medication regimen, may be more difficult with single-item measures. By using multiple probes, however, the assessor can triangulate in on the less accessible information. The logic of this approach is that each individual probe will contain some error and some truth. Because error is assumed to be random, when information is combined from different probes, the truth components should summate while the error components should regress toward zero.

There are two broad approaches to the development of multi-item instruments: classical test theory and item response theory. We briefly review both of these approaches in the next section.

Approaches to outcome assessment

Classical approaches

Methods based on classical test theory (CTT) (e.g. Nunnally 1978; Kline 2005 (Chapter 5); DeVellis 2006) assume that an observation (e.g. a score on some assessment tool) reflects two constituents: 1) the actual state or level of the phenomenon being observed (i.e. its 'true score') and 2) error (i.e. everything other than the true score that contributes to the nature of the observation). Moreover, the errors are assumed to be random. Accordingly, some will have a positive effect on the observed scores while others will have a negative effect; the net impact being close to zero when information is averaged across multiple observations.

The vast majority of measurement methodologies in use over the past several decades are based on CTT. This approach has its origins primarily in educational assessment such as ability testing (although the quantification of subjective sensory experiences in relation to the physical stimuli giving rise to them was also an area of active measurement development in the early twentieth century). Paralleling work in ability assessment, psychologists interested in non-intellective individual differences, such as personality characteristics, adopted similar measurement strategies. Most of the measurement approaches used to assess self-management outcomes are descended from these measurement approaches, particularly the use of self-administered questionnaires.

Self-administered, fixed-content questionnaires

Probably the most common CTT-based assessment methodology uses self-administered questionnaires comprising a fixed set of stimuli. These assessment tools are familiar to us all and we have already discussed some of the issues they raise. They consist of a series of verbal (e.g. questions or statements), numerical (e.g. numbers to circle) or pictorial (e.g. visual analogue scales) stimuli to which the examinee is asked to respond as a means of self-description. The most common format uses verbal statements or questions that the respondent is asked to evaluate by providing a response (e.g. expressing agreement with a descriptive statement, or answering a query). Often, questionnaires include multiple questions to assess a single variable and responses to these questions are combined to form an index or scale. Each index/scale is likely to have a fixed content. Thus, although a study design may call for different participants to be assessed on different variables (e.g. in a study of couples in which one spouse has a chronic illness, the partner with the illness may be assessed for medication adherence while the other partner is not), the items representing a given variable are usually the same for all cases in which that variable is assessed. This contrasts with adaptive assessment strategies that we will describe later.

When self-report by means of fixed-item assessment procedures is the data collection method, adhering to established principles of scale development can improve the quality of the instrument (see DeVellis 2003, especially Chapter 5). These principles include ensuring that individual items and response options are unambiguous and will be properly understood by respondents. As in all questionnaire design, the primary concerns should be that the indicators are reliable and that they correspond to the variables of interest. Moreover, they should represent the relevant *levels* of those variables for the research questions being addressed. Thus, for each variable to be assessed in a study, special attention should be paid to the range of the variable anticipated in the target population and the range of the variable covered by the items being used. For example, an instrument designed specifically for use with people having significant motor impairments may not work well in a sample that includes many individuals with only minor motor impairments. In this case, there may be few if any items differentiating among levels of motor performance among those with only minor impairments. Conversely, a motor performance measure (to continue with this example) intended for general populations may not provide sufficiently detailed information about individuals with significant impairments. One should also be mindful of potential ordering effects. For example, a set of items assessing affective state might yield different results depending on the items that immediately precede them. Asking a respondent, for example, to list their most serious health problems, greatest sources of dissatisfaction with care, or the most distressing aspects of their interpersonal circumstances might induce negative emotions that could carry over to the next set of items. In the process of questionnaire development, asking oneself, 'How might this questionnaire go wrong?' can be a useful device for detecting potential problems that could compromise the final instrument.

Clinician ratings

Another common type of assessment involves having clinicians rate individuals they have treated. There are a number of disease activity scales, for example, that can be used to obtain a physician's assessment concerning the status (e.g. in a state of exacerbation v. in remission) of a specific disease process. Indicators of this sort have many of the advantages and disadvantages of self-reports. The information may be observable or unobservable, a judgement or a sentiment, accurate or inaccurate, and subject to conflicting motivations or not. The professional training of the clinician may help to enhance accuracy and reduce the influence of competing motivations. On the other hand, if the rating is based on an interpretation of the patient's subjective states (such as pain, fatigue or emotional state), the clinician's report may be farther removed from the variable of interest than a self-report would be and thus may be less accurate (e.g. von Essen 2004). There is considerable evidence indicating that patient self-reports and clinician reports often diverge substantially. Also, because the physician may have access to less nuanced information about the patient's subjective states, classifications may be more course-grained than self-reports. On the other hand, an expert clinician may have a broader range of experience with different aspects of an illness and may understand underlying processes in ways that result in greater accuracy. When clinician ratings are obtained, it is very important to recognize that the variable being assessed (e.g. clinician perception of the patient's pain) may differ from the variable captured by a self-rating (e.g. patient's report of pain). Maintaining an awareness of the distinction may be very important in accurately assessing outcomes.

Proxy reports

Some types of clinician ratings (e.g. physician's judgement of patient pain) are part of a broader class of assessments that involve some individual serving as a proxy for the individual who is being assessed. In some cases, these reports from others are obtained when the person of interest cannot provide a self-report. This may be the case when the individual of interest is cognitively impaired, does not speak the language in which a questionnaire is written, or is too young to provide the information sought (e.g. Sneeuw et al. 1997). Although proxy reports may be the only means of collecting data in some situations, available evidence suggests that it is not necessarily equivalent to what a self-report from the patient would have revealed.

Behavioural/performance measure

Although questionnaires are probably the most widely used assessment tools, it is important not to overlook opportunities for the observation of actual behaviour. This approach bypasses some of the potential problems associated with self-report. For example, interpersonal relationships may exert a powerful influence on self-management outcomes. One strategy for capturing critical aspects of these relation-ships is by means of self-report, with measures of perceived social support serving as a common example. An alternative is to observe interactions more directly. One of us (RFD) for example, is currently conducting an investigation in which empathic accuracy (the extent to which an individual can correctly infer their spouse's unspoken thoughts and feelings) is a variable of interest (see DeVellis 2003 for an overview). The assessment procedure involves having individuals interact with one another while being video-taped. Each partner then views the tape of the interaction without their spouse present and is asked to indicate moments during the conversation when they experienced an unexpressed thought or feeling. When they identify such an instance, they are asked to describe their thoughts and feelings that were not expressed. In a second stage of the procedure, each spouse is shown a moment from the conversation when their partner experiences an unexpressed thought or feeling and are asked to infer what that thought or feeling was. The self-description and the partner's inferred description of each unexpressed thought and feeling are then coded for similarity by trained raters who are blinded to the design of the study. Raters' similarity judgements provide a behaviourally based indicator of empathic accuracy that avoids at least some of the shortcomings of self-report.

Modern measurement approaches

New measurement methodologies based on item response theory (e.g. Embretson and Reise 2000) are gaining wider recognition for the potential advantages they offer over classical measurement methods. In IRT approaches, parameters of individual items can be modelled in a way that is not dependent on the sample from which the data were collected. IRT is not a single approach but a family of approaches represented by different underlying models. One dimension across which IRT models differ is the number of item parameters that they assess. One common IRT approach, which includes Rasch modelling, is based on the estimation of a single parameter, often called the *difficulty* parameter. This usage is a legacy of the extensive work on IRT done in the context of ability testing. When measuring abilities, such as mathematical proficiency, with multiple items, one obvious item characteristic is item difficulty. Some items require more mathematical proficiency than others. By analogy, characteristics other than abilities assessed in educational realms can also be measured with graded items that differ in the strength of the attribute necessary for item endorsement. For example, 'I sometimes feel sad', is an affect-relevant item that requires relatively little sadness on the part of the respondent to garner an endorsement. On the other hand, 'I usually feel that life is not worth living' is an item requiring a considerably higher level of depressive affect to garner endorsement. A single-parameter IRT model would determine the 'difficulty' of items such as these by establishing how much of the attribute being measured (be it mathematical proficiency or depressive affect) a respondent must possess in order to have a 50 per cent likelihood of endorsing the item. Individual items can be represented by item characteristic curves (ICCs) that plot the likelihood of endorsement (Y axis) against the strength of the attribute being measured (X axis). By examining the ICCs for a pool of items, a subset of items can be selected to ensure that the precision of measurement is maintained across the full range of the attribute being assessed.

A second parameter often examined in IRT models is *discrimination*. This parameter represents the item's ability to differentiate with relatively little ambiguity between people who are low versus high on the attribute being measured and is associated with a steep ICC. A highly discriminating item, in essence, has a stronger relationship to (or is a better exemplar of) the attribute of interest, relative to a less discriminating item.

Another item parameter included in some IRT models concerns the extent to which people who are completely lacking in the attribute are inclined to endorse or 'pass' an item intended to tap that attribute. In an educational context, this amounts to getting a test item correct even if you really do not know the answer. Accordingly, this is often called the *guessing* parameter. In the context of health assessment, this parameter can represent a false positive. For example, the likelihood of someone without a particular illness checking off that illness on a list of co-morbidities could be represented by this guessing parameter. Although IRT models can differ in many more ways than the inclusion or exclusion of specific parameters, a more extensive discussion is beyond the scope of this chapter. Hambleton et al. (1991) give an overview of IRT that is among the more accessible descriptions of this approach to measurement.

Cross-sample comparisons

Measurement consistency across different studies or different samples within a study is desirable because it facilitates making direct comparisons from one set of findings to another. This, in turn, lends a collective continuity to the literature describing work in a given area. Under CTT, such comparisons may prove difficult. The first problem arises when different measures are used across samples to operationalize the same construct. Obviously, equating a score on Measure X to another score on Measure Y is problematic even if both measures purport to tap the same variable. Issues of calibration, sensitivity and score dispersion all can complicate comparisons of this type. Identifying the ideal measure of a variable, so that whenever that variable is assessed the same tool is used, would remedy some of these issues. Such a solution, however, is highly impractical. Different investigators may prefer different measures of the same construct for a variety of reasons.

Even when there is agreement regarding which measure to use for a given variable, cross-sample comparisons can pose problems. Under CTT, how measures perform is influenced by the samples themselves. For example, a measure might have low reliability in a sample where the range of values for the variable assessed is severely constrained but may have acceptable reliability on a more heterogeneous sample. That is, the same measurement tool may be highly error prone in one case but yet sufficiently reliable in the other. If a measurement instrument spans a sufficiently wide range of the underlying variable (e.g. physical ability levels suitable for everyone from elite athletes to individuals with severe chronic conditions) to be universally useful, then much of the information it yields in any given application may be worthless if certain items lie beyond the sample's range of capabilities. Items intended for athletes, for example, will be consistently too difficult for people with motor impairments. Thus, the 'one-tool-fits-all' approach, even if adopted will create its own problems.

IRT and adaptive testing

In fact, under IRT, one would not need to administer the full range of items to the two samples described in the preceding section in order to make cross-sample comparisons. One of the advantages of IRT approaches is that, with sufficient information, individual items can be directly tied to specific levels of the phenomenon being measured. For example, an item assessing depression can be calibrated so that the level of depression associated with a transition from not endorsing to endorsing that item can be established. This forms a basis for adaptive testing, in which items are chosen for their relevance to the specifics of the individual respondent. In a typical adaptive test, a respondent first answers a few probe items that determine coarsely where that person falls on the continuum of the attribute. Once a rough determination is made, subsequent items are automatically selected that successively target the precise level of the individual respondent. Each subsequent item is selected on the basis of the response to the previous item, targeting a lower level of difficulty if the previous item was not endorsed and a higher level if it was. The process continues until the information obtained constitutes a stable determination of the individual's location on the attribute continuum.

This process can be highly efficient, requiring each respondent to complete only a small subset of the total items, without encountering items that are substantially below or above the respondent's actual position on the attribute continuum. For example, a person whose functional status was essentially intact would not be required to answer multiple items about functional limitations. Conversely, someone with substantial functional impairment would not be asked questions about activities that were well beyond his or her capacity.

Another noteworthy aspect of adaptive testing is that identical items need not be administered before and after an intervention to determine improvement. In fact, it would not be uncommon when using adaptive testing for the post-intervention items to represent a higher level of ability than the pre-intervention assessment completed by the same individual. If the intervention succeeded, the ability level of that individual should have improved and the relevant items for assessing ability at the improved level would be different than those administered prior to the intervention. Because the items can be calibrated to ability, the amount of change in ability could be accurately gauged even though different items were administered on the two occasions. Of course, this approach can only succeed when the items have undergone sufficient pre-testing to ensure their accurate calibration relative to the underlying ability in question.

Patient Reported Outcomes Measurement Information System (PROMIS)

The PROMIS initiative, funded by the US National Institutes of Health (NIH), is a noteworthy effort to apply IRT methods to assessing health outcomes. PROMIS is a collaborative project involving the NIH in collaboration with researchers from Duke

University, Northwestern University, Stanford University, the University of North Carolina, the University of Pittsburgh, the University of Stony Brook and the University of Washington. Its goal is to develop item banks representing five broad domains of health-related outcomes: pain, fatigue, physical functioning, social functioning and emotional distress. The items comprising these banks have undergone extensive qualitative and quantitative evaluation. Recent papers describe the foundational work of the PROMIS team (e.g. Ader 2007; Cella et al. 2007). PROMIS will make these item banks available to researchers at little or no cost as a means of improving the quality and standardization of health outcomes assessment. PROMIS has also developed a computerized interface that investigators can use for the administration of items from the banks in either fixed-form or adaptive assessment configurations. The PROMIS initiative has been a sizeable undertaking and represents a major effort to identify, classify, evaluate, calibrate and disseminate items that can be used for assessing health-related patient-reported outcomes. Even this effort, however, has not been all inclusive. For example, PROMIS has focused primarily on end-points. Further work providing comparable information on items assessing more proximal outcomes remains to be done. The products of PROMIS and subsequent efforts that can build upon it will be a rich resource for investigators seeking tools for evaluating self-management and other types of interventions.

Conclusions

In summary, properly defining and operationalizing outcomes of self-management interventions is critical to any effort to evaluate their success. Approaching these tasks systematically is essential. Different types of outcome and their specific features must be recognized and measurement strategies should be compatible with those features. Thus, for example, if information is not readily accessible to respondents, it may be necessary to use a multi-item measurement strategy.

Attending to issues of careful measurement is important in many contexts but may be especially so in the context of self-management interventions because of certain features of the latter. For example, because self-management, by definition, is implemented largely by the person targeted for change, there may be less external scrutiny of the intervention process. There is potentially less observation by expert eyes, relative to interventions conducted under direct professional supervision. For example, rather than a therapist logging exercise hours, in the case of a self-management intervention, it is the patient who may be responsible for tracking exercise sessions. Thus, measures the participants fill out may be the primary or even the only source of information for certain important variables. A related feature of self-management interventions is their heavy reliance on self-report measures of outcomes. While these can work well when properly developed and used, special care may be required to achieve optimal validity, relative to methods such as direct observation. A key strength of self-management is that it gives greater control to the participant. In so doing, however, it may also increase opportunities for improper measurement. Appropriate care and the careful selection of measurement strategies can mitigate such errors.

Assessment approaches can make use of both classical and modern measurement theories and methods. Modern methods based on IRT are likely to increase in familiarity and popularity as they are used more widely. Efforts such as the PROMIS initiative can play an important role in fostering the adoption of items developed under IRT approaches and benefiting from the advantages that these approaches offer. At the same time, methods developed under CTT, if developed carefully and applied prudently, can continue to provide useful information for judging the impacts of self-management interventions.

References

Ader, D.N. (2007) Developing the Patient-Reported Outcomes Measurement Information System (PROMIS), *Medical Care*, 45(5) (Suppl. 1): S1–S2.

Ajzen, I. (1985) From intentions to actions: a theory of planned behavior, in J. Kuhl and J. Beckman (eds) *Action-control: From Cognition to Behavior* (pp. 11–39). Heidelberg: Springer.

Ajzen, I. (1991) The theory of planned behavior, *Organizational Behavior and Human Decision Processes*, 50(2): 179–211.

Cella, D.F. and Tulsky, D.S. (1990) Measuring quality of life today: methodological aspects, *Oncology*, 4(5): 29–38.

Cella, D., Yount, S., Rothrock, N., Gershon, R., Cook, K., Reeve, B., Ader, D., Fries, J.F., Bruce, B. and Rose, M. on behalf of the PROMIS Cooperative Group (2007) The Patient-Reported Outcomes Measurement Information System (PROMIS): progress of an NIH Roadman cooperative group during its first two years, *Medical Care*, 45(5) (Suppl. 1): S3–S11.

Crowne, D.P. and Marlowe, D. (1960) A new scale of social desirability independent of psychopathology, *Journal of Consulting Psychology*, 24: 349–54.

Crowne, D.P. and Marlowe, D. (1964) *The Approval Motive*. New York: John Wiley & Sons.

Curtin RB, Mapes D, Schatell D, Burrows-Hudson S. Self-management in ESRD: Exploring its domains and dimensions. *Nephrology Nursing Journal* 32(4):389–395, 2005

DeVellis, R.F. (2003) *Scale Development: Theory and Applications*. Thousand Oaks, CA: Sage Publications.

DeVellis, R.F. (2006) Classical test theory. *Medical Care*, 44(11) (Suppl. 3): S50–S59.

DeVellis, R.F., Lewis, M.A. and Sterba, K.R. (2003). Interpersonal and emotional processes in adjustment to chronic illness, in J. Suls and K. Wallston (eds) *Social Psychological Foundations of Health*. Oxford, UK: Blackwell Publishers.

Embreston, E.E., & Reise, S.P. (2000). Item response theory for psychologists. Mahwah, NJ: Lawrence Erlbaum Associates.

Ersek, M., Turner, J.A., Cain, K.C. and Kemp, C.A. (2004) Chronic pain self-management for older adults: a randomized controlled trial, *BMC Geriatrics*, 4: 7.

Fisher, E. B., Brownson, C. A., O'Toole, M. L., Shetty, G., Anwuri, V. V., & Glasgow, R. E. (2005). Ecological approaches to self-management: The case of diabetes. *American Journal of Public Health, 95*, 1523–1535.

Glasgow, R.E., Fisher, L., Skaff, M., Mullan, J. and Toobert, D.J. (2007) Problem solving and diabetes self-management investigation in a large, multiracial sample, *Diabetes Care*, 30: 33–37.

Gramzow, R.H. and Willard, G. (2006) Exaggerating current and past performance: motivated self-enhancement versus reconstructive memory, *Personality and Social Psychology Bulletin*, 32: 1114–25.

Hambleton, R.K., Swaminathan, H. and Rogers, H.J. (1991) *Fundaments of Item Response Theory*. Thousand Oaks, CA: Sage Publications.

Kline, T.J.B. (2005) *Psychological Testing: A Practical Approach to Design and Evaluation.* Thousand Oaks, CA: Sage Publications.

Koenigsberg, M.R., Bartlett, D. and Cramer, J.S. (2004) Facilitating treatment adherence with lifestyle changes in diabetes, *American Family Physician*, 69(2): 309–16.

Nunnally, J.C. (1978) *Psychometric Theory*. New York: McGraw-Hill.

Schmiege, S.J., Aiken, L.S., Sander, J.L. and Gerend, M.A. (2007) Osteoporosis prevention among young women: psychosocial models of calcium consumption and weight-bearing exercise. *Health Psychology*, 26: 577–87.

Sneeuw, K., Aaronson, N.K., Osoba, D., Muller, M., Hsu, M., Yung, W.K.A., Brada, M. and Newlands, E.S. (1997) The use of significant others as proxy raters of the quality of life of patients with brain cancer, *Medical Care*, 35(5): 490–506.

Tourangeau, R., Rips, L.J. and Rasinski, K. (2000) *The Psychology of Survey Response*. Cambridge: Cambridge University Press.

von Essen, L. (2004) Proxy ratings of patient quality of life: factors related to patient-proxy agreement, *Acta Oncologica*, 43(3): 229–34.

Wyer, R.S. (1980) The acquisition and use of social knowledge, *Personality and Social Psychology Bulletin*, 6: 558–73.

PART IV

Self-management in Specific Conditions

10 Diabetes

Frank J. Snoek, Timothy C. Skinner and Liz Steed

Introduction

This chapter reviews the role of self-management and behavioural interventions aimed at improving self-management in people, both youth and adults, with diabetes. A short introduction into the medical aspects of diabetes is provided, highlighting the central role of self-management as a means to attain adequate diabetes control and reduce health risks in the short and longer term.

Diabetes mellitus

Diabetes mellitus is a metabolic condition characterized by chronic hyperglycaemia (elevated blood glucose levels) resulting from defects in insulin secretion, insulin absorption or both. Hyperglycaemia is accompanied by acute symptoms like thirst, tiredness and a frequent need to urinate. Extremely high levels of blood glucose can lead to coma and ultimately death. Long-standing hyperglycaemia causes micro- and macro-vascular complications in the longer term, leading to dysfunction and failure of the organs, especially the heart, kidneys, eyes, blood vessels and nerves. Complications of diabetes have the effect of shortening lifespan by up to 10 years. At present there is no cure for diabetes. Two main types of diabetes are distinguished: type 1 ('juvenile') diabetes and type 2 ('adult-onset') diabetes, with the latter being the most common form of diabetes, accounting for 85 per cent of all diabetes in Western economically developed countries.

Type 1 diabetes is usually diagnosed before the age of 40, with incidence peaking during adolescence, and is the result of a total destruction of the beta cells in the pancreas that manufacture insulin, leading to absolute insulin deficiency. As a consequence exogenous insulin is essential for survival, either by subcutaneous injections or a subcutaneous insulin infusion pump. Type 1 diabetes is thought to be an auto-immune disease and is associated with an increased risk of other auto-immune diseases like Grave's disease and hypothyroidism.

In type 2 diabetes, at least in the early stages, insulin production is usually not fully lacking, but insufficient to keep blood glucose levels in the normal range. This is a result of insulin resistance (often related to being overweight) and/or insufficient insulin production. As a consequence, exogenous insulin may not be essential to survival in type 2 diabetes, hence early labels of 'non-insulin dependent diabetes', however increasingly insulin administration may be prescribed as an aid to improving glycaemic control. About half of type 2 diabetes patients are in need of insulin therapy after six years due to progressive loss of beta cell function (UKPDS 1995). Traditionally, type 2 diabetes has been seen primarily among individuals greater than 40 years of age with the highest incidence in persons over 60 years old. The changing demographic in Westernized societies, with greater obesity at younger ages, has, however, meant that in some instances type 2 diabetes has been diagnosed in childhood (Alberti et al. 2004), although this remains a minority of cases.

Treatment of diabetes

Treatment of both types of diabetes is aimed at normalizing blood glucose levels and management of cardiovascular risk factors by means of symptom monitoring, lifestyle changes, blood glucose lowering therapy (tablets and/or insulin injections) and medication aimed at normalizing lipids, triglycerides and blood pressure. In addition, as with all chronic illnesses, management includes helping individuals adjust to the role and emotional changes concomitant to the illness.

Particularly in type 2 diabetes, healthy eating and physical activity are core elements of the treatment plan, although this does not negate the importance of other features of the regimen including self-monitoring of blood glucose, foot-care inspection and taking medications including both insulin or hypoglycaemic agents. However, many people with type 2 diabetes find following treatment advice difficult as reflected through studies that show poor adherence in type 2 diabetes. For example, approximately 36 per cent of individuals report following their dietary plan only sometimes, rarely or never (Ruggiero et al. 1997), while 62 per cent of individuals eat less than the recommended five servings of fruit or vegetables a day (Nelson et al. 2002). Sixty-nine per cent of individuals report taking less exercise than recommended, with 31 per cent of these taking no physical activity at all (Nelson et al. 2002). For individuals prescribed insulin, only 17 per cent have been found to obtain sufficient testing strips to test daily as recommended (Evans et al. 1999), while 67 per cent of those taking all forms of treatment report testing less frequently than recommended (Karter et al. 2000). Adherence to medication, although typically conceived of as one of the better adhered to components of the diabetes management regimen, also demonstrates low levels of adherence. Prospective studies of adherence to oral hypoglycaemic agents report rates of 61–85 per cent and for insulin only 63 per cent. Typically, these rates decrease the longer the individual has been prescribed medication and the more complex and demanding the regimen (Cramer 2004).

Type 1 diabetes requires intensive insulin treatment, including frequent self-monitoring of blood glucose (finger pricks) and adjusting insulin to food intake, physical activity and changing circumstances (e.g. climate, stress). However, one of the difficulties for individuals with type 1 diabetes is that adhering to the regimen to reduce high blood glucose levels (hyperglycaemia) brings along the risk of low blood glucose levels (hypoglycaemia), that can seriously affect a persons' cognitive, emotional and social functioning. Hypoglycaemia has been identified as the main limiting factor in modern type 1 diabetes management and a significant worry for many patients on intensive insulin therapy and their families (Gold et al. 1997; Cryer 2002). To minimize the risk of hypoglycaemia patients need to take precautionary measures and respond effectively to lowering glucose levels when they are detected, either symptomatically or by checking blood sugars. Some patients may lack warning signs and are thus dependent on their partner, family members and colleagues to detect and correct hypoglycaemia in time with, for example, a fruit juice, glucose tablets or small snack.

Self-management interventions in adolescents with type 1 diabetes

There are two key features that distinguish self-management education programmes for adolescents with type 1 diabetes from adult studies: 1) the young person is growing through a period of rapid biological, psychological and social development. This means that the self-management skills of young people, along with their self-management goals, will change over relatively short periods of time; and 2) when working with adolescents, there is also the need to work with parental relationships and the wider family. The literature is fairly clear in documenting the importance of family factors in influencing the psychological and biomedical outcomes of care in this period (Skinner et al. 2005).

Given these challenges, it is not surprising that routine clinical care is largely inadequate for supporting young people in developing optimal coping skills, quality of life and glycaemic control. However, two systematic reviews of the literature of psychoeducation interventions for adolescents have some positive messages (Hampson et al. 2000; Murphy et al. 2006). The published studies would suggest that self-management programmes in adolescents do have positive effects for young people for both psychological and metabolic outcomes. Given that adolescence is frequently a time of declining metabolic control (as a result of a combination of physiological and behavioural factors), providing self-management programmes that enable young people to remain relatively stable through this key developmental period is a significant improvement on standard care, with some interventions managing to obtain reductions in metabolic control. The achievement of stability in glycaemia may go some of the way to explain why effect sizes in this area are at best moderate and in most cases small for measures of glycaemia (Hampson et al. 2000).

However, from this literature two broad approaches seem to stand out, in terms of self-management interventions. While both provide self-management education concerning carbohydrate counting, blood glucose monitoring, insulin adjustment, and so on, each combines additional components; one to equip the young person to self-manage effectively while managing peer relations and social pressures; and the other provides support for negotiating the changing family relations.

With regard to helping young people self-manage amid the social pressures of adolescence, the work of Margaret Grey and colleagues stands out (Grey et al. 2000). They have evaluated the impact of a coping skills training programme as an adjunct to self-management education for starting intensive insulin regimens (either multiple daily injections or insulin pump therapy). The programme covers social problem-solving, and conflict resolution skills using scenarios the adolescent generated as causing problems for the intensive management of their diabetes. The programme used a professional educator for the first few group sessions, and then moved on to using trained adolescents with diabetes to complete the programme. The results of the programme, evaluated using a randomized trial are very encouraging, showing improved glycaemic control and psychological outcomes both in the short term and over an extended follow-up period. Other groups are currently in the process of attempting to replicate this work.

Although peers are important in adolescence, young people still have to make the transition from either dependent child with parents primarily caring for diabetes, or from a healthy adolescent who is recently diagnosed, to a young person who may need to spend a period of time having an interdependent relationship with parents, before moving onto being independently responsible for their diabetes care. Whatever the start point in adolescents, this means that both young people and their parents need to receive effective training in diabetes-specific self-management. Perhaps more challenging though is the need for the parents and young people to develop skills to help them negotiate the transitioning of care progressively into the hands of the young adult.

The research in this area is remarkably consistent in demonstrating that greater responsibility for diabetes care activities (e.g. injecting insulin, deciding on insulin dose, remembering to monitor blood glucose) taken by the adolescent with diabetes, and the less parental involvement, the worse their control (Skinner et al. 2005). More detailed examination of parent and child perceptions of responsibility indicated that where no one was taking responsibility, the young person with diabetes was in worse diabetes control. This handing over of responsibility needs not only to be negotiated and managed, but also needs to match the maturity of the individual and their ability to take responsibility. These hypotheses have now been tested with intervention studies that specifically targeted this process of negotiating responsibility, combined with self-management education (Anderson et al. 1999; Anderson et al. 1998; Laffel et al. 2003; Murphy et al. 2007). These studies have demonstrated that this is an issue that could be readily integrated into normal diabetes care, and consultations without increasing diabetes-related conflict can be delivered in a group or individual format and can support improved glyceamic control and self-care.

Of particular note is that unlike the vast majority of research in the self-management of diabetes, this approach has been replicated by a second independent research group in the UK, the original studies being undertaken in the USA. The FACTS (Families, Adolescents and Children's Teamwork Study) project has demonstrated that the results were replicated, when the work is undertaken in a small district general hospital, compared to the large diabetes specialist research centre where the original investigations were undertaken (Murphy et al. 2007). Furthermore, the modest effects achieved in the FACTS study were obtained without the need for additional visits to hospital. In short, self-management programmes that provide both parents and young people with self-management skills, and develop family communication skills, appear to reduce family conflict, increase agreement on who is taking responsibility for diabetes care, and help maintain metabolic control in adolescents. The next step may be to combine the two approaches so that adolescents are progressively equipped with the skills to self-manage their diabetes, their parents and their peers.

Self-management interventions in adults with type 1 diabetes

While the incidence of type 1 diabetes is highest among adolescents, a substantial number of people receive the diagnosis of type 1 diabetes during adulthood, necessitating significant changes in lifestyle, sometimes accompanied by loss of work and social responsibilities. With the diagnosis comes the acute need to self-inject insulin three to five times daily to avoid keto-acidosis due to extremely high blood glucose levels which may lead to death. To enable patients to self-manage their diabetes from a technical perspective, they customarily receive information and instruction in most cases on an individual basis and from specialized nurses in an outpatient setting. Very little research has been done to clarify what is the best way to guide patients through this important first phase, taking individual differences into account. Providing structured (group) self-management education to patients following diagnosis may help to reduce initial stress and promote active coping, but convincing evidence is lacking (Spiess et al. 1995). Also, the logistics of organizing groups for newly diagnosed type 1 diabetes patients is complex, given the relatively low incidence of type 1 diabetes among adults. There may be less need for such interventions with more and more patients having access to the Internet where medical information is available and the technology also offers the opportunity to share experiences with others (Zrebiec and Jacobson 2001).

Although the majority of patients appear to initially adapt reasonably quickly to the fact that they have a chronic illness, patients with longer diabetes duration may have difficulties, suggesting that the demands of continuous self-management may become problematic over time. Structured group self-management education programmes have been developed to assist such patients to improve their adherence behaviours and emotional functioning. Rubin and colleagues at Hopkins University (USA) were among the first to add coping-oriented modules to an outpatient education programme, integrating techniques from cognitive behavioural therapy and relapse prevention. Participants showed improved emotional well-being and glycaemic control at six and twelve month follow-ups (Rubin et al. 1989). Building on a structured five-day inpatient group training developed by Berger and colleagues in Düsseldorf , the 'DAFNE' (Dose Adjustment For Normal Eating) trial was conducted in the UK, promoting flexible insulin therapy based on skills training. The results of this waitlist controlled study demonstrated improved glycaemic control as well as perceived quality of life following a five-day DAFNE course (DAFNE study group 2002). Bott et al. (2000) tested the effects of a similar five-day inpatient training programme that included psychosocial modules for type 1 diabetes patients with persistent poor glycaemic control. The intervention included group meetings that covered individual goal-setting, motivation and coping strategies. At follow-up, glycaemic control had not improved but patients did report feeling less externally controlled and had increased levels of diabetes self-efficacy.

A six-week cognitive-behavioural group programme developed by Snoek et al. (2001) specifically for poorly controlled type 1 diabetes patients found positive effects on self-efficacy, self-care behaviours and diabetes distress, but not on glycaemic control (Van der Ven et al. 2005).

To help patients cope with the problem of recurrent hypoglycaemia, Cox and his colleagues developed the Blood Glucose Awareness Training (BGAT), an eight-week psychoeducational group intervention that helps patients to become more aware of their hypoglycaemia symptoms, reduce the number of (severe) hypoglycaemic episodes and lower fear of low blood glucose levels (Cox et al. 1995). Following the development of BGAT Cox et al. have tested the efficacy of BGAT in controlled studies to show its long-term beneficial effects on glucose stability, psychosocial functioning and driving behaviour (Cox et al. 2001).

Self-management education for type 1 diabetes patients with advanced microvascular complications, such as neuropathy or retinopathy, so far has received little attention. There has been some work in the area of support groups for patients with visual impairment due to diabetic retinopathy, showing improved knowledge and use of visual aids and psychosocial functioning (Bernbaum et al. 1989; Caditz 1992). This may be an area which needs further research as these issues are particularly pertinent to patients with type 1 diabetes who are now living for longer durations.

Self-management interventions in type 2 diabetes

Management of type 2 diabetes may be less intensive than type 1 diabetes in that it does not necessarily require intensive insulin regimens. It is important to recognize, however, that for the older individual diagnosed with type 2 diabetes uptake of lifestyle and other changes occurs at a point in life when behavioural and coping patterns have been well established.

A large number of interventions have been developed in response to the difficulties in self-management that patients with type 2 diabetes report. These are summarized in a number of reviews (see Table 10.1 for examples of key reviews in recent years). The focus of these reviews has varied, with some focusing on specific outcomes; for example, glycaemic control, psychosocial outcomes (Steed et al. 2003; Ellis et al. 2004); and others considering issues such as the intervention setting; for example, community versus hospital (Norris et al. 2002a), type of intervention; for example, social support, psychotherapeutic approaches (Ismail et al. 2004; van Dam et al. 2005). Some reviews were not specific to type 2 diabetes but included this as one of several chronic illnesses (e.g. Newman et al. 2004); other reviews focused more on specific behaviours rather than self-management; for example, interventions to address adherence or weight loss (Norris et al. 2005; Vermiere et al. 2005) have also added to knowledge in this area.

Table 10.1

Name	Type of interventions and outcomes	Search strategy	Analysis	Studies	Conclusions
Jackson (2006)	Interactive computer-assisted technology Range outcomes	1966–2003, PM, PI, C, CL+ hand search	Descriptive	14 RCTs 3 CCTs 9 PPT	Mixed results in relation to HbA1c and other clinical outcomes. Some benefits in relation to health care utilization. More evaluation of new technologies is necessary
Deakin et al. (2005)	Group-based, patient-centred self-management Clinical, lifestyle, psychosocial outcomes	M, C, ERIC, ASSIA, AMED, Psychinfo, LILACS, NHS EED, BEI, BNI, SCI, NRR, Dissertation abstracts, conf. proc., ref. lists, experts	Meta-analysis and descriptive	8 RCT 3 CCT	Significant improvement in fasting blood glucose, glycated haemoglobin, knowledge, systolic blood pressure, body weight, diabetes medication at both short and long ~(12–14 month) follow-ups. Some evidence of improvement in self-empowerment, quality of life, skills and satisfaction but insufficient studies to confirm
van Dam et al. (2005)	Social support Interventions Range outcomes	1980–2003 M, CL, Eric, PI, E, ref. lists	Descriptive	6 RCTs	Few studies, with little reference to theory in studies. Some support for such interventions, especially where support is from peers/other patients rather than spouse or friend, except in weight loss. May be gender differences, and amount of support key

Table 10.1 – continued

Ismail et al. 2004	Psychological interventions (CBT, counselling, psychodynamic or interpersonal psychotherapy) Glycaemic control, blood glucose conc., weight loss, psychological distress	1966–2003 CL, ML E, PI, conf. proc., ref list	Meta-analysis	25 RCTs	Psychological interventions resulted in decreased glycated haemoglobin. No effect on current blood glucose concentrations or weight, positive effect on psychological distress. Number of sessions, duration inter-vention, duration follow-up not asso-ciated with change. Studies of moderate to poor quality. Majority of interventions based on CBT or moti-vational interviewing
Ellis et al. (2004)	Patient education Glycaemic control	1990–2000 ML, C, healthstar, ERIC, PI, SCI, CRISP	Meta-analysis and meta-regression	21 RCTs	Patient education significantly improved HbA1c. Interventions that were performed face to face, which used cognitive reframing or included exercise, had a larger decrease in HbA1c. Dose of intervention not sen-sitive to success or failure
Loveman et al. (2003)	Self-management (multi-component and specific) Clinical, QoL and cost-effectiveness at >12-month follow-up	1980–2002 CL, ML, E, SCI, web of science, DARE, HTA, PI, C, ref lists, experts	Descriptive	13 RCTs 3 CCTs	Positive effects of interventions on each type of outcome; however, lim-ited lasting effects. No clear charac-terization of what features of education may be beneficial. Unclear evidence on cost-effective-ness, however, where costs ~£500–600 per patient, benefits over time would have to be very modest to offer an attractive cost-effective profile

Table 10.1 – continued

Steed et al. (2003)	Self-management Psychosocial outcomes	1980–2000 ML, E, PL, ref. list	Descriptive	19 RCTs 2 CCTs 11 PPTs	Depression improved following interventions with cognitive component and when baseline levels of depression higher than in general population. Findings for quality of life mixed, although illness specific measures more sensitive to change than generic measures
Norris et al. (2002a)	Self-management in community settings Range outcomes	1966–2000 ML, Eric, C, Healthstar, CDP, CHID	Descriptive	6 RCTs 4 PPTs 1 R	For glycaemic control sufficient evidence to indicate effectiveness or self-mangement education in community settings for type 2 diabetes. Insufficient evidence to assess effectiveness of home or workplace interventions
Norris et al. (2002b)	Self-management (educational – didactic/collaborative; lifestyle, skills, coping) Glycaemic control	1980–1999 ML, ERIC, C, hand search	Meta-analysis	31 RCTs	Self-management education associated with improved glycaemic control, with studies of greater duration having a more significant effect. Age, baseline glycaemic control, treatment, number of contacts, group versus individual, provider, type intervention not significant. Effects tended to diminish over longer follow-up

Table 10.1 – continued

Norris et al. (2001)	Self-management (educational – didactic/ collaborative; lifestyle, skills, coping) Range of outcomes	1980–1999 ML, ERIC, C, handsearch	Descriptive	72 RCTs	Didactic interventions focusing on knowledge and information demonstrate positive effects on knowledge but mixed results on glycaemic control and blood pressure and no effect on weight. Collaborative interventions focusing on knowledge tend to demonstrate positive effects on glycaemic control in the short term and mixed results with follow-up over one year. Effects of collaborative interventions on lipids, weight and blood pressure mixed. Insufficient studies report theoretical basis to determine those with greatest efficacy; however, more exploration of this is recommended

Footnote

BEI – British Education Index, BNI – British Nursing Index, C – CINAML, CDP – Chronic Disease Prevention database, CL – Cochrane Library, E – EMBASE, M – Medline, NHS EED. NHS Economic Evaluation Database, NRR – National Research Register, PL – Psychlit, PI – Psychinfo, PM – PubMed, RCT – randomised controlled trial, CCT – Controlled Clinical trial, PPT – Pre-Post trial.

From this significant body of work, conclusions in relation to a number of factors important to self-management can be drawn. With respect to the impact of self-management interventions on outcome, there appears to be reasonable evidence that self-management interventions in type 2 diabetes positively affect glycaemic control, particularly when assessments are made in the short term (Norris et al. 2001; Loveman et al. 2003; Ellis et al. 2004). Findings tend to be less clear for other clinical outcomes such as weight loss, blood pressure, and so on. For psychosocial outcomes positive effects are found when appropriate interventions and measurement tools are used (Steed et al. 2003; Ismail et al. 2004). However, quality of life still appears to be a relatively infrequently assessed outcome with reviews by Vermiere et al. (2005), Norris et al. (2005) and Deakin et al. (2005) unable to draw conclusions due to too few studies assessing this outcome. Evaluation of how such different types of intervention relate to efficacy in reviews is dependent on the methodology and categorization within the review. However, Ellis 2004, who used a systematic taxonomy to categorize interventions (see Elasy et al. 2001 for description of taxonomy), reported that studies that included cognitive-reframing components had greater efficacy. This finding is similar to other reviews which have suggested that interventions based on social learning theory or use psychological approaches such as cognitive behavioural techniques have greater efficacy (Griffin et al. 1988; Ismail et al. 2004; Deakin et al. 2005). This contrasts to interventions that provide simple didactic information which appears insufficient to improve self-management (Deakin et al. 2005). The commonality between these types of intervention is that they are based on psychological theories of behaviour change and adjustment to illness (see Chapter 3).

An example of an intervention that is theoretically based is that by Steed et al. (2005). This uses Bandura's social cognitive theory (Bandura 1986) and Leventhal's self-regulatory theory (Leventhal et al. 1984) as a basis to suggest that targeting participants' beliefs about their illness and self-efficacy for self-management behaviours will result in an improvement in self-management. Techniques such as challenging beliefs, teaching problem-solving and patient-facilitated goal-setting are incorporated alongside basic skills training and group support. The intervention has been shown to significantly improve self-management behaviours, including diet and exercise and blood glucose monitoring, as well as quality of life. In addition, however, this study evaluated the process variables of illness beliefs and self-efficacy, both of which were significantly influenced by the intervention. As discussed in Chapter 8, inclusion of process variables is essential to explore the mechanisms through which change in self-management may occur, yet relatively few self-management interventions have included process measures to date.

Common themes and future directions for self-management interventions in diabetes

Content

Examination of self-management interventions from diabetes suggests that content has been very varied. For example, some interventions are based primarily on behavioural approaches such as skills training and self-monitoring (Pieber et al. 1995; Gruesser et al. 1996); others tend to include more cognitive components such as goal-setting, problem-solving and cognitive restructuring (Glasgow et al. 1996; Clark et al. 2004; Steed et al. 2005). Some label themselves as stress management interventions and focus on relaxation techniques either with (Surwit et al. 2002) or without (Jablon et al. 1997) cognitive components. Interventions also vary in their methods of delivery such as telephone support (Piette et al. 2000) or group interventions based mainly on the support received from peers (Gilden et al. 1992). Association of the content and focus of the interventions to the outcome assessed is not always clear. On one issue, however, there now appears to be consensus that simple didactic information provision in the format of traditional education programmes is insufficient to improve self-management (Deakin et al. 2005).

In type 2 diabetes there is evidence that basing interventions on theory is a helpful approach (see also Chapter 3). However, more work needs to be done on evaluation of theory in facilitating change in self-management interventions. For instance, it is not uncommon for studies to demonstrate that theoretical variables have changed (e.g. increased self-efficacy), and that outcome measures have changed (e.g decrease in HbA1c), and assert that the relevant theory has been supported. However, unless the researcher can demonstrate that the interventions used theory-promoting strategies as they were designed in the intervention, and that use of these strategies is related to changes in theoretical process variables; for example, self-efficacy, and that changes in such variables are predictive or mediate changes in outcome; for example, HbA1c (possibly through changes in behaviour), then it is inaccurate to assert that the intervention has demonstrated the theoretical mechanism of change and therefore supports the theory. The issue of attention controls is also seldom addressed and it may also be that similar effects could have been achieved through increased contact with the committed professionals delivering diabetes care. The issue of treatment fidelity is discussed in Chapter 6, however, with limited assessment of treatment fidelity in the diabetes area to date, care must be taken in asserting that we have evidence for the use of different theory in this work and greater use of fidelity checks, attention placebo control groups and mediating analysis must be implemented to progress this important area of work.

Delivery

While a lot of consideration has been given to the content of self-management interventions in diabetes, less focus has been given to the level of contact. In the self-management intervention literature in adolescents with diabetes, only two studies actually included a control group for the levels of contact between health care professionals and the adolescents with diabetes. It is important that in each of these studies the control groups showed improvements (Anderson et al. 1999; Wysocki et al. 2000). Furthermore, in another study it was demonstrated that the contact time may even be more important than content of the programme in determining the outcomes achieved (Howells et al. 2002). In type 2 diabetes interesting results have also been reported by the research group of Trento et al. (2004) who evaluated a low-intensity self-management intervention where groups of patients with type 2 diabetes came together once every three months for a 'systemic education approach' which incorporated education with groupwork, problem-solving, skills development, and so on. Over five years significant improvements relative to control participants were retained for glycaemic control and quality of life. These findings suggest that with some interventions it may not be intensity but the ongoing nature of the self-management intervention that leads to sustained benefits in diabetes.

In considering the literature on self-management, at least in type 2 diabetes, there appears to have been a shift towards more cost-effective, lower intensity interventions. For example, in a programme of studies over approximately two decades, the research team of Russell Glasgow has shifted from intensive weekly group interventions in the 1990s (Glasgow et al. 1992) to brief self-management interventions held 30 minutes prior to 6-monthly clinic visits or Internet-based programmes in recent years (Glasgow et al. 2005). The efficacy of the interventions by Trento and Glasgow show positive results, suggesting potential for these different approaches, which may be more cost-effective and easier to fit into clinical care than long-term intensive interventions.

A second issue related to delivery of self-management interventions in diabetes is the interventionist's skills and determining whether interventions with positive outcomes are due to the skills of the interventionist or the power of the intervention. The teamwork interventions developed by Barbara Anderson and now replicated by the FACTS group offers some insight into the role of skills of the interventionist (Anderson et al. 1999). This group have demonstrated that their interventions can be delivered effectively by qualified health care professionals and graduate students, suggesting the skill base required to work in this way can be trained. It should be noted that the researchers in this original study have assumed that the intervention was delivered in the way they intended on the basis of the outcomes they found, rather than using any form of treatment fidelity check. However, similar results were achieved by a second independent group, where the intervention was delivered by health care professionals (nurses, dietitians and adult physicians) who provided the routine diabetes care for these patients. Of note here though, as part of the training of the interventionist and as a treatment fidelity check, the groups were observed by the psychologist who provided the training to the delivery team. This observation included using 10-second event coding to examine the interaction that took place in the group sessions. Thus, using a CD player, with a single earpiece, the observer heard a beep every 10 seconds, whereupon they coded who was talking at that moment to get a very basic measure of the level of participant involvement in the session. This enabled the health care professionals to receive objective feedback on groups, and set a clear standard for the sessions.

Methodological issues for trial design

Numerous studies of self-management interventions in diabetes have been conducted and the use of systematic methodology to review these has to be commended. However, there is an increasing tendency of both reviews and studies to focus only on randomized controlled trials. Although often recommended as the gold-standard trial design, this is not the only appropriate methodology for evaluation of self-management interventions, as highlighted by Glasgow et al. (2003) and discussed in Chapter 8 of this book. The tendency to focus on randomized controlled trials (RCTs), use strict inclusion/exclusion criteria and commonly rely on a few computer databases for searches means that many reviews report results of very few studies relative to the number that have been published and this limited approach must be acknowledged. In addition, many reviews now use meta-analysis. Although a recognized analytical procedure, its appropriateness with self-management interventions where there is often gross heterogeneity must be questioned.

Studies continue to often be underpowered and frequently do not measure outcomes in the long term and this must be addressed. While assessment should include a range of outcomes to be comprehensive, this needs to be balanced with evaluating outcomes not directly the focus of the intervention. Psychosocial outcomes such as psychological well-being or quality of life are still relatively rarely assessed and few interventions consider the broader aspects of managing the emotional and role changes concomitant in living with diabetes. Additional focus on these areas would be of benefit.

Conclusions

The field of self-management in type 1 and type 2 diabetes can be considered to be well advanced compared to other illnesses. However, there is still much work in this illness area that needs to be developed. Specifically, greater focus on the process of self-management and how this relates to theory needs to be undertaken. As recommended by Newman et al. (2004), the publication of manuals may aid in this venture, as will assessments of treatment fidelity. Also, there is a need to consider ways of implementing self-management programmes in real life to optimize reach, with special reference to underserved populations (Glasgow et al. 2006a). Different approaches which have applicability to different populations may need to be looked at. For example, computer- and web-based self-management interventions have been tested successfully in type 2 diabetes and hold promise for the future as a means of providing self-management support to large communities at relatively low health care costs (Lorig et al. 2006; Glasgow et al. 2006b). In progressing the field it may be that research designs directly comparing two types of self-management intervention are needed and this should be considered for the next generation of self-management interventions in diabetes.

References

Alberti, G., Zimmet, P., Shaw, J., Bloomgarden, Z., Kaufman, F. and Silink, M. (2004) Type 2 diabetes in the young: the evolving epidemic (The International Diabetes Federation Consensus Workshop), *Diabetes Care*, 27: 1798–811.

Anderson, B.J., Wolf, F.M., Bukhart, M.T., Cornell, R.G. and Bacon, G.E. (1989) Effects of peer-group intervention on metabolic control of adolescents with IDDM: randomized outpatient study, *Diabetes Care*, 2: 179–83.

Anderson, B.J, Joyce, H., Brackeyy, J. and Laffel, L.M.B. (1999) An office-based intervention to maintain parent–adolescent teamwork in diabetes management, *Diabetes Care*, 22: 713–21.

Anderson, R.J., Freedland, K.E., Clouse, R.E. and Lustman, P.J. (2001) the prevalence of co-morbid depression in adults with diabetes: a meta-analysis, *Diabetes Care*, 24: 1069–78

Bandura, A. (1986) *Social Foundations of Thought and Action*. Englewood Cliffs, NJ: Prentice Hall.

Bernbaum, M., Albert, S.G., Bruscca, S.R., Drimmer, A., Duckro, P.N., Cohen, J.D., Trindade, M.C. and Silverberg, A.B. (1989) *Diabetes Educator*, 15: 325–30.

Bott, U., Bott, S., Hemmann, D. and Berger, M. (2000) Evaluation of a holistic treatment and teaching programme for patients with type 1 diabetes who failed to achieve their therapeutic golas under intensified insulin therapy, *Diabetic Medicine*, 17: 635–43.

Caditz, J. (1992) An education-suppport group program for visually impaired people with diabetes, *Journal of Visual Impairment and Blindness*, 96: 81–83.

Clark, M., Hampson, S.E., Avery, L., Simpson, R. (2004) Effects of a tailored lifestyle self-management intervention in patients with type 2 diabetes, *British Journal of Health Psychology*, 9: 365–79.

Cox, D.J., Gonder-Frederick, L.A., Polonsky, W.H., Schlundt, D., Kovatchev, B. and Clarke, W. (2001) Blood Glucose Awareness Training (BGAT-2): long-term benefits, *Diabetes Care*, 24: 637–42.

Cox D, Gonder-Frederick L, Polonsky W, Schlundt D, Julian D, Clarke W. A (1995) multicenter evaluation of blood glucose awareness training-II. Diabetes Care, Apr;18:523–8

Cramer, J.A. (2004) A systematic review of adherence with medications for diabetes, *Diabetes Care*, 27: 1218–24.

Cryer, P.E. (2002) Hypoglycaemia: the limiting factor in the glycaemic management of type 1 and type II diabetes, *Diabetologia*, 45: 937–48.

DAFNE study group (2002) Training in flexible, intensive management to enable dietary freedom in people with type 1 diabetes: dose adjustment for normal eating (DAFNE) randomised controlled trial, *British Medical Journal*, 325(7367): 746.

Deakin, T., McShane, C.E., Cade, J.E. and Williams, RDRR (2005) Group based training for self-management strategies in people with type 2 diabetes, *Cochrane Database of Systematic Reviews*, Issue 2. CD Number CD003417.

Elasy, T.A., Ellis, S.E. and Brown A. (2001) A taxonomy for diabetes educational interventions, *Patient Education and Counselling*, 43: 121–27.

Ellis, S.E., Speroff, T., Dittus, R.S., Brown, A., Pichert, J.A. and Elasy, T.A. (2004) Diabetes patient education: a meta-analysis and meta-regression, *Patient Education and Counselling*, 52: 97–105.

Evans, J.M.M., Newton, R.W., Ruta, D.A., MacDonald, T.M., Stevenson, R.J. and Morris, A.D. (1999) Frequency of blood glucose monitoring in relation to glycaemic control: observational study with diabetes database, *British Medical Journal*, 319: 83–86.

Gilden, J.L., Hendryx, M.S., Clar, S., Casia, C. and Singh, S.P. (1992) Diabetes support groups improve health care of older diabetic patients, *Journal of American Geriatrics Society*, 40: 147–50.

Glasgow, R.E., Toobert, D.J. and Hampson, S.E. (1996) Effects of a brief office-based intervention to facilitate diabetes dietary self-management, *Diabetes Care*, 19: 835–42.

Glasgow, R.E. (2003) Translating research to practice: lessons learned, areas for improvement, and future directions, *Diabetes Care*, 26: 2451–56.

Glasgow, R.E., Nutting, P.A., King, D.K., Nelson, C.C., Cutter, G., Gaglio, B., Rahm, A.K. and Whitesides, H. (2005) Randomised effectiveness trial of a computer-assisted intervention to improve diabetes care, *Diabetes Care*, 28: 33–39.

Glasgow, R.E., Nelson, C.C., Strycker, L.A. and King, D.K. (2006a) RE-AIM metrics to evaluate diabetes self-management support interventions, *American Journal of Preventive Medicine*, 30: 67–73.

Glasgow, R.E., Strycker, L.A., King, D.K., Toobert, D.J., Rahm, A.K., Jex, M. and Nutting, P.A. (2006b) Robustness of a computer-assisted self-management intervention across patient characteristics, health care settings and intervention staff, *American Journal of Managed Care*, 12: 137–45.

Glasgow, R. E., Toobert, D. J., Hampson, S. E., Brown, J. E., Lewinsohn, P. M., Donnelly, J. (1992) Improving Self-Care Among Older Patients With Type II Diabetes: The 'Sixty Something ...' Study. *Patient Education and Counseling*, 19: 61–74.

Gold, A.E., Deary, J.L. and Frier, B.M. (1997) Hypoglycaemia and non-cognitive aspects of psychological function in insulin-dependent (type 1) diabetes mellitus (IDDM), *Diabetic Medicine*, 14: 111–18.

Grey, M., Boland, E.A., Davidson, M., Li, J. and Tamborlane, W.V. (2000) Coping skills training for youth with diabetes mellitus has long-lasting effects on metabolic control and quality of life, *Journal of Pediatrics*, 137: 107–13.

Griffin, S., Kinmouth, A.L., Skinner, C. and Kelly, J. (1998) *Educational and Psychosocial Intervention for Adults with Diabetes*. London: British Diabetic Association.

Grigsby, A.B., Anderson, R.J., Freedland, K.E., Clouse, R.E. and Lustman, P.J. (2002) Prevalence of anxiety in adults with diabetes: a systematic review, *Journal of Psychosomatic Research*, 53: 1053–60.

Gruesser, M., Hartmann, P., Schlottmann, N. and Joergens, V. (1996) Structured treatment and teaching programme for type 2 diabetic patients on conventional insulin treatment: evaluation of reimbursement policy, *Patient Education and Counseling*, 29: 123–30.

Hampson, S.E., Skinner, T.C., Hart, J., Storey, L., Gage, H., Foxcroft, D., Kimber, A., Cradock, S. and McEvilly, A.E. (2000) Behavioral interventions for adolescents with type 1 diabetes: how effective are they? *Diabetes Care*, 23: 1416–22.

Howells, L., Wilson, A.C., Skinner, T.C., Newton, R., Morris, A.D. and Greene, S.A. (2002) A randomized control trial of the effect of negotiated telephone support on glycaemic control in young people with type 1 diabetes, *Diabetic Medicine*, 19: 643–48.

Ismail, K., Winkley, K. and Rabe-Hasketh, S. (2004) Systematic review and meta-analysis of randomised controlled trials of psychological interventions to improve glycaemic control in patients with type 2 diabetes, *The Lancet*, 363: 1589–97.

Jablon, S.L., Naliboff, B.D., Gilmore, S.L. and Rosenthal, M.J. (1997) Effects of relaxation training on glucose tolerance and diabetic control in type II diabetes, *Applied Psychophysiology Biofeedback*, 22: 155–69.

Jackson, C.L., Bolen, S., Brancati, F.L., Batts-Turner, M.L. and Gary, T.L. (2006) A systematic review of interactive computer-assisted technology in diabetes care: interactive information technology in diabetes care, *Journal of General Internal Medicine*, 21: 105–10.

Karter, A.J., Ferrara, A., Darbinian, J.A., Ackerson, L.M. and Selby, J.V. (2000), Self-monitoring of blood glucose: language and financial barriers in a managed care population with diabetes, *Diabetes Care*, 23: 477–83.

Laffel, L.M.B., Vangsness, L., Connell, A., Goebel-Fabbri, A., Butler, D. and Anderson, B.J. (2003) Impact of ambulatory, family-focused teamwork intervention on glycemic control in youth with type 1 diabetes, *Journal of Pediatrics*, 142: 409–16.

Leventhal, H., Nerenz, D.R. and Steele, D.F. (1984) Illness representations and coping with health threats, in A. Baum and J. Singer (eds) *A Handbook of Psychology and Health* (pp. 219–52). Hillsdale, NJ: Lawrence Erlbaum Associates.

Lorig, K., Ritter, P.L., Laurent, D.D. and Plant, K. (2006) Internet-based chronic disease management: a randomized controlled trial, *Medical Care*, 44: 964–71.

Loveman, E., Cave, C., Green, C., Royle, P., Dunn, N. and Waugh, N. (2003) The clinical and cost-effectiveness of patient education models for diabetes: a systematic review and economic evaluation, *Health Technology Assessments*, 7(22).

Murphy, H.R., Rayman, G. and Skinner, T.C. (2006) An update on the effects of psycho-educational interventions for children and young people with type 1 diabetes, *Diabetic Medicine*, 23, 935–43.

Murphy, H., Wadham, C., Rayman, G. and Skinner, T.C. (2007) Approaches to integrating paediatric diabetes care and structured education: experiences from the Families, Adolescents, and Children's Teamwork Study (FACTS), *Diabetic Medicine*, 24, 1261–68.

Nelson, K.M., Reiber, G. and Boyko, E.D.J. (2002) Diet and exercise among adults with type 2 diabetes. Findings from the Third National Health and Nutrition Examination Survey (NHANES III), *Diabetes Care*, 25: 1722–28.

Newman, S., Steed, L. and Mulligan, K. (2004) Self-management interventions for chronic illness, *Lancet*, 364: 1523–37.

Norris, S.L, Nichols, P.J., Caspersen, C.J., Glasgow, R.E., Engelgau, M.M. et al. (2002b) Increasing diabetes self-management education in community settings: a systematic review, *American Journal of Preventive Medicine*, 22: 39–66.

Norris, S.L., Engelgau, M.M. and Venkat Narayan, K.M. (2001) Effectiveness of self-management training in type 2 diabetes: a systematic review of randomized controlled trials, *Diabetes Care*, 24: 561–87.

Norris, S.L., Lau, J., Smith, S.J., Schmid, C.H. and Engelgau, M.M (2002a) Self-management education for adults with type 2 diabetes: a meta-analysis of the effect on glycaemic control, *Diabetes Care*, 25: 1159–71.

Norris, S.L., Zhang, X., Avenell, A., Gregg, E., Brown, T.J., Schmid, C.H. and Lau, J. (2005) Long-term non-pharmacological weight loss interventions for adults with type 2 diabetes mellitus, *Cochrane Database of Systematic Reviews*, Issue 2. CD number CD005270.

Pieber, T.R., Holler, A., Siebenhofer, A., Brunner, G. A., Semlitsch, B., Schattenberg, S., Zapotoczky, H., Rainer, W. and Krejs, G.J. (1995) Evaluation of a structured teaching and treatment programme for type 2 diabetes in general practice in a rural area of Austria, *Diabetic Medicine*, 12: 349–54.

Piette, J.D., Weinberger, M. and McPhee, S.J. (2000) The effect of automated calls with telephone nurse follow up on patient-centred outcomes of diabetes care: a randomised, controlled trial, *Medical Care*, 4: 783–91.

Rubin, R.R., Peyrot, M. and Saudek, C.D. (1989) The effect of a diabetes education programme incorporating coping skills training on emotional well-being and diabetes self-efficacy, *Diabetes Educator*, 19: 210–14.

Ruggiero, L., Glasgow, R.E., Dryfoos, J.M., Rossi, J.S., Prochaska, J.O., Orleans, C.T., Prokhorov, A.V., Rossi, S.R., Greene, G.W., Reed, G.R., Dpharm, K.K., Chobanian, L. and Johnson, S. (1997) Diabetes self-management: self-reported recommendations and patterns in a large population, *Diabetes Care*, 20: 568–76.

Skinner, T.C., Murphy, H. and Huws-Thomas, M.V. (2005) Diabetes in adolescents, in F.J. Snoek and T.C. Skinner *Psychology in Diabetes Care* (2nd edn). (pp. 27–51) Chichester: John Wiley and Sons.

Snoek, F.J., Van der Ven, N.C.W., Lubach, C.H.C., Chatrou M., Ader, H.J., Heine, R.J. and Jacobson, A.M. (2001) Effects of cognitive behavioural group training (CBGT) in adults with poorly controlled insulin-dependent diabetes: a pilot study, *Patient Education and Counseling*, 51: 143–48.

Spiess K, Sachs G, Pietschmann P, Prager R. (1995) A program to reduce onset distress in unselected type I diabetic patients: effects on psychological variables and metabolic control. *Eur J Endocrinol*, 132: 580–586.

Steed, L., Cooke, D. and Newman, S. (2003) A systematic review of psychosocial outcomes following education, self-management and psychological interventions in diabetes mellitus, *Patient Education and Counselling*, 51: 5–15.

Steed, L., Lankester, J., Barnard, M., Earle, K., Hurel, S. and Newman, S. (2005) Evaluation of the UCL Diabetes Self-Management Programme (UCL-DSMP) in patients with type 2 diabetes and microalbuminuria: a randomised controlled trial, *Journal of Health Psychology*, 10: 261–276.

Surwit, R.S., van Tilburg, M.A., Zucker, N., McCaskill, C.C., Parekh, P., Feinglos, M.N., Edwards, C.L., Williams, P. and Lane, J.D. (2002) Stress management improves long-term glycemic control in type 2 diabetes, *Diabetes Care*, 25: 30–34.

Trento, M., Passera, P., Borgo, E., Tomalino, M., Bajardi, M., Cavallo, F. and Porta, M. (2004) A 5-year randomized controlled study of learning, problem solving ability, and quality of life modifications in people with type 2 diabetes managed by group care, *Diabetes Care*, 27: 670–75.

UKPDS Group (1995) UK prospective diabetes study 16: overview of six years' therapy of type 2 diabetes: a progressive disease, *Diabetes*, 44: 1249–58.

van Dam, H.A., van der Horst, F.G., Knoops, L., Ryckman, R.M., Crebolder, H.F.J.M. and van den Borne, B.H.W. (2005) Social support in diabetes: a systematic review of controlled intervention studies, *Patient Education and Counselling*, 59: 1–12.

Van der Ven, N.C.W., Hogenelst, M.H.E., Van Iperen, A., Tromp-Wever, A.M.E., Vriend, A., Van der Ploeg, H.M., Heine, R.J. and Snoek, F.J. (2005). Short-term effects of cognitive behavioural group training (CBGT) in adult type 1 diabetes patients in prolonged poor glycaemic control: a randomised controlled trial, *Diabetic Medicine*, 22: 1619–23.

Vermiere, E., Wens, J., Van Royen, P., Biot, Y., Hearnshaw, H. and Lindenmeyer, A. (2005) Interventions for improving adherence to treatment recommendations in people with type 2 diabetes mellitus, *Cochrane Database of Systematic Reviews*, 2. CD number CD003638.

Wysocki, T., Harris, M.A., Greco, P., Bubb, J., Danda, C.E. and Harvey, L.M. et al. (2000) Randomized, controlled trial of behavior therapy for families of adolescents with insulin-dependent diabetes mellitus, *Journal of Pediatric Psychology*, 25: 23–33.

Zrebiec, J. and Jacobson, A.M. (2001) What attracts patients with diabetes to an internet support group? A 21-month longitudinal study, *Diabetic Medicine*, 18: 154–58.

11 Rheumatoid arthritis

Jerry C. Parker and Eric S. Hart

Introduction

Rheumatoid arthritis (RA) is an autoimmune disease that leads to symmetric polyarticular pain and joint inflammation. At the pathophysiological level, RA is the result of chronic and progressive autoimmune-mediated inflammation of the synovial membrane, which deprives the surrounding joints of the lubrication needed for a smooth range of motion. This breakdown in lubrication is associated with painful swelling, stiffness and tenderness of joint structures. The autoimmune dysfunction in RA often produces systemic manifestations and tissue damage of nonarticular organs which can give rise to co-morbid ocular, vascular, dermatologic and respiratory complications. It is one of the most common inflammatory rheumatic diseases and sources of disability in the USA. Although several environmental and biological factors have been hypothesized to contribute to the onset of RA, the etiology remains largely unknown.

The diagnosis of RA can be difficult due to the variability in presentation and the lack of specificity of radiological and serologic tests. The systemic nature and the nonarticular co-morbidities, along with the lack of exclusivity of histological and radiological alterations observed during clinical evaluation, makes the unequivocal classification of RA difficult during the early stages of the disease process. The lack of pathognomonic indicators on clinical examination, especially within the first months of onset, can add uncertainty to the diagnosis. The American College of Rheumatology criteria for RA requires that the constellation of inflammatory symptoms must be present for several weeks prior to diagnosis.

Prevalence and demographics of RA

Due to the variability in clinical presentation and the individual differences found among persons with RA, prevalence estimates have remained an area of controversy. Specifically, inconsistent diagnostic criteria and uncertainty surrounding early stage

RA have caused difficulty in the estimation of the course and occurrence of this disease. Accurate estimates have been further complicated by the fact that individuals with rheumatic symptoms often do not seek medical attention. Nevertheless, RA is estimated to be one of the most common rheumatologic and musculoskeletal diseases in the USA. Lawrence et al. (1998) reported that definite RA occurs in 10 per 10,000 American adults, which corresponds to approximately 2.1 million persons nationwide. The incidence for women is significantly higher than for men.

Functional implications for RA in everyday life

Clinical assessments of RA often have limited predictive utility for daily functional status. Functional status refers to an individual's capacity to adequately negotiate the challenges of daily living; RA can be challenging for many individuals who may experience physical limitations.

Interestingly, psychological variables have emerged as factors which can be related to functional status and morbidity in RA. Scharloo et al. (1999) found that coping styles and perception of illness were correlated with variations in health outcome. Specifically, illness perception and coping style were found to predict functional variables such as number of hospitalizations, level of fatigue and degree of anxiety. Scharloo et al. (1999) also found that the perception that RA has 'disabling consequences' was associated with higher utilization of outpatient services.

A significant percentage of persons with RA encounter emotional challenges in addition to a variety of physical limitations, although the association between psychological variables and disease course remains unclear. For example, Parker et al. (1988a) did not find a significant correlation between pain and medical variables, but they reported that pain was correlated with age, income and specific psychological variables.

Implications of depression in RA

Depression has become a major health concern in the USA; epidemiological studies have estimated the prevalence of depression to be 5–12 per cent in males and 10–25 per cent in females (American Psychiatric Association 1994). Depression is one of the most common psychological manifestations in RA, occurring in as much as 17–27 per cent of the population (Creed and Ash 1992). Depression in RA has significant societal implications because symptoms frequently produce negative health consequences, functional limitations and higher utilization of health services (Katz and Yelin 1993). Unfortunately, the somatic symptoms of depression are easily confounded with the RA disease process itself. Therefore, depression is sometimes not recognized by clinicians as an independent source of distress, but the relatively high incidence of depression in RA conveys the importance of addressing emotional distress in comprehensive approaches to disease management.

Several factors complicate estimates of the base rate of depression in an RA population. Early studies, which employed dependent measures that lacked sensitivity and specificity, frequently produced inflated estimates of occurrence. DeVellis (1995) described several methodological problems in the study of depression in RA. Specifically, the author stated that criterion contamination is a major obstacle in the study of depression in RA because many of the commonly used measures are artificially impacted by the presence of somatic symptoms. Thus, conclusions regarding the presence of depressive symptoms within the context of RA may be biased by disease manifestations such as pain and fatigue. Temporal factors also are a potential problem when studying depression in RA; DeVellis (1995) stated that assessing depressive symptoms in persons with RA during a relatively brief time interval, such as during the previous week, is insufficient because the Diagnostic and Statistical Manual (DSM) requires that symptoms be present for at least two weeks. Another methodological challenge in the estimation of depression in RA pertains to sampling strategy; clinic-based samples may include only those individuals who have adequate access to medical care, may over-represent individuals with more severe rheumatic disease, or may lack appropriate comparison groups of individuals with medical conditions (DeVellis 1995).

A meta-analysis of depression in RA conducted by Dickens et al. (2002) found that depression is significantly more common in persons with RA as compared to healthy individuals and is associated with pain intensity. Wright et al. (1998) found that younger individuals with RA are at higher risk for developing symptoms of depression than are older individuals. The authors suggested that the higher depression levels in younger persons might be associated with higher levels of stress, such as job-related pressures or child-rearing responsibilities.

Psychoneuroimmunologic implications on RA

Advances in the study of neuroimmunology have provided important insights into the role of physiological processes in various disease presentations. As a result, the interaction among psychological, immunological and endocrine variables and their relationship to the onset and progression of RA has been given substantial attention in recent years. The heterogeneity of disease characteristics (i.e. seropositive v. seronegative) has resulted in many challenges for studying RA pathophysiology at the cellular and hormonal level (Ader et al. 1991); a single pathogenesis may not be discernible, and the degree of joint destruction often varies in individual cases (Ader *et al.* 1991). Research on the impact of stress on immunological and neuroendocrine processes has offered novel hypotheses regarding the pathways that may be involved in the onset and progression of RA.

Animal and human studies have found that the HPA (hypothalamic-pituitary-adrenal) axis is activated in response to environmental stressors that may be biological, physiological, or social in origin. Activation of the HPA axis elicits a cascade of events that mediate a fight or flight response. Cash and Wilder (1991) offer a dynamic interpretation of this interrelation; the authors indicate that the hypothalamus produces corticoid releasing hormone (CRH), which leads to an activation of the sympathetic-adrenal-medullary axis. Activation of the sympathetic-adrenal-medullary axis prompts the release of adrenocorticotropic hormone (ACTH) into the blood stream. Cortisol is then produced as ACTH stimulates the adrenal cortex. Down-regulation of CRH and ACTH occurs by feedback mechanisms when cortisol levels rise. Because CRH is secreted following immune activation, an effect on the inflammatory process occurs that is mediated by cytokines such as interleukin 1 and 6. In general, a dysregulation involving the endocrine and immune systems is believed to play a pivotal role in RA.

Rogers and Fozdar (1996) describe the extravascular immune complex hypothesis, which suggests an interaction between antigens and antibodies in synovial tissues and in the synovial fluid around the cartilage. Specifically, the authors state that the antigens found in the synovial tissues are thought to be by-products of the inflammatory process and are constituents of articular tissue such as collagen, cartilage, fibrinogen and fibrin. The interaction between the antibodies and antigens causes a change in vascular permeability which leads to an accumulation of cellular blood elements. Enzymes are then released leading to inflammation of the synovial elements and joint damage.

The sympathetic-adrenal-medullary (SAM) system also has been identified as playing a pivotal role in RA. Several studies have indicated that the SAM system in persons with RA is abnormal in comparison with healthy controls. Receptor densities have been found to decrease in response to elevated ligand levels. Specifically, a significant decrease in beta-2 receptor density on peripheral blood mononuclear cells may indicate patterns of sympathetic hyperactivity secondary to stressors (Huyser and Parker 1998).

The implication of these studies are that management of stress activators, whether physiological, social or psychological, are important targets in self-management.

Additional challenges for persons with RA

RA frequently requires the management of physical and economic challenges. From an economic perspective, the chronic symptoms of RA can lead to sizeable financial burdens. Indirect costs, such as decreased wages, are not only limited to the advanced stages of RA. Merkesdal et al. (2001) found high indirect annual costs were associated with even the early stages of RA, essentially equalling those associated with the later stages. The authors suggested that early intense vocational rehabilitation as an adjunct to medication may offset some of these costs.

Because there is no known cure for RA, self-management of symptoms is important for enhancing daily functioning. The implications of enhanced daily functioning (e.g. continued employment and ability to participate in enjoyable activities) can lead to improved quality of life. Overall, employing specific strategies for managing the potential consequences of RA is crucial for comprehensive care.

Review of self-management interventions in RA

A meta-analysis by Warsi et al. (2003) offers several conclusions regarding the overall usefulness of self-management education programmes. The authors suggest that participation in self-management programmes results in a small, yet significant, impact on levels of pain and disability. The literature on self-management programmes for persons with RA has focused primarily on patient education, therapeutic writing (self-expression), pain management, stress management, depression management and the Arthritis Self-Management Programme (ASMP). In general, self-management programmes have been shown to have long-term benefits and may lead to decreases in medical costs; self-management programmes have been recommended in the US National Arthritis Action Plan as an important component of comprehensive rheumatologic care.

Traditional patient education

Traditional patient education programmes are typically designed to encourage behavioural change and to promote healthy living. The general intent of patient education programmes is to provide information to persons with RA regarding ways to modify or adjust essential daily activities to circumvent limitations associated with the disease process. Riemsma et al. (2004) cited several studies that support the benefits of educational programmes as evidenced by improvements in pain, functional status and psychological well-being; those programmes that also incorporated behavioural interventions revealed the greatest benefits.

A study by Parker et al. (1984) was one of the first to use a randomized controlled trial to examine the effects of patient education in a cohort of persons with RA; the patient education programme consisted of information regarding RA disease process, common therapies/medications, joint protection, energy conservation and unproven treatment methods. Results from this study were surprising because RA patient education programmes did not offer significant advantages when compared to a control group. Interestingly, a paradoxical effect also was observed in that persons with RA who participated in the education programme reported an increase in pain and a greater impairment of physical activity at a three-month follow-up; fortunately, this adverse effect did not persist at the six-month follow-up. The authors suggested that an emphasis on rest and joint protection, in particular, might promote sensitization to the experience of pain.

Brus et al. (1998) examined the impact of patient education on adherence with treatment regimens in persons with recent onset RA; the authors found that adherence with sulphasalazine therapy was high in their sample, but not related to participation in patient education programmes. Education programmes were found to correlate with adherence with physical exercise regimens and prescriptions for ergonomic measures. No effect was found on the health status of persons with recent onset RA. Conversely, Fries et al. (1997) examined the efficacy of a mail-delivered arthritis management programme in a randomized study and found improvements in physical function, pain, joint count, global vitality, doctor visits and sick days; medical care utilization also decreased as a result of the programme. Helliwell et al. (1999) examined the influence of a 12-month trial of a patient education programme on radiographic changes in RA. The hypothesis was that improved knowledge would increase the use of joint protection techniques, result in decreased joint damage, and thereby, lead to improved functionality. Although no significant improvement was found on measures of radiographic progression, the authors stated that there was a trend in favour of the education programme.

Therapeutic writing (self-expression) programmes

Therapeutic writing programmes are based on the premise that improvements in emotional and physical well-being can be achieved through guided expression of stressful life events. However, research on the utility of expressive writing as an intervention for psychosocial aspects of RA has produced variable results. Studies that support the influence of expressive writing programmes are particularly intriguing because such interventions appear to be cost-efficient and capable of overcoming financial and geographic limitations. Broderick et al. (2004) evaluated the usefulness of a self-expression programme distributed in a video-tape format to persons with RA. The video-tape presented a rationale for the self-expression programme along with specific instructions on implementing exercises at home. A video-tape format was selected by the authors because video-tapes are cost-effective, minimize extensive involvement of treatment professionals, allow for self-administration, and provide an opportunity to reach a large number of people. Results from this study were encouraging with regard to feasibility and adherence, but disappointing from the stand-point of providing empirical support for overall effectiveness.

Wetherell et al. (2005) studied the effect of a home-based emotional disclosure programme on psychological and physical outcomes for persons with RA; participants were asked to disclose (by either writing or talking) personal traumatic experiences. A comparison group was developed in which participants were instructed to disclose relatively benign events of their day. This study was unique with regard to participant recruitment because it did not exclude persons with RA who were limited in their ability to write for extended periods of time due to joint damage. Thus, selection bias was minimized by the opportunity to choose either written or verbal expression. This study was additionally unique because it included measures of disease activity. Interestingly, the programme was found to produce deterioration in mood at one-week post-intervention, which was sustained for six subsequent weeks. However, significant improvement in mood was demonstrated following 10 weeks of exposure to the programme.

Smyth et al. (1999) compared the effect of a self-expression programme on symptom reduction in persons with RA and asthma. They found that both groups demonstrated significant improvements in health status at a four-month follow-up; 47 per cent of the sample met criteria for clinically relevant improvement. The programme was found to have different effects for persons with asthma versus RA. Specifically, participants with asthma improved at two-week follow-up, while participants with RA showed improvement at four-week follow-up. Accordingly, the authors suggested that the mechanisms for improvement may be different for the two diseases and related to a differential immune response. A complementary study by Stone et al. (2000) attempted to determine potential psychological mediators of the positive health effects of self-expression programmes, but they concluded that the underlying mechanism remains largely unknown.

Pain management programmes

Pain has long been considered a significant source of disability and emotional distress for persons with RA. Thus, there is no surprise that significant attention has been given to research on both pharmacological and non-pharmacological interventions to manage the consequences of chronic pain. Keefe et al. (2005) stated that examination of the psychological implications of pain is especially important with persons with chronic medical illnesses because traditional biomedical interventions have several limitations and/or side-effects. In addition, some persons with RA pain experience only a minimal response to medical intervention, which may leave pain inadequately managed.

Surprisingly, pain in RA has not consistently been found to be directly correlated with disease activity which suggests a possible influence of psychological factors. Keefe et al. (2005) summarized the literature on the psychological aspects of chronic pain and concluded that pain catastrophizing (i.e. an exaggerated and disproportionate response to pain) is associated with poor adjustment to pain. Bradley et al. (1987) examined the impact of a social support group on pain behaviours in persons with RA and found that participation in a support group resulted in significant reductions in pain behaviour and disease activity. Trait anxiety also was reduced at six months post-treatment. The authors stated that relaxation training appeared to be the most beneficial aspect of the intervention.

Pain management interventions are focused on minimizing the emotional sequelae of chronic pain through the establishment of effective coping strategies. Keefe et al. (2005) stated that interventions for RA pain typically involve coping skills training and emotional disclosure. Coping skills training is usually aimed at increasing the available personal resources for managing pain and improving perceptions of control. Emotional disclosure paradigms focus on encouraging emotional expression of stressful life events; this 'processing' of stressful events is thought to result in decreased pain.

Over the past 40 years, the field of psychology has witnessed an emergence of cognitive-behavioural interventions to treat a myriad of sources of emotional distress. In general, the cognitive-behavioural approach is focused on uncovering beliefs that are held about one's self, others and the world in general. These core perceptions are thought to mediate emotional and behavioural responses as a person goes about the tasks of daily living. In pain management, cognitive-behavioural interventions are designed to assist in developing greater perceptions of control and self-efficacy regarding the experience of pain.

Brown et al. (1989) found that cognitive-behavioural management programmes may significantly reduce the use of passive pain coping strategies as a means of managing chronic arthritis pain. Although a single cognitive-behavioural approach to pain management in RA does not exist, some similarities across programmes are common. Parker et al. (1993) described that cognitive-behavioural interventions for pain management typically include three essential elements: 1) an educational phase; 2) a skills-acquisition phase; and 3) a maintenance phase. Whereas the educational phase provides the conceptual information regarding the psychological aspects of pain, the skills-acquisition phase assists in the development of appropriate coping behaviours by establishing positive attitudes and realistic expectations. Specific cognitive-behavioural treatment paradigms often incorporate relaxation training, coping skills enhancement, communication training, assertiveness training and problem-solving. During the maintenance phase, persons experiencing pain learn to apply their new skills to the challenges of daily life. In a review of cognitive-behavioural approaches to pain management, Parker et al. (1993) concluded that the literature supported the value of integrating cognitive-behavioural interventions as a component of comprehensive rheumatologic care.

Stress management programmes

Stress, defined as a demand upon an organism to respond to environmental changes, may have important implications on the course of RA. In general, there appears to be a paradoxical relationship between acute versus chronic stress and disease activity. Interestingly, minor short-term stressors have been found to cause disease exacerbations, while chronic stressors have been shown to be related to an improvement in RA symptoms. To explain the differential influence of acute versus chronic stress, Huyser and Parker (1998) suggest that dramatic increases in cortisol may result from certain major stressors (i.e. death of a loved one), which prompts the paradoxical effect of decreased RA symptoms. Conversely, minor stressors may not result in sufficient cortisol release to counteract the sympathetic-mediated inflammatory responses.

Stress management training is frequently incorporated into treatment programmes for persons with RA. Stress management programmes are frequently based on cognitive-behavioural principles, in which persons develop skills to make realistic appraisals of their abilities to effectively manage change and stressors in their daily lives. In RA, stress appears to be partially related to perception of limited control over an unpredictable disease process. In addition, the long-term disability associated with RA often produces financial pressures and anxiety. In comparison to other treatment modalities, stress management programmes can often be presented in ways that de-emphasize psychopathology or mental illness (Parker et al. 1995). Thus, due to this more acceptable connotation, persons with RA are often highly receptive to stress management interventions.

Parker et al. (1995) studied the long-term effects of stress management on disease outcome in RA. The authors designed a randomized controlled trial in which participants were assigned to a stress management group, an attention control group (i.e. general patient education), or a standard care control group. The intervention groups were exposed to 10 weeks of treatment and a 15-month maintenance phase. Participants in the stress management programme demonstrated the highest treatment adherence; they reported improvements in helplessness, self-efficacy, coping, pain and health status. Participants in the stress management group also experienced decreased pain and lower-extremity impairment immediately post-intervention. The 15-month follow-up revealed sustained improvements on measures of helplessness and self-efficacy. Rhee et al. (2000) found that decreases in pain and depression following stress management programmes were mediated by enhanced coping strategies (confidence in the ability to manage pain), reduced helplessness and higher self-efficacy.

Depression management programmes

Management of depression in RA appears to be important in order to improve long-term outcomes and to reduce the secondary impact on pain and disability (Parker and Slaughter 2004). In addition to biological and immunological variables, social influences also have been found to contribute to the onset of depression in RA. Dickens et al. (2003) found that social difficulties were predictive of depression in persons with RA. In addition, coping style also has been shown to be an important mediator of depression in RA. Parker et al. (1988b) found that coping styles such as wish-fulfilling fantasy (i.e. unrealistic recovery expectations) and self-blame were related to significant emotional distress, whereas cognitive restructuring was associated with less depression and reduced perceptions of helplessness. Similarly, Brown et al. (1989) found that the use of passive pain coping strategies in the presence of high-intensity pain was associated with the most severe levels of depression over time for persons with RA.

Studies of the additive efficacy of combined psychopharmacological and psychological interventions for the treatment of depression have been equivocal, although positive results have been found with specific subgroups of persons with depression. Lenze et al. (2002) found that combined medication treatment (nortriptyline) and psychotherapy for late-life depression was more likely to help maintain social adjustment than either treatment offered by itself. In addition, Hollon et al. (2005) found that combined treatment was superior to monotherapy for both adult and geriatric depression. Combination treatment for depression also has been shown to result in significant medical cost-offset due to fewer hospitalizations and less absence from work (Burnand et al. 2002).

Combined psychopharmacological and psychological interventions have not consistently been found to produce additive benefits for depression in RA. Parker et al. (2003) hypothesized that a combined cognitive-behavioural/pharmacologic treatment programme would have a beneficial impact on psychosocial well-being, health status, pain and disease activity for persons with RA and that a combination of treatment modalities would be more effective than either intervention alone. Surprisingly, Parker et al. (2003) found that, in the acute phase of treatment, medication intervention alone was equally as effective as combined pharmacological/psychological intervention for persons with RA; the benefits of medication remained at a 15-month follow-up, including significant improvements on measures of helplessness, self-efficacy, psychological distress, perceived life stress, anxiety, coping and fatigue.

Self-help (self-management programme)

Cost-effective treatments are important for all chronic diseases. Socio-economic research on RA has identified the financial burdens associated with prolonged disability. In response to the need for inexpensive and effective treatments, Lorig et al. (1985) examined the utility of the ASMP on multiple disease outcome variables. The ASMP was developed at the Stanford Arthritis Center and is a community-based patient education programme. This patient education programme was developed as a result of an assessment of the needs of persons with RA; the ASMP content covers the general nature of arthritis, appropriate uses of medication, exercise, relaxation techniques, joint protection, nutrition, interaction of patients with physicians and evaluation of nontraditional treatments. The ASMP is designed to be presented by trained lay people (Lorig et al. 1985).

Lorig et al. (1985) hypothesized that persons with RA would be able to learn important principles for managing RA and that the use of self-management techniques would result in improved physical functioning, less pain and lower health care costs. In addition, the ASMP was expected to be cost-effective and widely available, resulting in less dependency on health professionals. The authors report that they chose the ASMP approach because it 'approximates attributes assumed to be desirable in health education for persons with chronic illness: voluntary participation, group learning, teaching by trained lay persons, and applicability to a broad range of patients' (Lorig et al. 1985: 684). The ASMP was found to lead to an increase in RA knowledge and the adoption of taught behaviours. Participants in the programme also experienced a decrease in pain; the beneficial effects remained at a 20-month follow-up.

The ASMP is one of the leading arthritis patient education programmes in the world serving thousands of persons with RA each year. Modifications to the programme have included the implementation of a more extended 'introduction' component. This modification has resulted in improvements on measures of arthritis knowledge and has encouraged persons with RA to seek other Arthritis Foundation services (Lorig et al. 1998). Research on the cost-effectiveness of the ASMP has revealed significant savings as a result of decreased physician visits (Kruger et al. 1998).

Critical assessment of self-management approaches

Outcome research on the effectiveness of self-management programmes for persons with RA is encouraging. However, support for the efficacy of some approaches has been confounded by methodological limitations. For example, the small sample sizes found in many studies have limited the conclusiveness and generalizability of the results. In addition, dropout rates are a major obstacle when studying chronic disease and are especially problematic in the context of RA due to the associated physical discomfort and disability. Such factors, in addition to the diagnostic ambiguity of early-stage RA, pose methodological challenges. Overall, randomized trials and longitudinal designs have produced the most definitive results regarding the utility of self-management in RA.

Effective coping strategies appear to be one of the greatest predictors of programme success. Research has shown that passive coping styles result in higher levels of depression and pain intensity (Parker et al. 1988b; Brown et al. 1989). Self-management programmes that focus on active coping, such as cognitive restructuring and relaxation training, appear to be more helpful than passive approaches that do not encourage the application of learned skills. O'Leary et al. (1988) found that cognitive-behavioural treatments for RA result in enhanced self-efficacy, reduced pain/joint inflammation and improved psychosocial functioning. In their study, individuals who simply received literature on managing RA, as opposed to direct cognitive-behavioural intervention, did not experience a significant benefit.

Overall, the preponderance of evidence suggests that self-management programmes for RA are generally helpful for reducing the emotional challenges commonly associated with the disease. Therefore, persons with RA may benefit from the use of self-management strategies as components of a comprehensive programme of rheumatologic care. Clearly, reductions in pain and disability can lead to improved quality of life; self-management programmes also appear to help offset the cumulative direct and indirect costs associated with RA.

Practical implications for self-management techniques

The success of self-management programmes for RA is based on several factors. First, specific skills sets of the facilitator and participant are required for different programmes. For example, programmes focused on stress and depression management frequently involve strategies which require facilitators to have adequate training in cognitive-behavioural interventions. In addition, success is contingent upon participants motivation and ability to implement learned strategies in their daily life. Second, adequate financial resources are often required for many programmes; self-management programmes typically require nominal, yet potentially significant, fees for materials such as workbooks and instructor costs. Given that RA can lead to sizeable economic demands as a result of direct and indirect medical costs, additional treatment fees may not be feasible for some persons. Therefore, cost-effectiveness is an important consideration for programme development. Finally, physical limitations have been found to impact participant performance and programme adherence in programmes that employ measures requiring sustained effort or a high degree of geographic mobility.

Future directions for research and practice

Physical disability and mobility limitations can reduce the ability of persons with RA to participate in treatment outcome studies, so future research might examine the development of self-management programmes for persons with RA who have severe physical limitations. Specifically, Internet-based delivery systems may help to overcome the major accessibility challenges.

From a methodological stand-point, randomized controlled trials have much to offer to the study of self-management interventions. Without randomization, comparison groups can differ on many potentially confounding variables. Similarly, sample sizes must be adequate in order for the literature to evolve in a definitive manner. Non-randomized designs may be useful in some contexts, but randomized trials with a sufficient number of participants will be critically important for future research on the effectiveness of self-management interventions.

The socio-economic impact of RA will be another important area for future research. Studies of self-management programmes that include examination of medical cost-offset will be highly advantageous. Evaluation of the cost-effectiveness of self-management programmes will be particularly crucial for improving access and third-party reimbursement for psychosocial interventions. In general, the outcome literature has consistently supported the efficacy of self-management programmes as viable adjunctive components of comprehensive rheumatologic care, but additional well-designed research continues to be needed.

References

Ader, R., Felten, D.L. and Cohen, N. (eds) (1991) *Psychoneuroimmunology* (2nd edn). San Diego: Academic Press, Inc.

American Psychiatric Association (1994) *Diagnostic and Statistical Manual of Mental Disorders* (4th edn). Washington, DC: American Psychiatric Association.

Bradley, L.A., Young, L.D., Anderson, K.O., Turner, R.A., Agudelo, C.A., McDaniel, L.K., Pisko, E.J., Semble, E.L. and Morgan, T.M. (1987) Effects of psychological therapy on pain behavior of rheumatoid arthritis patients: treatment outcome and six-month follow-up. *Arthritis and Rheumatism*, 30(10): 1105–14.

Broderick, J.E., Stone, A.A., Smyth, J.M. and Kaell, A.T. (2004) The feasibility and effectiveness of an expressive writing intervention for rheumatoid arthritis via home-based videotaped instructions, *Annals of Behavioral Medicine*, 27(1): 50–59.

Brown, G.K., Nicassio, P.M. and Wallston, K.A. (1989) Pain coping strategies and depression in rheumatoid arthritis, *Journal of Consulting and Clinical Psychology*, 57(5): 652–57.

Brus, H.L.M., van de Laar, M., Taal, E., Rasker, J.J. and Wiegman, O. (1998) Effects of patient education on compliance with basic treatment regimens and health in recent onset active rheumatoid arthritis, *Annals of the Rheumatic Diseases*, 57: 146–51.

Burnand, Y., Anderioli, A., Kolatte, E., Venturini, A. and Rosset, N. (2002) Psychodynamic psychotherapy and clomipramine in the treatment of major depression, *Psychiatric Services*, 53: 585–90.

Cash, J.M. and Wilder, R.L. (1991) Stress, depression, and rheumatoid arthritis, *Contemporary Internal Medicine*, 3(5): 13–16.

Creed, F. and Ash, G. (1992) Depression in rheumatoid arthritis: aetiology and treatment, *International Review of Psychiatry*, 4: 23–34.

DeVellis, B.M. (1995) The psychological impact of arthritis: prevalence of depression, *Arthritis Care & Research*, 8(4), 284–89.

Dickens, C., McGowan, L., Clark-Carter, D. and Creed, F. (2002) Depression in rheumatoid arthritis: a systematic review of the literature with meta-analysis, *Psychosomatic Medicine*, 64: 52–60.

Dickens, C., Jackson, J., Tomenson, B., Hay, E. and Creed, F. (2003) Association of depression and rheumatoid arthritis, *Psychosomatics*, 44: 209–15.

Fries, J.F., Carey, C. and McShane, D.J. (1997) Patient education in arthritis: randomized controlled trial of a mail-delivered program, *The Journal of Rheumatology*, 24: 1378–83.

Helliwell, P.S., O'Hara, M., Holdsworth, J., Hesselden, A., King, T. and Evans, P. (1999) A 12-month randomized controlled trial of patient education on radiographic changes and quality of life in early rheumatoid arthritis, *Rheumatology*, 38: 303–08.

Hollon, S.D., Jarrett, R.B., Nierenberg, A.A., Thase, M.E., Trivedi, M. and Rush, A.J. (2005) Psychotherapy and medication in the treatment of adult and geriatric depression: which monotherapy or combined treatment? *Journal of Clinical Psychiatry*, 66: 455–68.

Huyser, B. and Parker, J.C. (1998) Stress and rheumatoid arthritis: an integrative review, *Arthritis Care & Research*, 11: 135–45.

Katz, P.P. and Yelin, E.H. (1993) Prevalence and correlates of depressive symptoms among persons with rheumatoid arthritis, *Journal of Rheumatology*, 20(5): 790–96.

Keefe, F.J., Abernethy, A.P. and Campbell, L.C. (2005) Psychological approaches to understanding and treating disease-related pain, *Annual Review of Psychology*, 56: 601–30.

Kruger, J., Helmick, C.G., Callahan, L.F. and Haddix, A. (1998) Cost-effectiveness of the arthritis self-help course, *Archives of Internal Medicine*, 158: 1245–49.

Lawrence, R.C., Helmick, C.G., Arnett, F.C., Deyo, R.A., Felson, D.T., Giannini, E.H., Heyse, S.P., Hirsch, R., Hochberg, M.C., Hunder, G.G., Liang, M.H., Pillemer, S.R., Steen, V.D. and Wolfe, F. (1998) Estimates of the prevalence of arthritis and selected musculoskeletal disorders in the United States, *Arthritis & Rheumatism*, 41(5): 778–99.

Lenze, E., Dew, M., Mazumdar, S., Begley, A., Cornes, C., Miller, M.D., Imber, S.D., Frank, E., Kupfer, D.J. and Reynolds, C.F. (2002) Combined pharmacology as maintenance treatment for late-life depression: effects on social adjustment, *American Journal of Psychiatry*, 159: 466–68.

Lorig, K., Lubeck, D., Kraines, R.G., Seleznick, M. and Holman, H.R. (1985) Outcomes of self-help education for patients with arthritis, *Arthritis & Rheumatism*, 28(6): 680–85.

Lorig, K., Gonzalez, V.M., Laurent, D.D., Morgan, L. and Laris, B.A. (1998) Arthritis self-management program variations: three studies, *Arthritis Care & Research*, 11(6): 448–54.

Merkesdal, S., Ruof, J., Schöffski, O., Bernitt, K., Zeidler, H. and Mau, W. (2001) Indirect medical costs in early rheumatoid arthritis, *Arthritis & Rheumatism*, 44(3): 528–34.

O'Leary, A., Shoor, S., Lorig, K. and Holman, H.R. (1988) A cognitive-behavioral treatment for rheumatoid arthritis, *Health Psychology*, 7(6): 527–44.

Parker, J C. and Slaughter, J.R. (2004) Depression, in E.W. St. Clair, D.S. Pisetsky and B.F. Haynes (eds) *Rheumatoid Arthritis* (pp. 517–25). Philadelphia: Lippincott, Williams & Wilkins.

Parker, J.C., Singsen, B.H., Hewett, J.E., Walker, S.E., Hazelwood, S.E., Hall, P.J., Holsten, D.J. and Rodon, C.M. (1984) Educating patients with rheumatoid arthritis: a prospective analysis, *Archives of Physical Medicine and Rehabilitation*, 65: 771–74.

Parker, J.C., Frank, R.G., Beck, N.C., Smarr, K.L., Buescher, K.L., Phillips, L.R., Smith, E.I., Anderson, S.K. and Walker, S.E. (1988a) Pain management in rheumatoid arthritis patients: a cognitive-behavioral approach, *Arthritis & Rheumatism*, 31(5): 593–601.

Parker, J.C., McRae, C., Smarr, K.L., Beck, N.C., Frank, R.G., Anderson, S.K. and Walker, S.E. (1988b) Coping strategies in rheumatoid arthritis, *The Journal of Rheumatology*, 15(9): 1376–83.

Parker, J.C., Iverson, G.L., Smarr, K.L. and Stucky-Ropp, R.C. (1993) Cognitive-behavioral approaches to pain management in rheumatoid arthritis, *Arthritis Care & Research*, 6(4): 207–12.

Parker, J.C., Smarr, K.L., Buckelew, S.P., Stucky-Ropp, R.C., Hewett, J.E., Johnson, J.C., Wright, G.E., Irvin, W.S. and Walker, S.E. (1995) Effects of stress-management on clinical outcomes in rheumatoid arthritis, *Arthritis & Rheumatism*, 38(12): 1807–18.

Parker, J.C., Smarr, K.L., Slaughter, J.R., Johnston, S.K., Priesmeyer, M.L., Donovan, J., Hanson, K., Wright, G.E., Hewett, J.E., Hewett, J.E., Irvin, W.S., Komatireddy, G.R. and Walker, S.E. (2003) Management of depression in rheumatoid arthritis: a combined pharmacologic and cognitive-behavioral approach, *Arthritis Care & Research*, 49: 766–77.

Rhee, S.H., Parker, J.C., Smarr, K.L., Petroski, G.F., Johnson, J.C., Hewett, J.E., Wright, G.E., Multon, K.D. and Walker, S.E. (2000) Stress management in rheumatoid arthritis: what is the underlying mechanism? *Arthritis Care & Research*, 13(6): 435–42.

Riemsma, R., Taal, E., Kirwan, J.R. and Rasker, J.J. (2004) Systematic review of rheumatoid arthritis patient education, *Arthritis & Rheumatism*, 51(6): 1045–59.

Rogers, M.P. and Fozdar, M. (1996) Psychoneuroimmunology of autoimmune disorders, *Advances in Neuroimmunology*, 6: 169–77.

Scharloo, M., Kaptein, A.A., Weinman, J.A., Hazes, J.M.W., Breedveld, F.C. and Rooijmans, H.G.M. (1999) Predicting functional status in patients with rheumatoid arthritis, *Journal of Rheumatology*, 26(8): 1686–93.

Smyth, J.M., Stone, A.A., Hurewitz, A. and Kaell, A. (1999) Effects of writing about stressful experiences on symptom reduction in patients with asthma or rheumatoid arthritis: a randomized trial, *Journal of the American Medical Association*, 281(14): 1304–09.

Stone, A.A. and Smyth, J.M. (2000) Structured writing about stressful events: exploring potential psychological mediators of positive health effects, *Health Psychology*, 19(6): 619–24.

Warsi, A., LaValley, M.P., Wang, P.S., Avorn, J. and Solomon, D.H. (2003) Arthritis self-management education programs: a meta-analysis of the effect on pain and disability, *Arthritis & Rheumatism*, 48(8): 2207–13.

Wetherell, M.A., Byrne-Davis, L., Dieppe, P., Donovan, J., Brookes, S., Byron, M., Vedhara, K., Horne, R., Weinman, J. and Miles, J. (2005) Effects of emotional disclosure on psychological and physiological outcomes in patients with rheumatoid arthritis: an explanatory home-based study, *Journal of Health Psychology*, 10(2): 277–85.

Wright, G.E., Parker, J.C., Smarr, K.L., Johnson, J.C., Hewett, J.E. and Walker, S.E. (1998) Age, depressive symptoms, and rheumatoid arthritis, *Arthritis & Rheumatism*, 41(2): 298–305.

12 Asthma

Jane R. Smith

Asthma as a chronic illness

Definition and diagnosis

Asthma is recognizable by its pathological, physiological and clinical characteristics (Global Initiative for Asthma (GINA) 2006). In terms of pathology, asthma is a chronic inflammatory disorder of the airways, the causes and mechanisms of which are complex, variable and not fully understood (GINA 2006). Inflammation makes the airways hypersensitive such that they periodically narrow in response to certain internal or external 'triggers', such as allergens, irritants or infections (National Asthma Education and Prevention Program (NAEPP) 2007). Measures of respiratory function, such as those obtained from patient-held peak expiratory flow (PEF) meters, can demonstrate whether the resultant airflow obstruction is variable over time and improves spontaneously or on treatment with medications that open up the airways (British Thoracic Society and Scottish Intercollegiate Guideline Network (BTS and SIGN) 2003). These episodes of airflow obstruction constitute the main physiological feature of asthma and lead to clinical symptoms of breathlessness, wheeze, chest tightness and cough (GINA 2006). Asthma is usually diagnosed when symptoms tend to be variable, intermittent, worse at night and provoked by triggers (BTS and SIGN 2003). If uncontrolled, symptoms can result in an asthma attack. Asthma as a chronic illness is thus characterized by episodes of symptoms interspersed with periods of reduced or no symptoms.

Classification and assessment

Asthma was traditionally classified into four levels of severity: intermittent, and mild, moderate and severe persistent (GINA 2006; NAEPP 2007), according to the degree and variability of airflow obstruction, and the frequency and impact of symptoms and attacks before treatment, and/or the treatment 'step' (see below) required to minimize these. However, severity classifications have proved difficult to use, can be inconsistent, and change as asthma varies over time (Graham 2006). Thus, there has been a shift towards classifying and monitoring asthma in terms of disease control, which reflects suppression or minimization of the manifestations of the disease needed to reduce current impairments and prevent future risks (NAEPP 2007). Respiratory function and patient-reported outcomes, assessed via key questions about recent symptoms and their impact (Royal College of Physicians 1999) or validated scales incorporating such questions (see Revicki and Weiss 2006), are increasingly used together for monitoring control. This is in line with the goal of treatment being to achieve asthma control, considered as near-normal respiratory function, minimal or no symptoms and impact on functioning, and no attacks (BTS and SIGN 2003; GINA 2006; NAEPP 2007).

Impact

An estimated 300 million people worldwide have asthma, with the highest prevalence in the UK, Australasia and north America where it affects 11–16 per cent of the population (Masoli et al. 2004), and up to 12 per cent of adults (Janson et al. 2001). Figures suggest an increasing global prevalence, which may have peaked in the mid to late 1990s in some Western countries (Anderson et al. 2007). Globally, more than 15 million disability-adjusted life years (DALYs) are lost due to asthma annually, accounting for 1 per cent of the total, making asthma the twenty-fifth leading cause of DALYs lost, and comparable to diabetes in terms of its health burden (Masoli et al. 2004). Health care and societal costs attributable to asthma are estimated at nearly £2.5, $12 and €17.7 billion in the UK, the USA and Europe, respectively (Loddenkemper et al. 2003; Masoli et al. 2004).

A majority of patients have suboptimal asthma control and around 40 per cent have moderate to severe disease resulting in daily symptoms and frequent restrictions to activities (Rabe et al. 2004). In less than 10 per cent of patients, disease remains severe and uncontrolled with severe attacks despite intensive treatment (Masoli et al. 2004) and is so-called 'difficult' asthma. Although rare, asthma deaths represent a major cause of preventable mortality and globally account for about 1 in 250, or 250,000 deaths annually (Masoli et al. 2004). Up to 9 per cent of asthma patients are hospitalized each year in Western countries, small numbers require intensive care for near-fatal asthma, and a further quarter attend for emergency or unscheduled health care (Rabe et al. 2004). Ethnic minorities, low socio-economic groups and those with coexisting psychosocial problems are over-represented in asthma mortality and morbidity statistics (Masoli et al. 2004). It is proposed that mortality and morbidity could be reduced with improved management.

Medical management

Evidence-based international (GINA 2006) and national (e.g. BTS and SIGN 2003; NAEPP 2007) guidelines provide advice for clinicians involved in the medical care of asthma patients. Key recommendations relate to the use of two main types of medication effective in improving respiratory function, controlling symptoms, and preventing and treating attacks. These are commonly delivered via inhalers to act directly on the lungs while minimizing side-effects and include: 1) reliever or rescue medications which rapidly open up the airways during attacks and are used by all patients as needed for relieving symptoms; for example, short-acting beta$_2$-agonists; and 2) preventer or controller medications taken daily, primarily to reduce underlying inflammation; for example, inhaled cortico-steroids (ICS). For chronic asthma, a stepwise approach is recommended whereby the dose, frequency of administration and number of preventer medications are 'stepped-up' with increasing severity or until asthma control is achieved and subsequently 'stepped-down' to identify the minimum required to maintain control in light of potential side-effects and patient goals.

Self-management of asthma

Importance

The need for patients to take an active role in management and engage in self-management is inherent in asthma, not least because the as-needed use of relievers relies on patient judgement and effective long-term treatment depends on regular use of preventer medications (Partridge 1997). Indeed, one of the earliest references to 'self-management' is purported to have been made in a paper on asthma in the 1970s (Lorig and Holman 2003). In the most recent international guidelines the need for clinicians to communicate effectively, in order to develop and work in a partnership with patients in guiding and strengthening self-management, is seen to underpin all other aspects of management (GINA 2006).

Key features and components

In common with some other conditions (e.g. diabetes, see Chapter 10), and unlike others (e.g. arthritis, see Chapter 11), asthma self-management tends to be defined from a clinical perspective, focusing on the patient's role in effective medical management in terms of performance of behaviours important for controlling asthma. In addition to appropriate use of medications, these cover self-monitoring of asthma to recognize deterioration and guide prevention and management of attacks, avoidance or control of triggers, performance of general health-promoting behaviours and regular contact and effective communication with clinicians (Wilson 1993).

A central component, sometimes considered synonymous with asthma self-management (Fishwick et al. 1997) or referred to as guided self-management (Lahden-suo 1999), focuses on patients identifying and responding to worsening asthma according to an agreed written 'action' or 'self-management' plan. Action plans provide specific individualized instructions on actions to take (e.g. initiating or increasing the dose of particular medications, seeking urgent medical care) within several 'zones' of worsening asthma defined on the basis of symptoms, reliever use and/or PEF (Fishwick et al. 1997). Self-management plans sometimes also incorporate advice regarding other aspects of daily management (e.g. triggers). Guidelines increasingly recommend adaptation of plans according to a patient's disease severity, ability to perceive symptoms, goals and capability or preferences for independence (BTS and SIGN 2003; GINA 2006; NAEPP 2007). However, a one-size-fits-all approach tends to predominate in practice (Kolbe 2002).

Patient management behaviours and influences on performance

There is a history of in-depth research on asthma self-management in children (e.g. Clark et al. 1980), but little is applicable to adults given the role of carers in asthma management in younger children and issues pertinent to adolescents. Given the focus on behaviours supporting effective medical management, most research in adults has explored medication use. More limited study of other behaviours and influences on their performance has largely been undertaken in the context of other behaviour and morbidity surveys or trials evaluating treatments, relying on responses to simple questions regarding their execution and/or information from selected and motivated patients. Evidence from some recent and large studies is discussed below.

Medication use

Overuse of reliever medications appears common (Rabe et al. 2004) regardless of asthma severity (Marks et al. 2007) or concurrent prescription of preventers (Partridge et al. 2006). However, much of this, and its relationship to adverse outcomes, may reflect uncontrolled asthma resulting from underuse of preventers (Williams et al. 2004). Use of preventer medications appears highest in Western Europe, where they are still only used by less than 30 per cent of patients at all levels of severity (Rabe et al. 2004). Some underuse likely stems from prescribed treatment being misaligned with guidelines (Canonica et al. 2007). However, poor patient adherence to preventers, consistently found to be less than 50 per cent even among patients discharged from hospital, has long been recognized and is reviewed in depth elsewhere (Bender et al. 1997; Schmier and Leidy 1998).

Research has not identified consistent relationships between socio-demographic, socio-economic or personality characteristics and adherence in asthma (Schmier and Leidy 1998). Treatment and clinician/consultation factors, including simplified regimens (Schmier and Leidy 1998), appropriate inhaler technique (Cochrane et al. 2000) and regular contact and a good relationship with clinicians (Corsico et al. 2007), appear important in reducing unintentional poor adherence (Horne 2006). However, despite most patients having been shown how to use inhalers (Canonica et al. 2007; Marks et al. 2007) up to 40 per cent have poor technique (Cochrane et al. 2000). Individual psychosocial factors interact in complex ways to influence intentional poor adherence (Bender et al. 1997; Schmier and Leidy 1998). Beliefs consistent with the medical viewpoint of asthma being a chronic, rather than episodic, condition, with potentially serious consequences, relate to greater adherence to preventers (Halm et al. 2006), both directly and via their influence on patients' beliefs about medications (Horne and Weinman 2002). Doubts over the necessity of preventers when symptom-free or asthma is perceived as mild, and concerns regarding side-effects and steroid dependency are associated with poor adherence (Horne and Weinman 2002). These concerns may be driven by non-specific negative beliefs about asthma medications (Osman et al. 1993) or medicines in general, likely influenced by educational, social and cultural factors (Horne 2006). Side-effects are experienced and relate to the use and dose of ICS (Horne 2006) but, despite being far outweighed by benefits from asthma medications (GINA 2006), over 70 per cent of patients and 40 per cent of physicians in one survey reported never or rarely discussing side-effects (Canonica et al. 2007).

That illness beliefs and evaluation of pros (e.g. symptom relief) and cons (e.g. side-effects) appear to influence adherence to preventers is consistent with several models of health-related behaviour (Chapter 3). As Leventhal's self-regulatory model recognizes, emotional representations of illness (Jessop et al. 2004) and depression (Bender et al. 1997) are also important. More proximal influences on behaviour, such as self-efficacy and readiness to change, are beginning to be explored in relation to asthma medication adherence (Schmaling et al. 2000).

Use of action plans

In Australia, where use of action plans has been widely promoted, surveys from one state suggest that ownership peaked at 42 per cent in 1994, dropping to 21 per cent in 2003 (Wilson et al. 2006), a figure supported by a concurrent national survey (Marks et al. 2007). Provision of plans by clinicians is low but their use by patients appears even lower. For example, in one survey only half of the 11 per cent of Canadian patients with a written plan used it (Fitzgerald et al. 2006). Studies of patients with persistent and moderate to severe asthma in the USA found ownership to be slightly higher, but it is unclear whether the associations found between ownership and use of plans and asthma control persist when other factors are controlled for (Schatz et al. 2006; Peters et al. 2007). Low uptake is perhaps not surprising given qualitative studies highlighting mixed views among patients and clinicians about action plans and guided self-management (Jones et al. 2000; Douglass et al. 2002).

Self-monitoring and managing attacks

In an international survey, ownership of peak flow meters to support self-monitoring and implementation of action plans was highest in the UK at 40 per cent and ownership and regular use were 28 per cent and 8 per cent, respectively in the USA and across Western Europe (Rabe et al. 2004), with similar patterns in Australia (Marks et al. 2007). Although high usage (89 per cent) was achieved in a trial where data were recorded electronically and guided use of preventers (Reddel et al. 2002), their poor uptake outside research settings has led to a shift towards symptom-based plans (BTS and SIGN 2003). However, there appears to be little research on symptom monitoring. Although one survey found that two-thirds of patients could recognize early warning signs of worsening asthma, most commonly through increased symptoms, the most common response was initially to increase use of reliever rather than preventer medications (Partridge et al. 2006). This is despite one study suggesting that nearly three-quarters of patients reported being told to increase the latter (Hyland 1997). In another study, management errors, including inappropriate medication use and delays in contacting medical services, were common in the face of attacks resulting in hospitalization and associated with patients' social, economic and psychological characteristics (Kolbe et al. 1998). As research on health-related behaviours acknowledges, there are discrepancies between patients' knowledge and behaviour in relation to attack management and various psychosocial factors are differentially associated with knowledge, behaviour and the degree of discrepancy between them (Kolbe 2002).

Trigger avoidance and control

Links between asthma control or attacks and triggers are clearly established (GINA 2006). However, some triggers (e.g. pollens, climatic conditions) cannot easily be avoided, common measures to reduce exposures (e.g. dust mite and pet allergen control) appear ineffective and even those that are effective (e.g. influenza vaccination) do not appear to improve asthma outcomes (GINA 2006). Given the impact of triggers, the lack of patient-level research is surprising, with most taking place alongside broader studies using unstructured assessment via simple questions. A small study found that significantly more patients with severe asthma compared to those with mild asthma were sensitized and exposed to dust mite, dog and cat allergens; that is, kept pets to which they were allergic (Tunnicliffe et al. 1999). In another study 74 per cent of patients knew or avoided their triggers and this was associated with asthma control one year later in univariate but not in multivariate analyses (Schatz et al. 2006). One study found that over 90 per cent of patients with severe asthma were able to identify their triggers, with animals, dust mites, climatic conditions, pollen, smoke and stress mentioned by over 20 per cent, but differences in reported triggers were apparent between those with uncontrolled and well-controlled disease (e.g. stress more common among the former) (Smith et al. 2005a). These findings are broadly in line with those from a recent study on the development and validation of an asthma trigger inventory (Ritz et al. 2006), which will facilitate future research on the topic.

Other health-promoting behaviours

Exposure to smoke is a common asthma trigger, and smoking is associated with severity, poor control and the inefficacy of preventer medications (GINA 2006).

Despite this, nearly 20 per cent of adults with asthma in developed countries smoke (Rabe et al. 2004). Clinical and demographic factors are associated with ever smoking and delayed cessation in asthma (Eisner et al. 2000) but there appears to be little research on psychosocial influences. The importance of exercise and obesity in asthma is increasingly recognized (GINA 2006), but many patients experience limitations on physical activity (Rabe et al. 2004), increasing numbers are obese (Laforest et al. 2006; Wilson et al. 2006) and little is known about influences on these behaviours specifically among those with asthma.

Contact and communication with health professionals

Suboptimal performance of self-management behaviours may reflect difficulties patients experience in implementing actions agreed with clinicians. However, across various surveys 11 per cent of patients were not seeing any clinician about their asthma (Canonica et al. 2007), 19 per cent had not discussed their asthma with a doctor since diagnosis (Bellamy and Harris 2005) and two-thirds had failed to attend asthma clinics at some point, mostly because they did not perceive they had asthma or that it was sufficiently severe to warrant check-ups (Gruffydd-Jones et al. 1999). In another study, 23 per cent of patients seeing clinicians reported that no time was spent discussing successful self-management; however, those reporting more discussion were more adherent (Canonica et al. 2007). Elsewhere, 37 per cent of patients surveyed did not report symptoms to their clinician; this concerned 68 per cent of clinicians and 55 per cent wanted patients to be more forthcoming (Bellamy and Harris 2005). There are thus patient and clinician factors contributing to difficulties with communicating and working in partnership to achieve effective asthma management.

Summary of issues surrounding asthma self-management

Empirical and theoretical developments are increasing understanding of some self-management behaviours among adults with asthma, particularly medication adherence. Despite their importance (Kolbe 2002), particularly in certain groups (Wilson 1993), research on other behaviours and their combined and relative influence on outcomes is limited. In one study, an increasing number of self-management strategies was associated with improved long-term asthma control, but medical management (e.g. medications dispensed) appeared more important than patient self-management. However, the inclusion of specialist care under medical management may have masked the influence of patient strategies which are more likely advocated by specialists, and assessment of patient self-management was limited (Schatz et al. 2006). There is currently a lack of validated measures of many patient self-management behaviours and their psychological correlates thus limiting knowledge on effective management and its global predictors as a whole. More work is needed in this area and some studies are currently under way.

Even when patient self-management behaviours have been assessed and controlled for, socio-demographic and severity characteristics remain independent predictors of asthma control (Laforest et al. 2006; Schatz et al. 2006). Furthermore, in line with broader definitions of self-management considered in this book, patient motivation for asthma treatment and self-management does not necessarily match the goals of medical management directed towards asthma control. Instead, it may be influenced by personal life goals and the effects of asthma on valued activity, with which taking medications, avoiding triggers, and so on may be at odds (Osman et al. 1993; Steven et al. 2002). This highlights the need for a conceptualization of asthma self-management which goes beyond medical aspects and considers adapting to everyday life and roles with asthma and its management and coping with the emotional consequences of these (Lorig and Holman 2003). Unlike in some other conditions (e.g. arthritis, see Chapter 11) there is a limited and fairly isolated literature on coping with asthma (Barton et al. 2003). This is despite: 1) large decrements in quality of life and high levels of psychological morbidity among those with severe asthma, who face the threat or reality of its significant adverse consequences and must engage in complex and intense management activities (Smith and Harrison 2007); and 2) growing evidence that stress can impact directly on symptom perception and asthma disease processes via psychoneuroimmunological pathways (Wright et al. 1998). As represented in Figure 12.1, these aspects are important to consider in supporting asthma self-management.

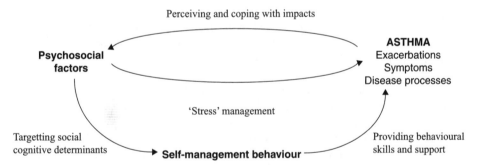

Figure 12.1 Relationships between psychosocial factors and asthma and potential points for intervention to improve self-management

Asthma self-management interventions

Definitions and types

Interventions to support asthma self-management in children, not reviewed here, appeared in the early 1980s. Adult programmes have continued to proliferate since their inception in the late 1980s. Due to their number, individual programmes will not be reviewed. Instead, observations and findings from reviews and key discussion papers focused on asthma self-management interventions in adults, or which consider relevant interventions in mixed ages or diseases but comment on asthma self-management in adults separately, are discussed. In line with a broad conceptualization of self-management, any interventions that assist patients in managing, adapting to and/or coping with asthma and its consequences, are considered. These are sometimes referred to as psychoeducational interventions (Devine 1996; Smith et al. 2005b) to reflect potential overlap and integration between education and training in self-management behaviours and interventions targeting specific psychosocial factors resulting from or impacting on asthma and its management (see Figure 12.1).

In line with divisions between recent Cochrane reviews in the field and distinctions made in a review by the author (Smith et al. 2005b; Smith et al. 2007), education, guided self-management, psychosocial and mixed or multifaceted interventions, are initially distinguished. The latter sometimes include adjunctive physical therapies (e.g. medical treatment, exercise) or environmental control measures (e.g. physical or chemical methods to reduce triggers); however, interventions working primarily at physical or environmental levels are not discussed. Furthermore, alternative therapies, such as yoga, are only considered when reviewed on the basis that they were deemed to be working primarily at a psychological level (e.g. as relaxation techniques).

Educational interventions

Early programmes primarily comprised education aimed at increasing patients' knowledge of asthma and its management on the assumption that this would lead to behaviour changes resulting in improved outcomes. Educational interventions have used various techniques to convey information (e.g. verbal, written) and facilitate learning (e.g. discussion, skills training, role-play). Recommended components matching core knowledge (e.g. nature of asthma, medications) and skills (e.g. inhaler use) are summarized in guidelines (BTS and SIGN 2003; GINA 2006).

A narrative review of 18 early asthma education programmes in adults (Clark and Nothwehr 1997) involving random assignment and adequate samples concluded that they showed effects on a range of health and psychological outcomes. However, a systematic review summarizing the content and methods applied in 94 studies highlighted that asthma education for adults was highly variable and generally poorly described and reported (Sudre et al. 1999). It is therefore perhaps not surprising that when a later Cochrane review examined 12 randomized controlled trials (RCTs) of limited, information-only education, few benefits were identified (Gibson et al. 2002). On the basis that one included study showed reductions in emergency visits for those previously attending the emergency department, a later Cochrane review examined effects of asthma education among this group. The analysis of 12 RCTs showed effects on admissions and attendance for scheduled follow-up, but, conflictingly, not on subsequent emergency visits or other outcomes that were assessed by small numbers of studies (Tapp et al. 2007). An earlier narrative review (Fitzgerald and Turner 1997) recognized the potential for education to improve outcomes for a range of high-risk asthma patients but emphasized integrating interventions with optimal medical care and follow-up in an effort to overcome potential psychosocial barriers to attendance and education in such groups. A review of 16 mainly educational interventions to improve adherence in asthma identified some successful programmes, but similarly highlighted that poorly adherent patients are least likely to participate and remain in studies, likely biasing results (Bender et al. 2003).

Guided self-management interventions

Asthma education has increasingly incorporated use of self-monitoring and/or action plans, and these guided self-management interventions have recently become synonymous with asthma self-management education. A narrative review of 15 programmes incorporating PEF or symptom-based guidelines for self-adjustment of medications concluded that although several showed improvements across various outcomes, the two of highest quality showed little effect (Van Der Palen et al. 1998). In contrast, meta-analyses from a Cochrane review of 36 RCTs demonstrated that guided self-management improved a range of health-related outcomes (Gibson et al. 2003). In line with identifying evidence to support Australian guideline recommendations to 'educate and review regularly', relevant interventions incorporated education plus one or more of self-monitoring, medical review and/or use of a written action plan, with 15 'optimal' interventions including all components generally showing the greatest effects. These findings underpin recommendations on self-management education in current guidelines (BTS and SIGN 2003; GINA 2006; NAEPP 2007), although their generalizability to routine practice in a range of contexts or patient groups, is far from clear (Fay et al. 2000).

   Further reviews have begun to explore the effective components of guided self-management. Another Cochrane review (Powell and Gibson 2002) compared the 15 optimal guided self-management interventions identified above to modified interventions or control groups receiving regular medical review as a minimum. In qualitative syntheses and limited meta-analyses, adjustment of medication by medical review or self-adjustment according to a plan, and self-monitoring based on PEF or symptoms, appeared largely equivalent. In a further review of these studies (Gibson and Powell 2004), meta-analyses of small numbers showed that individualized, complete action plans based on both predicted or personal best PEF reduced admissions, but only those based on personal best improved other outcomes. Inclusion of more action points or presentation in a 'traffic light' format did not consistently improve effects, but there were insufficient studies to permit conclusions about other features, particularly in symptom-based plans. It is unclear how potential effects of other differences between the interventions incorporating the different plans were considered. However, these were eliminated in a Cochrane review of seven RCTs, which provided no consistent evidence that provision of written individualized plans in isolation improved outcomes, and highlighted conflicting results regarding PEF versus symptom-based plans (Toelle and Ram 2004).

Psychosocial interventions

Prior to improved understanding of its pathophysiology and pharmacology, asthma was considered largely psychosomatic in origin so there is a history of using psychological interventions in asthma. However, most have evolved separately from interventions aimed at improving patient self-management behaviours. A discussion paper on psychological approaches published soon after the first asthma guidelines concluded that relaxation and psychoeducation, in particular, may be useful adjuncts to medical treatment in asthma (Lehrer et al. 1992). A broader review (Devine 1996) of various psychoeducational interventions (education, behavioural and cognitive therapies, counselling) in adults with asthma, found positive impacts on physiological, health and psychological outcomes in meta-analyses of 31 studies (58 per cent randomized, 77 per cent with control groups). A descriptive review of hypnosis and asthma highlighted some positive effects among uncontrolled and non-randomized studies, but results from RCTs were equivocal (Hackman et al. 2000). Conclusions from more recent systematic reviews of RCTs are similarly more cautious.

A systematic (Ernst 2000) and Cochrane review (Holloway and Ram 2004), respectively examined six and seven RCTs of breathing retraining techniques, which sometimes combine physiotherapeutic and psychotherapeutic components or form part of broader interventions. Both concluded that although some studies showed beneficial effects in certain patients, there was insufficient evidence to draw firm conclusions. A systematic review (Huntley et al. 2002) examining relaxation techniques in asthma found across nine RCTs that only two of mental and muscular relaxation showed significant effects. Limited meta-analyses from a Cochrane review (Yorke et al. 2006) of various psychotherapeutic interventions (classified as relaxation, biofeedback, cognitive-behavioural therapy) for asthma in adults evaluated in 15 small and poor-quality studies showed limited effects on clinical and psychological outcomes.

Multifaceted and mixed interventions

Numerous multifaceted approaches, such as primary care-based clinics, have evolved to support implementation of asthma guidelines and self-management. However, reviews of these generally identify a paucity of good quality research (Eastwood and Sheldon 1996; Ram et al. 2002). In a review of a range of self-management interventions, including 18 recent RCTs in asthma alongside 45 in diabetes and arthritis, over half the asthma interventions, and frequently those incorporating education with use of an action plan, consistently showed significant effects on asthma outcomes (Newman et al. 2004). A systematic review by the author (Smith et al. 2005b; Smith et al. 2007) investigated the effects of psychoeducational interventions, including multifaceted programmes incorporating enhanced medical care or other adjunctive components alongside guided self-management and/or psychosocial support, in patients with severe or difficult asthma. Syntheses of results from 17 studies suggested that largely positive effects on self-management behaviours, statistically significant effects on health outcomes from several individual studies and small but potentially important pooled effects on admissions, quality of life and psychological morbidity, were mainly confined to the short term and did not appear to extend to high-risk patients in whom multiple factors complicate management.

Nature of interventions and use of theory

The reviews by Newman et al. (2004) and Smith et al. (2007) explored similarities and differences between a range of self-management interventions in more depth than has been done, for example, in Cochrane reviews which have tended to focus on the efficacy, rather than effectiveness, of specific interventions. Smith et al. (2007) observed almost as much variation (e.g. in terms of content, delivery and approaches used) across interventions classified as being of the same type as between different types, and there was often overlap between types. This challenges distinctions made between Cochrane reviews and highlights that some multifaceted interventions, particularly important for at-risk groups, fall between these reviews (Smith et al. 2005b). Further observations parallel conclusions from the review by Newman et al. (2004), namely that asthma programmes tend to be briefer, less theory-based and have narrower objectives that are focused on medical management, rather than lifestyle and emotional aspects, than self-management interventions in other conditions. Further reviews, which do not consider asthma interventions separately, make similar observations (Barlow et al. 2002a, 2002b).

Guided self-management incorporating interactive education is the best researched and consistently most effective self-management approach identified to date for asthma. However, since interventions commonly incorporate regular medical review, it is difficult to distinguish whether enhanced medical care or patient self-management improves outcomes. For this and other reasons, the need for further high-quality research is a recurring theme. Many reviews (Clark and Nothwehr 1997; Sudre et al. 1999; Gibson et al. 2002; Bender et al. 2003; Gibson et al. 2003; Yorke et al. 2006) highlight limitations to approaches based on improving knowledge and advocate enhancing interventions through consideration of psychosocial factors that influence behaviour change and incorporate theories or techniques to address these. Recommendations on clinician–patient communication in recent international guidelines reflect sound psychological principles, but that theory may otherwise be important is intimated only in a statement that 'social and psychological support may also be required to maintain positive behavioral change' (GINA 2006: 51). However, this reinforces the focus on performance of behaviours important for medical management to the exclusion of other aspects of self-management.

The dominance of the narrow conceptualization and prescriptive approach to asthma self-management is interestingly at odds with early psychologically based work in the field, carried forward by some recent commentators in asthma (e.g. Clark and Gong 2000) and chronic disease generally (e.g. Lorig and Holman 2003). This recognizes that most aspects of asthma self-management are unique to individuals and situations, due to the individual nature, variability and complexity of asthma, and changing personal circumstances and goals (Clark and Gong 2000). Thus, rather than a prescribed set of behaviours or actions in the face of an attack, self-management can be viewed as requiring dynamic, independent decision-making and problem-solving, best conceptualized in terms of a self-regulatory model where future actions are guided by individual evaluations of previous behaviour and its associated outcomes. The importance of patients' perceptions of control (e.g. self-efficacy) in self-regulatory processes, possibly independent of their effects on specific behaviours, and the potential for psychopathology to interfere with these, is also acknowledged (Lorig and Holman 2003).

The above points towards a more holistic and flexible approach to supporting asthma self-management that, as a minimum, individually considers each of the pathways by which psychosocial factors and asthma interact (see Figure 12.1). Increasing overlap between different intervention types suggests that an alternative classification in light of these pathways may be a useful precursor to further research. Given its central function in many of the more effective interventions, guided self-management is likely to remain a core component. However, this may need to be accompanied by use of psychoeducational theories and techniques to facilitate related behavioural changes, and address other psychosocial factors resulting from or impacting on asthma. For example, emotional consequences of living with severe disease or recurrent exacerbations, and patients' coping with them, may be helpful to address prior to attempts at behaviour change. Optimization of medical care along-side any interventions in multifaceted, multidisciplinary programmes may be promising approaches. These might target key issues (e.g. stress management) in selected patients (e.g. those with high anxiety) or address multiple factors and be individualized to needs among broader groups of complex patients. Since at-risk patients in particular often fail to attend health care facilities, interventions tied to opportunistic contacts in emergency, primary care or community settings may also be desirable. Future research could usefully build on the wider range of, sometimes innovative, programmes excluded from many reviews because they have not been evaluated via controlled studies (Smith et al. 2005b).

Summary and areas for future research

Asthma is a complex and variable condition in which self-management is multifaceted but key to ensuring effective adoption of medical treatment by patients and to reducing its sometimes substantial impact. Most descriptive studies of, and interventions to support, asthma self-management focus on behaviours important in medical management, commonly medication use. Further research is needed to develop measures that would allow assessment of broader aspects of asthma self-management and its psychosocial correlates. Research could then extend to examining influencing factors and highlight the potential role for theory in designing future interventions. Lessons can be learned from other conditions which place greater emphasis on coping with lifestyle and emotional consequences of illness. Particularly for those with severe disease, addressing these may reduce direct effects of stress on symptoms and exacerbations, and might need to precede efforts to improve patient self-management behaviours (Barnes 1998). Work elsewhere on the importance of control, self-efficacy and enablement in coping with life and illness (Haughney et al. 2007) has implications for asthma and it is proposed that self-management plans may help patients to develop these attributes (Ruhl and Price 2004).

Positively in asthma, self-management is central to most medical guidelines. However, there is a need for work on integrating recommendations made on the basis of systematic reviews of RCTs in selected and motivated patients, into clinical practice. In other words, the real-life effectiveness of strategies to support self-management, and their acceptability to patients and health professionals, need further evaluation. Guidelines have shifted towards a more patient-centred, individu-alized approach by recommending consideration, negotiation and agreement of patient goals (Barnes 1998) and the need for assessment of patients' desire for and ability to control their management (Hyland 1997; Caress et al. 2005). Work on how self-management plans might be individualized is already under way (Horne et al. 2007). Research indicating that higher preferences for participation in decision-making are associated with lower adherence in asthma (Schneider et al. 2007) also points to a possible need for acceptance by clinicians of less than optimal asthma control among patients for whom achieving this reduces their quality of life in other ways.

References

Anderson, H.R., Gupta, R., Strachan, D.P. and Limb, E.S. (2007) 50 years of asthma: UK trends from 1955 to 2004, *Thorax*, 62(1): 85–90.

Barlow, J., Wright, C., Sheasby, J., Turner, A. and Hainsworth, J. (2002a) Self-management approaches for people with chronic conditions: a review, *Patient Education and Counseling*, 48(2): 177–87.

Barlow, J., Sturt, J. and Hearnshaw, H. (2002b) Self-management interventions for people with chronic conditions in primary care: examples from arthritis, asthma and diabetes, *Health Education Journal*, 61(4): 365–78.

Barnes, G.R. (1998) Delivery of patient education in asthma management, *European Respiratory Review*, 8(56): 267–69.

Barton, C., Clarke, D., Sulaiman, N. and Abramson, M. (2003) Coping as a mediator of psychosocial impediments to optimal management and control of asthma, *Respiratory Medicine*, 97(7): 747–61.

Bellamy, D. and Harris, T. (2005) Poor perceptions and expectations of asthma control: results of the International Control of Asthma Symptoms (ICAS) survey of patients and general practitioners, *Primary Care Respiratory Journal*, 14(5): 252–58.

Bender, B., Milgrom, H. and Rand, C. S. (1997) Nonadherence in asthmatic patients: is there a solution to the problem? *Annals of Allergy, Asthma and Immunology*, 79(3): 177–85.

Bender, B., Milgrom, H. and Apter, A. (2003) Adherence intervention research: what have we learned and what do we do next? *Journal of Allergy and Clinical Immunology*, 112(3): 489–94.

British Thoracic Society and Scottish Intercollegiate Guideline Network (2003) British guideline on the management of asthma, *Thorax*, 58(Suppl. 1): 1i–83i.

Canonica, G.W., Baena-Cagnani, C.E., Blaiss, M.S. et al. (2007) Unmet needs in asthma: Global Asthma Physician and Patient (GAPP) survey: global adult findings, *Allergy*, 62(6): 668–74.

Caress, A.L., Beaver, K., Luker, K., Campbell, M. and Woodcock, A. (2005) Involvement in treatment decisions: what do adults with asthma want and do they get? Results of a cross sectional survey, *Thorax*, 60(3): 199–205.

Clark, N.M. and Gong, M. (2000) Management of chronic disease by practitioners and patients: are we teaching the wrong things? *British Medical Journal*, 320: 572–75.

Clark, N.M. and Nothwehr, F. (1997) Self management of asthma by adult patients, *Patient Education and Counseling*, 32(Suppl.): S5–S20.

Clark, N.M., Feldman, C.H., Freudenberg, N. et al. (1980) Developing education for children with asthma through study of self-management behavior, *Health Education Quarterly*, 7(4): 278–97.

Cochrane, M.G., Bala, M.V., Downs, K.E., Mauskopf, J. and Ben-Joseph, R.H. (2000) Inhaled corticosteroids for asthma therapy – patient compliance, devices, and inhalation technique, *Chest*, 117(2): 542–50.

Corsico, A.G., Cazzoletti, L., de Marco, R. et al. (2007) Factors affecting adherence to asthma treatment in an international cohort of young and middle-aged adults, *Respiratory Medicine*, 101(6): 1363–67.

Devine, E.C. (1996) Meta-analysis of the effects of psychoeducational care in adults with asthma, *Research in Nursing and Health*, 19: 367–76.

Douglass, J., Aroni, R., Goeman, D. et al. (2002) A qualitative study of action plans for asthma, *British Medical Journal*, 324: 1003–05.

Eastwood, A.J. and Sheldon, T.A. (1996) Organisation of asthma care: what difference does it make. A systematic review of the literature, *Quality in Health Care*, 5: 134–43.

Eisner, M.D., Yelin, E.H., Katz, P.P. et al. (2000) Predictors of cigarette smoking and smoking cessation among adults with asthma, *American Journal of Public Health*, 90(8): 1307–11.

Ernst, E. (2000) Breathing techniques: adjunctive treatment modalities for asthma? A systematic review, *European Respiratory Journal*, 15(5): 969–72.

Fay, J.K., Jones, A. and Lahdensuo, A. (2000) Guided self management of asthma, *British Medical Journal*, 320: 249.

Fishwick, D., D'Souza, W. and Beasley, R. (1997) The asthma self-management plan system of care: what does it mean, how is it done, does it work, what models are available, what do patients want and who needs it? *Patient Education and Counseling*, 32(Suppl.): S21–S33.

Fitzgerald, J.M. and Turner, M.O. (1997) Delivering asthma education to special high risk groups, *Patient Education and Counseling*, 32(Suppl.): S77–S86.

Fitzgerald, J.M., Boulet, L.P., McIvor, R.A., Zimmerman, S. and Chapman, K.R. (2006) Asthma control in Canada remains suboptimal: the Reality of Asthma Control (TRAC) study, *Canadian Respiratory Journal*, 13(5): 253–59.

Gibson, P.G. and Powell, H. (2004) Written action plans for asthma: an evidence-based review of the key components, *Thorax*, 59(2): 94–99.

Gibson, P.G., Powell, H., Coughlan, J. et al. (2002) Limited (information only) patient education programs for adults with asthma, *Cochrane Database of Systematic Reviews*, Issue 1, No. CD001005.

Gibson, P.G., Powell, H., Coughlan, J. et al. (2003) Self-management education and regular practitioner review for adults with asthma, *Cochrane Database of Systematic Reviews*, Issue 3, No. CD001117.

Global Initiative for Asthma (2006) *GINA Global Strategy for Asthma Management and Prevention* (www.ginasthma.com/).

Graham, L.M. (2006) Classifying asthma, *Chest*, 130(Suppl. 1): 13S–20S.

Gruffydd-Jones, K., Nicholson, I., Best, L. and Connell, E. (1999) Why don't patients attend the asthma clinic? *Asthma in General Practice*, 7(3): 36–38.

Hackman, R.M., Stern, J.S. and Gershwin, M.E. (2000) Hypnosis and asthma: a critical review, *Journal of Asthma*, 37(1): 1–15.

Halm, E.A., Mora, P. and Leventhal, H. (2006) No symptoms, no asthma: the acute episodic disease belief is associated with poor self-management among inner-city adults with persistent asthma, *Chest*, 129: 573–80.

Haughney, J., Cotton, P., Rosen, J.P. et al. (2007) The use of a modification of the Patient Enablement Instrument in asthma, *Primary Care Respiratory Journal*, 16(2): 89–92.

Holloway, E. and Ram, F.S.F. (2004) Breathing exercises for asthma, *Cochrane Database of Systematic Reviews*, Issue 1, No. CD001277.

Horne, R. (2006) Compliance, adherence, and concordance: implications for asthma treatment, *Chest*, 130 (Suppl. 1): 65S–72S.

Horne, R. and Weinman, J. (2002) Self-regulation and self-management in asthma: exploring the role of illness perceptions and treatment beliefs in explaining non-adherence to preventer medication, *Psychology and Health*, 17(1): 17–32.

Horne, R., Price, D., Cleland, J., et al. (2007) Can asthma control be improved by understanding the patient's perspective? BMC Pulmonary Medicine, 7:8. http://www.biomedcentral.com/1471-2466/718.

Huntley, A., White, A.R. and Ernst, E. (2002) Relaxation therapies for asthma: a systematic review, *Thorax*, 57(2): 127–31.

Hyland, M.E. (1997) How do patients operate self-management plans? *Asthma in General Practice*, 5(1): 11–13.

Janson, C., Anto, J., Burney, P. et al. (2001) The European Community Respiratory Health Survey: what are the main results so far? *European Respiratory Journal*, 18(3): 598–611.

Jessop, D.C., Rutter, D.R., Sharma, D. and Albery, I.P. (2004) Emotion and adherence to treatment in people with asthma: an application of the emotional Stroop paradigm, *British Journal of Psychology*, 95(2): 127–47.

Jones, A., Pill, R. and Adams, S. (2000) Qualitative study of views of health professionals and patients on guided self management plans for asthma, *British Medical Journal*, 321: 1507–10.

Kolbe, J. (2002) The influence of socioeconomic and psychological factors on patient adherence to self-management strategies: lessons learned in asthma, *Disease Management and Health Outcomes*, 10(9): 551–70.

Kolbe, J., Vamos, M., Fergusson, W. and Elkind, G. (1998) Determinants of management errors in acute severe asthma, *Thorax*, 53(1): 14–20.

Laforest, L., Van Ganse, E., Devouassoux, G. et al. (2006) Influence of patients characteristics and disease management on asthma control, *Journal of Allergy and Clinical Immunology*, 117(6): 1404–10.

Lahdensuo, A. (1999) Guided self management of asthma – how to do it, *British Medical Journal*, 319: 759–60.

Lehrer, P.M., Sargunaraj, D. and Hochron, S.M. (1992) Psychological approaches to the treatment of asthma, *Journal of Consulting and Clinical Psychology*, 60(4): 639–43.

Loddenkemper, R., Gibson, G.J. and Sibille, Y. (eds) (2003) *European Lung White Book: the First Comprehensive Survey of Respiratory Health in Europe*. Sheffield: European Respiratory Society and European Lung Foundation.

Lorig, K.R. and Holman, H.R. (2003) Self-management education: history, definition, outcomes, and mechanisms, *Annals of Behavioral Medicine*, 26(1): 1–7.

Marks, G.B., Abramson, M.J., Jenkins, C.R. et al. (2007) Asthma management and outcomes in Australia: a nation-wide telephone interview survey, *Respirology*, 12(2): 212–29.

Masoli, M., Fabian, D., Holt, S. and Beasley, R. (2004) *Global Burden of Asthma: Report Developed for the Global Initiative for Asthma* (www.ginasthma.com/).

National Asthma Education and Prevention Program (2007) Expert Panel Report 3 (EPR 3): guidelines for the diagnosis and management of asthma – summary report, *Journal of Allergy and Clinical Immunology*, 120(Suppl. 5): S94–S138.

Newman, S., Steed, L. and Mulligan, K. (2004) Self-management interventions for chronic illness, *The Lancet*, 364: 1523–37.

Osman, L.M., Russell, I.T., Friend, J.A., Legge, J.S. and Douglas, J.G. (1993) Predicting patient attitudes to asthma medication, *Thorax*, 48(8): 827–30.

Partridge, M.R. (1997) Self-management in adults with asthma, *Patient Education and Counseling*, 32(Suppl.): S1–S4.

Partridge, M.R., van der Molen, T., Myrseth, S.E. and Busse, W.W. (2006) Attitudes and actions of asthma patients on regular maintenance therapy: the INSPIRE study. BMC Pulmonary Medicine, 6:13. http://www.biomedcentral.com/1471-2466/6/13.

Peters, S.P., Jones, C.A., Haselkorn, T. et al. (2007) Real-world Evaluation of Asthma Control and Treatment (REACT): findings from a national web-based survey, *Journal of Allergy and Clinical Immunology*, 119(6): 1454–61.

Powell, H. and Gibson, P.G. (2002) Options for self-management education for adults with asthma, *Cochrane Database of Systematic Reviews*, Issue 3, No. CD004107.

Rabe, K.F., Adachi, M., Lai, C.K. et al. (2004) Worldwide severity and control of asthma in children and adults: the global asthma insights and reality surveys, *Journal of Allergy and Clinical Immunology*, 114(1): 40–47.

Ram, F.S.F., Jones, A. and Fay, J.K. (2002) Primary care based clinics for asthma. *Cochrane Database of Systematic Reviews*, Issue 1, No. CD003533.

Reddel, H.K., Toelle, B.G., Marks, G.B. et al. (2002) Analysis of adherence to peak flow monitoring when recording of data is electronic, *British Medical Journal*, 324: 146–47.

Revicki, D. and Weiss, K.B. (2006) Clinical assessment of asthma symptom control: review of current assessment instruments, *Journal of Asthma*, 43(7): 481–88.

Ritz, T., Steptoe, A., Bobb, C., Harris, A.H.S. and Edwards, M. (2006) The Asthma Trigger Inventory: validation of a questionnaire for perceived triggers of asthma, *Psychosomatic Medicine*, 68(6): 956–65.

Royal College of Physicians (1999) *Measuring Clinical Outcome in Asthma: a Patient-focused Approach*. London: Royal College of Physicians.

Ruhl, R. and Price, D. (2004) Patients' perceptions of well-being using a guided self-management plan in asthma, *International Journal of Clinical Practice*, 58(Suppl. 141): 26–32.

Schatz, M., Zeiger, R.S., Vollmer, W.M., Mosen, D. and Cook, E.F. (2006) Determinants of future long-term asthma control, *Journal of Allergy and Clinical Immunology*, 118(5): 1048–53.

Schmaling, K.B., Afari, N. and Blume, A.W. (2000) Assessment of psychological factors associated with adherence to medication regimens among adult patients with asthma, *Journal of Asthma*, 37(4): 335–43.

Schmier, J.K. and Leidy, N.K. (1998) The complexity of treatment adherence in adults with asthma: challenges and opportunities, *Journal of Asthma*, 35(6): 455–72.

Schneider, A., Wensing, M., Quinzler, R., Bieber, C. and Szecsenyi, J. (2007) Higher preference for participation in treatment decisions is associated with lower medication adherence in asthma patients, *Patient Education and Counseling*, 67(1–2): 57–62.

Smith, J.R. and Harrison, B.D.W. (2007) Psychosocial factors in severe asthma in adults, in S.L. Johnstone and P.M. O'Byrne (eds) *Exacerbations of Asthma* (pp. 321–40). Abingdon: Informa Healthcare.

Smith, J.R., Mildenhall, S., Noble, M. et al. (2005a) Clinician-assessed poor compliance identifies adults with severe asthma who are at risk of adverse outcomes, *Journal of Asthma*, 42(6): 437–45.

Smith, J.R., Mugford, M., Holland, R. et al. (2005b) A systematic review to examine the impact of psycho-educational interventions on health outcomes and costs in adults and children with difficult asthma, *Health Technology Assessment*, 9(23): 1–182.

Smith, J.R., Mugford, M., Holland, R., Noble, M.J. and Harrison, B.D.W. (2007) Psycho-educational interventions for adults with severe or difficult asthma: a systematic review, *Journal of Asthma*, 44(3): 219–41.

Steven, K., Morrison, J. and Drummond, N. (2002) Lay versus professional motivation for asthma treatment: a cross-sectional, qualitative study in a single Glasgow general practice, *Family Practice*, 19(2): 172–77.

Sudre, P., Jacquemet, S., Uldry, C. and Perneger, T.V. (1999) Objectives, methods and content of patient education programmes for adults with asthma: systematic review of studies published between 1979 and 1998, *Thorax*, 54: 681–87.

Tapp, S., Lasserson, T.J. and Rowe, B.H. (2007) Education interventions for adults who attend the emergency room for acute asthma, *Cochrane Database of Systematic Reviews*, Issue 3, No. CD003000.

Toelle, B.G. and Ram, F.S.F. (2004) Written individualised management plans for asthma in children and adults, *Cochrane Database of Systematic Reviews*, Issue 1, No. CD002171.

Tunnicliffe, W.S., Fletcher, T.J., Hammond, K. et al. (1999) Sensitivity and exposure to indoor allergens in adults with differing asthma severity, *European Respiratory Journal*, 13(3): 654–59.

Van Der Palen, J., Klein, J.J., Zielhuis, G.A. and van Herwaarden, C.L. (1998) The role of self-treatment guidelines in self-management education for adult asthmatics, *Respiratory Medicine*, 92: 668–75.

Williams, L.K., Pladevall, M., Xi, H. et al. (2004) Relationship between adherence to inhaled corticosteroids and poor outcomes among adults with asthma, *Journal of Allergy and Clinical Immunology*, 114(6): 1288–93.

Wilson, D.H., Adams, R.J., Tucker, G. et al. (2006) Trends in asthma prevalence and population changes in South Australia, 1990–2003, *Medical Journal of Australia*, 184(5): 226–29.

Wilson, S.R. (1993) Patient and physician behaviour models related to asthma care, *Medical Care*, 31(Suppl.): MS49–MS60.

Wright, R.J., Rodriguez, M. and Cohen, S. (1998) Review of psychosocial stress and asthma: an integrated biopsychosocial approach, *Thorax*, 53: 1066–74.

Yorke, J., Fleming, S.L. and Shuldham, C.M. (2006) Psychological interventions for adults with asthma, *Cochrane Database of Systematic Reviews*, Issue 1, No. CD002982.

13 Coronary artery disease

Nancy E. Schoenberg, Debra K. Moser, Kathleen Mulligan and Serap Osman

Overview

Coronary artery disease (CAD) is a chronic condition in which there is a narrowing of the coronary arteries due to a build up of fatty deposits, called plaque. The process by which plaque builds up in the arteries is called atherosclerosis. Coronary artery disease can cause angina, due to the narrowed arteries preventing a sufficient flow of blood and oxygen to the heart. Myocardial infarction (heart attack) occurs when there is a complete blockage of the coronary artery. Coronary artery disease tends to develop over the course of many years, and therefore ascertaining causes of individual cases of CAD is extremely difficult. However, there are many known common risk factors for developing atherosclerosis, which include smoking, suboptimal dietary intake, being overweight, excessive drinking, a sedentary lifestyle, hypercholesterolemia and hypertension, as well as hereditary factors, age and gender (Gaziano et al. 2008).

Coronary artery disease is a leading cause of mortality and morbidity in the developed world. For example, in 2004, CAD caused approximately 452,300 deaths in the USA and it is currently the single leading cause of death in the USA. An estimated 15,800,000 individuals in the USA have a history of myocardial infarction (MI), angina or both (American Heart Association 2006). In the UK, approximately 1 million people (4 per cent of males and 2 per cent of females) have suffered a MI and over 1.3 million have or have had angina (Allender et al. 2007). CAD is not only a disease of the developed world however; global trends in CAD indicate that between 1990–2020, the greatest increases in CAD mortality will be in the developing world (World Health Organization 2004). Disparities in the global context are likely to emerge given unequal access to health care and other resources. Within individual countries, the effects of CAD may also differ between social groups. In the USA, for example, coronary artery disease-related mortality is 29 per cent higher among African Americans than whites (American Public Health Association 2006). In the UK, the first Whitehall study identified that social position plays a significant role in heart disease mortality; Marmot and colleagues identified an inverse association between employment status and mortality from heart disease (Marmot et al. 1984). In subsequent studies by this group, the inverse social gradient in CAD incidence and mortality was found to be attributable to the psychosocial work environment as well as coronary risk factors, including smoking and early life circumstances (Marmot et al 1997).

There are some indications that the incidence of CAD in developed countries is declining (e.g. Hu et al. 2000; Davies et al. 2007); however, the overall burden and impact of CAD is projected to increase (Yusuf et al. 2001). This may be related to a recent trend in the increased likelihood of survival following cardiac events (Hu et al. 2000; Davies et al. 2007). Globally, approximately 20 million people survive MI and strokes each year (World Health Organisation 2003). Those with CAD currently have a longer life expectancy than in years past. For example, from 1990 to 1997, deaths from CAD in the USA dropped by 11.4 per cent (National Institutes of Health 1999). Prolonged life expectancy is attributable to several factors, including improved therapies, an overall decline in risk factors and enhanced management of co-morbidities (Cooper et al. 2000). While research has documented an overall reduction of risk factors – including intake of dietary saturated fat, serum cholesterol, smoking rates and hypertension – other risk factors, including total caloric intake and the prevalence of obesity and type 2 diabetes appear to be increasing dramatically, and these are likely to contribute to an increase in prevalence of CAD. In addition, the ageing of the population, as discussed in Chapter 1, is likely to exacerbate the situation. This raises new challenges in managing CAD. Data from the World Health Organization (WHO) indicate that the number of healthy life-years lost, expressed as disability-adjusted life-years (DALYs), attributable to CAD on a global basis is projected to rise from approximately 47 million in 1990 to 82 million by the year 2020 (World Health Organization 2004).

Management of CAD

The aims of medical treatment of CAD are to prolong life, relieve symptoms and prevent further cardiac events. The main intervention strategies are revascularization, either through coronary artery bypass graft surgery or percutaneous coronary interventions, and pharmacological therapy. Prevention of future deterioration (commonly referred to as secondary prevention) focuses on the identification, treatment and rehabilitation of those who have previously experienced acute events or been diagnosed with CAD. The ultimate goal of secondary prevention is reduction of recurrence, prevention of invasive medical procedures, and enhancement of the quality and duration of life (Cooper et al. 2000). Guidelines for secondary prevention have been published by professional organizations around the world (e.g. De Backer et al. 2003, Smith et al. 2006, National Heart Foundation of Australia, and the Cardiac Society of Australia and New Zealand 2007). The specific goals listed below for secondary prevention have been established by the American College of Cardiology, the American Heart Association and the National Institutes of Health (Smith et al.

2006). These overall goals are supported by global health organizations, including WHO, although specific recommendations may differ.

1 Complete smoking cessation.
2 Reduce blood pressure to less than 140/90 mm Hg, or 130/80 mm Hg for those with diabetes or chronic kidney disease.
3 Increase lipid management: reducing LDL cholesterol to under 100 mg/dL.
4 Increase physical activity to 30 minutes per day, 7 days per week.
5 Improve weight management: maintain a body mass index of 18.5–24.9 kg/m² and a waist circumference of <40 inches for men and < 35 inches for women.
6 Ensure diabetes management: maintain $HbA_{1C} < 7\%$.
7 Improve medication taking as directed including: antiplatelet and antico-agulants, renin-angiotensin-aldosterone system blockers, beta blockers and the influenza and pneumococcal vaccinations.

Other important goals include helping patients learn how to monitor symptoms of acute cardiac ischemia and to respond appropriately to their symptoms.

It is estimated that more than half of deaths and disability stemming from CAD can be avoided through secondary prevention. An example of the advantages to be gained in secondary prevention is the Scandinavian Simvastatin Survival Study (4S) where those who successfully followed a lipid-lowering regimen experienced a 35 per cent reduction in coronary-associated mortality after a 5.4-year follow-up (Pedersen et al. 1994). Similarly, Grover and colleagues have estimated that for those with cardiovascular disease, reduction of risk factors is estimated to increase life expectancy by up to two years (Grover et al. 1998). However, despite compelling evidence of the capacity to contain costs, improve symptom experience, increase overall quality of life, reduce future interventional procedures (angioplasty, bypass grafting) and in-crease survival by preventing subsequent CAD occurrences, most research suggests a limited uptake of these secondary prevention strategies. Missed opportunities for optimal secondary prevention include underuse of medications and undertreatment of hyperlipidemia. Cooper and colleagues estimate that fewer than 50 per cent of patients in the UK will undergo adequate risk assessment, treatment and maintenance (Cooper et al. 2000).

Self-management of CAD

While optimizing medical care is essential to secondary prevention, it is also vital to recognize the role of the individual in managing his or her condition. The goals of secondary prevention listed above incorporate clinical targets that are dependent on patients adopting and maintaining recommended behaviours, such as smoking cessation, adherence to medication, eating a healthy diet and taking regular exercise. Most chronic cardiac care is done in the home by patients and their families, and self-management is therefore the foundation upon which such secondary prevention efforts are built.

Self-management of CAD does not, however, involve only changes in health behaviours, and it is important to recognize that managing the emotional effect of CAD also forms part of self-management. A life-threatening event such as a heart attack can have a significant emotional impact and may involve many life changes, such as in working life and leisure pursuits as well as impacting on close relationships. The emotional impact of experiencing a heart attack has been shown in many studies, which have found increased rates of anxiety and depression following a MI (Lane et al. 2003). Furthermore, these are not restricted to the period immediately following the MI but may persist into the longer term (Lane et al. 2002).

Self-management of CAD can be seen to be complex and optimal self-management may be influenced by many factors, including knowledge and beliefs about both CAD and self-management regimens. In a study by Haugbølle et al. (2002), 44 per cent of patients with angina were unaware of a relationship between lifestyle factors and angina, an issue likely to influence performance of health behaviours. Furze and colleagues found that people with fewer accurate beliefs about angina, such as believing angina to be a mini heart attack, were less physically active than those with beliefs that converged with biomedicine (Furze et al. 2005). Byrne et al. (2005), however, found only a weak association between illness beliefs and health behaviours, which the researchers considered may have been partly explained by their sample's low level of illness identity (i.e. few perceived symptoms). The association between beliefs about medication and adherence was a little stronger. Greater medication adherence was reported by those with a stronger belief in the necessity of their medication and with fewer concerns about taking medications.

Patients' perceptions of their risk of further cardiac events have been found to be incongruent with their actual clinical risk (Broadbent et al. 2006). In patients who had experienced a MI, higher perceived risk was associated with a longer perceived duration of their heart condition, more severe perceived consequences of the MI on their lives, lower perceptions of personal control, less belief that treatment would be helpful, a poorer understanding of their condition, greater emotional distress about the MI, less belief in their own ability to reduce risk and a greater perception of a need to restrict activities. It might be expected that patients' perception of their risk of future events would influence their adherence to recommended treatment and lifestyle changes.

Other factors influential in CAD self-management include cognitive performance, symptom experience, co-morbidity including mental health status, social support and the self-management regimen itself. Occasionally forgetting to take medication was reported by 50 per cent of patients in the study by Haugbølle et al. (2002), while others intentionally adjusted their dose, for example, to try to reduce side-effects. Depression and anxiety often go unrecognized and untreated (Huffman et al. 2006) which also has implications for self-management. For example, depression has been associated with non-adherence to medication among outpatients with stable CAD (Gehi et al. 2005). In Gehi and colleagues' study, self-reported non-adherence to medication was 14 per cent in those with depression, compared with 5 per cent among those who were not depressed. Depressed patients were twice as likely as the non-depressed to report forgetting to take their medication (18 per cent v. 9 per cent) and deciding to skip their medication (9 per cent v. 4 per cent). In addition, because those who have experienced CAD tend also to have a common cluster of co-morbid conditions like diabetes, hypertension and obesity, self-management regimes often are complex and sometimes competing (Schoenberg et al. 2003). Having three or more medications is associated with reduced adherence (Dunbar-Jacobs et al. 2003). Many different factors have also been found to influence patients' participation in interventions to enhance secondary prevention. These interventions are reviewed below.

Interventions to enhance self-management of CAD

Coronary artery disease differs from most other illnesses discussed in this book in that there is an established approach in some countries that is aimed at changing patients' health behaviours through the provision of cardiac rehabilitation programmes. While traditional cardiac rehabilitation programmes were exercise-based, current guidelines consider that they should not consist solely of exercise but be multifaceted and multidisciplinary and aimed at overall cardiac risk reduction. Guidelines have been published regarding the recommended core components of cardiac rehabilitation (e.g. Balady et al. 2007; British Association for Cardiovascular Rehabilitation 2007), which parallel the recommendations for secondary prevention outlined above. It is recommended that cardiac rehabilitation programmes 'optimize cardiovascular risk reduction, foster healthy behaviors and compliance with these behaviors, reduce disability, and promote an active lifestyle' (Balady et al. 2007). Hence the core components are wide-ranging and incorporate recommendations for medical review and treatment as well as behavioural and psychosocial intervention.

Cardiac rehabilitation has been shown to reduce mortality and the risk of further coronary events and to be a cost-effective treatment (Ades 2001; Bittner and Sanderson 2006). However, a large proportion of patients who are considered eligible for cardiac rehabilitation programmes do not attend them. For example, a survey of provision in the UK between 1998–2004 found that only one-third of patients eligible for cardiac rehabilitation attended a programme (Bethell et al. 2007). Similar rates have been found in Australia (Bunker et al. 1999) and the USA (Centers for Disease Control and Prevention 2008).

A number of factors have been identified that predict non-attendance at cardiac rehabilitation, which include demographic, medical and psychosocial factors (Cooper et al. 2002). Older patients, women, less-educated patients and those who experience greater deprivation are less likely to attend (Cooper et al. 2002; Jackson et al. 2005). Endorsement of cardiac rehabilitation by the patient's physician is very important for increasing attendance (Cooper et al. 2002; Jackson et al. 2005) and patients are more likely to attend programmes if they are easily accessible. High social support is also likely to increase attendance (Jackson et al. 2005). Patients' beliefs about their illness and about rehabilitation are also important. For example, Cooper et al. (2007) found differences in beliefs between attenders and non-attenders of cardiac rehabilitation. Patients who attended were more likely than non-attenders to believe that cardiac rehabilitation was necessary and to understand its role, whereas patients who thought cardiac rehabilitation was suitable for a younger, more active person were less likely to attend. French et al (2006) concluded that patients who had had a MI who felt they understood their condition and who viewed it as controllable, symptomatic, and with severe consequences, were more likely to attend cardiac rehabilitation. These findings suggest that to optimize patient outcomes requires a commitment on several levels, from the patient and his or her family, the health care provider, and the health care environment. Few studies have evaluated interventions to increase attendance at cardiac rehabilitation (Beswick et al. 2005) but successful interventions include one based on the Theory of Planned Behaviour (see Chapter 3) (Wyer et al. 2001) and coordination of care after hospital discharge (Jolly et al. 1999).

Another important issue is the extent to which those people who attend cardiac rehabilitation programmes actually put into practice the advice they are given. While these programmes have been shown to improve outcomes, greater practice of the recommended behaviours may bring about further improvements. However, adherence to cardiac rehabilitation is also poor with only about one-third of participants maintaining attendance after six months (Daly et al. 2002). Some of the reasons for non-adherence reported in a qualitative study by Jones et al. (2007) included other health conditions that affect patients' ability to exercise, difficulty in travelling to the programme, and stopping once they felt better.

Inclusion of more psychologically based self-management techniques may encourage greater performance of the behaviours recommended in cardiac rehabilitation. For example, Carlson et al. (2000) compared a programme incorporating exercise and traditional education with a programme based on self-efficacy theory to encourage home exercise and improved nutrition. Continued participation over six months was higher in the latter programme, as were rates of independent exercise. In a review of interventions to improve adherence in cardiac rehabilitation, Beswick et al. (2005) concluded that programmes using motivational and self-management strategies showed some promise in promoting lifestyle change. A programme developed by Lewin et al. (1992) aimed to overcome some of the barriers to uptake and adherence to cardiac rehabilitation by offering a home-based comprehensive rehabilitation programme. This included education, exercise, relaxation and stress management. It also included techniques to help deal with intrusive and distressing thoughts, panic, anxiety, depression and undue illness behaviour. The programme resulted in fewer admissions to hospital, fewer physician visits and better psychological adjustment.

The extent to which cardiac rehabilitation programmes have incorporated self-management techniques, however, is highly variable. While several programmes include psychological components such as stress management (Clark et al. 2005), techniques to promote health behaviour change are not necessarily included. Exercise typically is addressed in a supervised programme while other lifestyle behaviours often are addressed using a more traditional education format.

The more successful attempts to promote health behaviour change tend to be rooted in a theoretically based approach. For example, in the management of cardiac risk factors after coronary artery bypass graft surgery, Allen (1996) conducted a randomized clinical trial of an intervention to help patients decrease dietary fat intake, quit or decrease smoking, and increase exercise. The intervention was a behavioural programme based on social cognitive theory and it was administered in the home two weeks after discharge with regular follow-up. After one year, patients in the intervention group decreased their fat intake, while those in the usual care control group demonstrated an increase. The prevalence of smoking decreased from 24 per cent at baseline to 8 per cent at one year in the intervention group, with little change in the control group, while the quit rate was 64 per cent in the intervention group, compared with 55 per cent in the control group.

Another example of theory-based designs to improve CAD self-management is the MULTIFIT intervention, based on social cognitive theory, in which nurse case-management directed at improving a number of cardiac risk factors post acute MI (smoking, dietary intake, exercise, lipid-lowering drug therapy), was successful in increasing smoking cessation, lowering lipid levels and improving functional capacity (DeBusk, 1994; DeBusk 1996; Miller et al. 1996).

Other interventions have adopted a cognitive-behavioural approach. Moore et al. (2005, 2007) evaluated a cognitive-behavioural intervention for refractory angina. This intervention involved identification of misconceptions and associated maladaptive behaviours (i.e. those which increase the risk of MI), challenging patients' beliefs and offering evidence-based alternative explanations for their symptoms. All patients set a personal objective, received stress management advice and relaxation training and agreed to undertake a graduated home exercise programme. In a pre-post comparison of the 12 months prior to and following enrolment, the intervention was found to improve quality of life, and to reduce angina frequency, anxiety, depression and hospital admissions.

One intervention based on the self-regulatory model (see Chapter 3) aimed to alter participants' perceptions of their MI (Petrie et al. 2002). Compared with the control group, intervention participants had a stronger belief that their illness could be controlled and maintained lower levels of distress about symptoms. They also were less likely to believe that their illness would have serious consequences and last a long time or indefinitely. Intervention group participants returned to work earlier than those in the control group and reported a lower rate of angina symptoms at the three-month follow-up. There were no significant differences between the groups in rehabilitation attendance.

Most interventions that address secondary prevention of CAD are multicomponent programmes that target several aspects of self-management. However, a programme that requires special mention is the Enhancing Recovery in Coronary Heart Disease Patients (ENRICHD) Randomized Trial (Berkman et al. 2003). Depression and low perceived social support after MI are associated with higher morbidity and mortality; therefore, this study examined whether mortality and recurrent MI were reduced by treatment of depression and low perceived social support. The intervention involved cognitive behaviour therapy (CBT) and, in those patients who scored highly on a depression scale, initiation of anti-depressant medication. Improvements in depression and perceived social support were found but these did not translate into improvements in event-free survival. However, intervention patients whose depression responded to treatment were at lower risk of late mortality (≥6 months after MI) than those whose depression did not improve (Carney et al. 2004).

These examples demonstrate the variety of approaches to improving outcomes for CAD that come under the heading cardiac rehabilitation. With an intervention as complex as cardiac rehabilitation, the mechanism(s) by which successful outcomes are achieved are not necessarily clear. A meta-analysis by Clark et al. (2005) concluded that secondary prevention programmes reduce the risk of subsequent MI and mortality; however, the optimal mix of intervention, including duration and frequency remains unclear.

Some of the challenges to improve self-management of CAD involve exploring different ways to improve uptake and adherence to cardiac rehabilitation. It is also important to explore the suitability of other models of delivering interventions to enhance self-management that may be more attractive to those participants who currently choose not to attend existing programmes.

Community-based interventions

Public health programmes offer an additional way in which self-management of CAD could be supported. A community-based focus to encourage secondary prevention moves away from the high-risk, individual focused and clinically based approach towards public health interventions where the population becomes the basis for primary prevention strategies through targeted improvement in risk factors for CAD. Epidemiological evidence, combined with demographic trends and some successful outcomes from these population-based studies, provide compelling rationales for this focus. The most frequently occurring and modifiable risk factors for CAD-related morbidity and mortality are lifestyle factors which are often shaped by environmental determinants and/or policies; thus, addressing secondary prevention from the community level may be particularly helpful.

Community-based interventions targeting secondary prevention and self-management of coronary heart disease range from government-led campaigns that focus on salt reduction, community-wide nutritional interventions that target components of risk reduction (e.g. in Mauritius, the government has spearheaded a campaign to encourage the use of soy instead of palm oil), attempts to encourage consumers to switch back to more traditional rather than processed foods, government mandates to limit salt content or transfats in the food industry, and government labelling of food products that provide information about sodium and fat content (World Health Organization 2004).

Since the 1970s, there have been a number of public health community-level interventions aimed at primary and secondary prevention of cardiovascular disease, some of which provide empirical evidence of community-wide behavioural change (Stone et al 1997). More than three decades' worth of community prevention trials suggest that organizing communities, educating through mass and direct education, providing screenings for risk factors, and changing environments through local programmes and policies can change behaviours (Pearson et al. 2001). For example, in response to having the highest heart attack rate globally, the North Karelia Project

(Finland) used local worksite approaches, national media broadcasts that have targeted smoking and offered guidance about health, and national 'quit and win' contests. After one decade of the project, CVD mortality declined by 55 per cent and 68 per cent for men and women, respectively, primarily attributable to dramatic dietary changes (Sorenson et al. 1998). Unfortunately, many of these programmes often lack published data including their details and effectiveness (Cooper et al. 2000). As one researcher lamented, 'Our review of community prevention trials, however, revealed inadequate information about how program components achieved their effects' (Schooler et al. 1997).

Conclusions and future directions

Our review of research on CAD self-management leads us to several conclusions. First, providers and patients must be proactive in their initial management of cardiovascular disease, attending to both primary prevention and acute health concerns. However, secondary prevention and self-management of chronic conditions promise to occupy an ever growing component of CAD prevention and management.

Medical management and self-management of CAD increasingly takes place within the context of controlling multiple chronic conditions over a prolonged period among diverse populations. At least 63 per cent of older adults have at least two chronic conditions and acknowledging the complexities of these sometimes competing regimens is important in optimizing self-management. The benefits of secondary prevention programmes need to reach beyond a small selection of eligible patients and encompass those from more socio-economically, ethnically and nationally diverse groups. Finally, creating and sustaining partnerships with health care providers, families and patients is key, for example, through shared decision-making. These cannot be viewed as add-ons or 'by the way' messages during patient counselling.

Approaches to improve participation in cardiac rehabilitation programmes are needed as are ways of supporting self-management for those who would prefer not to attend these programmes. Although we have discussed self-management, decisions made outside of the clinical environment are heavily shaped by household setting, access to resources like healthy foods and safe exercise locations, and larger policies like smoking bans. Addressing multiple levels of health influences holds promise for secondary prevention and improved self-management for coronary artery disease.

References

Ades, P.A. (2001) Cardiac rehabilitation and secondary prevention of coronary heart disease, *The New England Journal of Medicine*, 345(12): 892–902.

Allen, J.K. (1996) Coronary risk factor modification in women after coronary artery bypass surgery, *Nursing Research*, 45(5): 260–65.

Allender, S., Peto, V., Scarborough, P., Boxer, A. and Rayner, M. (2007) *Coronary Heart Disease Statistics*. London: British Heart Foundation.

American Heart Association (2006) *Cardiovascular Disease Statistics* (www.american-heart.org).

American Public Health Association (2006) (Publication no. http://www.apha.org/NPHW/facts/Heart-PHW04_Facts.pdf).

Balady, G.J., Williams, M.A., Ades, P.A., Bittner, Ve., Comoss, P., Foody, J.M., Franklin, B., Sanderson, B. and Southard, D. (2007) Core components of cardiac rehabilitation/secondary prevention programs: 2007 update: a scientific statement from the American Heart Association Exercise, Cardiac Rehabilitation, and Prevention Committee, the Council on Clinical Cardiology; the Councils on Cardiovascular Nursing, Epidemiology and Prevention, and Nutrition, Physical Activity, and Metabolism; and the American Association of Cardiovascular and Pulmonary Rehabilitation, *Circulation*, 115(20): 2675–82.

Berkman, L.F., Blumenthal, J., Burg, M., Carney, R.M., Catellier, D., Cowan, M.J., Czajkowski, S.M., DeBusk, R., Hosking, J., Jaffe, A., Kaufmann, P.G., Mitchell, P., Norman, J., Powell, L.H., Raczynski, J.M. and Schneiderman, N. (2003) Effects of treating depression and low perceived social support on clinical events after myocardial infarction: the Enhancing Recovery in Coronary Heart Disease Patients (ENRICHD) Randomized Trial, *JAMA*, 289(23): 3106–16.

Beswick, A.D., Rees, K., West, R.R., Taylor, F.C., Burke, M., Griebsch, I., Taylor, R.S., Victory, J., Brown, J. and Ebrahim, S. (2005) Improving uptake and adherence in cardiac rehabilitation: literature review, *Journal of Advanced Nursing*, 49(5): 538–55.

Bethell, H.J., Evans, J.A., Turner, S.C., & Lewin, R.J. (2007) The rise and fall of cardiac rehabilitation in the United Kingdom since 1998. Journal of Public Health, 29, (1): 57–61.

Bittner, V. and Sanderson, B. (2006) Cardiac rehabilitation as secondary prevention center, *Coronary Artery Disease*, 17(3): 211–18.

British Association for Cardiac Rehabilitation (2007) Standards and Core Components for Cardiac Rehabilitation (www.bcs.com/documents/affiliates/bacr/BACR%20Standards%202007.pdf).

Broadbent, E., Petrie, K.J., Ellis, C. J., Anderson, J., Gamble, G., Anderson, D. and Benjamin, W. (2006) Patients with acute myocardial infarction have an inaccurate understanding of their risk of a future cardiac event, *Internal Medicine Journal*, 36(10): 643–47.

Bunker, S., McBurney, H., Cox, H. and Jelinek, M. (1999) Identifying participation rates at outpatient cardiac rehabilitation programs in Victoria, Australia, *Journal of Cardiopulmonary Rehabilitation*, 19(6): 334–38.

Byrne, M., Walsh, J. and Murphy, A.W. (2005) Secondary prevention of coronary heart disease: patient beliefs and health-related behaviour, *Journal of Psychosomatic Research*, 58(5): 403–15.

Carlson, J.J., Johnson, J.A., Franklin, B.A. and VanderLaan, R.L. (2000) Program participation, exercise adherence, cardiovascular outcomes, and program cost of traditional versus modified cardiac rehabilitation, *The American Journal of Cardiology*, 86(1): 17–23.

Carney, R.M., Blumenthal, J.A., Freedland, K.E., Youngblood, M., Veith, R.C., Burg, M.M., Cornell, C., Saab, P.G., Kaufmann, P.G., Czajkowski, S.M. and Jaffe, A.S. (2004) Depression and late mortality after myocardial infarction in the Enhancing Recovery in Coronary Heart Disease (ENRICHD) study, *Psychosomatic Medicine*, 66(4): 466–74.

Centers for Disease Control and Prevention (2008) Receipt of outpatient cardiac rehabilitation among heart attack survivors – United States, 2005, *MMWR Morbidity and Mortality Weekly Report*, 57(4): 89–94.

Clark, A.M., Hartling, L., Vandermeer, B. and McAlister, F.A. (2005) Meta-analysis: secondary prevention programs for patients with coronary artery disease, *Annals of Internal Medicine*, 143(9): 659–72.

Cooper, A.F., Jackson, G., Weinman, J. and Horne, R. (2002) Factors associated with cardiac rehabilitation attendance: a systematic review of the literature, *Clinical Rehabilitation*, 16(5): 541–52.

Cooper, A.F., Weinman, J., Hankins, M., Jackson, G. and Horne, R. (2007) Assessing patients' beliefs about cardiac rehabilitation as a basis for predicting attendance after acute myocardial infarction, *Heart*, 93(1): 53–58.

Cooper, R., Cutler, J., Desvigne-Nickens, P., Fortmann, S.P., Friedman, L. and Havlik, R. et al. (2000) Trends and disparities in coronary heart disease, stroke, and other cardiovascular diseases in the United States, *Circulation*, 102: 3137–47.

Daly, J., Sindone, A.P., Thompson, D.R., Hancock, K., Chang, E. and Davidson, P. (2002) Barriers to participation in and adherence to cardiac rehabilitation programs: a critical literature review, *Progress in Cardiovascular Nursing*, 17(1): 8–17.

Davies, A.R., Smeeth, L. and Grundy, E.M. (2007) Contribution of changes in incidence and mortality to trends in the prevalence of coronary heart disease in the UK: 1996-2005, *European Heart Journal*, 28(17): 2142–47.

De Backer, G., Ambrosioni, E., Borch-Johnsen, K., Brotons, C., Cifkova, R., Dallon-geville, J., Ebrahim, S., Faergeman, O., Graham, I., Mancia, G., Manger-Cats, V., Orth-Gomer, K., Perk, J., Pyorala, K., Rodicio, J.L., Sans, S., Sansoy, V., Sechtem, U., Silber, S., Thomsen, T. and Wood, D. (2003) European guidelines on cardiovascular disease prevention in clinical practice. Third Joint Task Force of European and Other Societies on Cardiovascular Disease Prevention in Clinical Practice, *European Heart Journal*, 24(17): 1601–10.

DeBusk, R.F. (1996) MULTIFIT: a new approach to risk factor modification, *Cardiology Clinics*, 14(1): 143–57.

DeBusk, R.F., Miller, N.H., Superko, H.R., Dennis, C.A., Thomas, R.J., Lew, H.T. et al. (1994) A case-management system for coronary risk factor modification after acute myocardial infarction, *Annals of Internal Medicine*, 120(9): 721–29.

Dunbar-Jacobs, J., Bohachick, P., Mortimer, M., Sereika, S. and Foley, S. (2003) Medication adherence in persons with cardiovascular disease, *Journal of Cardiovascular Nursing*, 18(3): 209–18.

French, D.P., Cooper, A. and Weinman, J. (2006) Illness perceptions predict attendance at cardiac rehabilitation following acute myocardial infarction: a systematic review with meta-analysis, *Journal of Psychosomatic Research*, 61(6): 757–67.

Furze, G., Lewin, R.J., Murberg, T., Bull, P. and Thompson, D.R. (2005) Does it matter what patients think? The relationship between changes in patients' beliefs about angina and their psychological and functional status, *Journal of Psychosomatic Research*, 59(5): 323–29.

Gaziano, J.M., Manson, J.E. and Ridker, P.M. (2008) Primary and secondary prevention of coronary heart disease, in P. Libby et al. (eds) *Braunwald's Heart Disease: A Textbook of Cardiovascular Medicine* (8th edn) (pp. 1057–84), Philadelphia PA: Elsevier Saunders.

Gehi, A., Haas, D., Pipkin, S. and Whooley, M.A. (2005) Depression and medication adherence in outpatients with coronary heart disease: findings from the Heart and Soul Study, *Archives of Internal Medicine*, 165(21): 2508–13.

Grover, S.A., Paquet, S., Levington, C., Coupal, L. and Zowall, H. (1998) Estimating the benefits of modifying risk factors of cardiovascular disease, *Archives of Internal Medicine*, 158: 655–62.

Haugbolle, L.S., Sorensen, E.W. and Henriksen, H.H. (2002) Medication- and illness-related factual knowledge, perceptions and behaviour in angina pectoris patients, *Patient Education and Counseling*, 47(4): 281–89.

Hu, F.B. et al. (2000) Trends in the incidence of coronary heart disease and changes in diet and lifestyle in women, *The New England Journal of Medicine*, 343(8): 530–37.

Huffman, J.C., Smith, F.A., Blais, M.A., Beiser, M.E., Januzzi, J.L. and Fricchione, G.L. (2006) Recognition and treatment of depression and anxiety in patients with acute myocardial infarction, *The American Journal of Cardiology*, 98(3): 319–24.

Jackson, L., Leclerc, J., Erskine, Y. and Linden, W. (2005) Getting the most out of cardiac rehabilitation: a review of referral and adherence predictors, *Heart*, 91(1): 10–14.

Jolly, K., Bradley, F., Sharp, S., Smith, H., Thompson, S., Kinmonth, A.L. and Mant, D. (1999) Randomised controlled trial of follow up care in general practice of patients with myocardial infarction and angina: final results of the Southampton Heart Integrated Care Project (SHIP). The SHIP Collaborative Group, *British Medical Journal of Clinical Research*, 318(7185): 706–11.

Jones, M., Jolly, K., Raftery, J., Lip, G.Y. and Greenfield, S. (2007) DNA may not mean 'did not participate': a qualitative study of reasons for non-adherence at home- and centre-based cardiac rehabilitation, *Family Practice*, 24(4): 343–57.

Lane, D., Carroll, D., Ring, C., Beevers, D.G. and Lip, G.Y.H. (2002) The prevalence and persistence of depression and anxiety following myocardial infarction, *British Journal of Health Psychology*, 7(1): 11–21.

Lane, D., Carroll, D. and Lip, G.Y.H. (2003) Anxiety, depression, and prognosis after myocardial infarction: is there a causal association? *Journal of the American College of Cardiology*, 42(10): 1808–10.

Lewin, B., Robertson, I.H., Cay, E.L., Irving, J.B. and Campbell, M. (1992) Effects of self-help post-myocardial-infarction rehabilitation on psychological adjustment and use of health services, *The Lancet*, 339(8800): 1036–40.

Marmot, M.G., Shipley, M.J. and Rose, G. (1984) Inequalities in death – specific explanations of a general pattern? *The Lancet*, 1(8384): 1003–06.

Marmot, M.G., Bosma, H., Hemingway, H., Brunner, E. and S.S. (1997). Contribution of job control and other risk factors to social variations in coronary heart disease incidence, *The Lancet*, 350: 235–39.

Miller, N.H., Warren, D. and Myers, D. (1996) Home-based cardiac rehabilitation and lifestyle modification: the MULTIFIT model, *Journal of Cardiovascular Nursing*, 11(1): 76–87.

Moore, R.K., Groves, D., Bateson, S., Barlow, P., Hammond, C., Leach, A.A. and Chester, M.R. (2005) Health related quality of life of patients with refractory angina before and one year after enrolment onto a refractory angina program, *European Journal of Pain*, 9(3): 305–10.

Moore, R.K., Groves, D.G., Bridson, J.D., Grayson, A.D., Wong, H., Leach, A., Lewin, R.J. and Chester, M.R. (2007) A brief cognitive-behavioral intervention reduces hospital admissions in refractory angina patients, *Journal of Pain and Symptom Management*, 33(3): 310–16.

National Heart Foundation of Australia and the Cardiac Society of Australia and New Zealand (2007) Reducing Risk in Heart Disease 2007: A summary guide for preventing cardiovascular events in people with coronary heart disease, National Heart Foundation of Australia and the Cardiac Society of Australia and New Zealand.

National Institutes of Health (1999) National conference explores CVD trends (electronic version), NIH Record, 51.

Pearson, T.A., Wall, S., Lewis, C., Jenkins, P., Nafziger, A. and Weinehall, L. (2001) Describing the 'Black Box' of community intervention: lessons from community-wide cardiovascular disease prevention programs in the United States and Sweden, *Scandavian Journal of Public Health*, 29 (Suppl. 56): 69–78.

Pedersen, T., Kjekshus, J. and Berg, K. et al. (1994) Randomized trial of cholesterol lowering in 4444 patients with coronary heart disease: the Scandinavian Simvastatin Survival Study (4S), *The Lancet*, 344: 1383–89.

Petrie, K.J., Cameron, L.D., Ellis, C.J., Buick, D. and Weinman, J. (2002) Changing illness perceptions after myocardial infarction: an early intervention randomized controlled trial, *Psychosomatic Medicine*, 64(4): 580–86.

Schoenberg, N., Drew, E. and Peters, J. (2003) Unraveling the mysteries of timing: emically-derived explanations for time to treatment for women with cardiac symptoms, *Social Science and Medicine*, 56: 271–84.

Schooler, C., Farquhar, J.W., Fortmann, S.P. and Flora, J.A. (1997) Synthesis of findings and issues from community prevention trials, *Annals of Epidemiology*, S7: S54–S68.

Smith, K.M., Harkness, K. and Arthur, H.M. (2006) Predicting cardiac rehabilitation enrollment: the role of automatic physician referral, *European Journal of Cardiovascular Prevention and Rehabilitation*, 13(1): 60–66.

Sorenson, G., Emmons, K., Hunt, M. and Johnston D. (1998) Implications of the results of community intervention trials, *Annual Review of Public Health*, 19: 379–416.

Stone, E.J. and Pearson, T.A. (eds) (1997) Community trials for cardiopulmonary health: directions for public health practice, policy, and research, *Annals of Epidemiology*, S7: S1–S124.

World Health Organization (2003) Cardiovascular Disease. www.who.int/hpr/NPH/docs.gs_cvd.pdf.

World Health Organization (2004) Atlas of heart disease and stroke (www.who.int/cardiovascular_diseases/resources/atlas/en/print.html).

Wyer, S.J., Earll, L., Joseph, S., Harrison, J., Giles, M. and Johnston, M. (2001) Increasing attendance at a cardiac rehabilitation programme: an intervention study using the theory of planned behaviour, *Coronary Health Care*, 5(3): 154–59.

Yusuf, S., Reddy, S., Ounpuu, S. and Anand, S. (2001) Global burden of cardiovascular diseases: part I: general considerations, the epidemiologic transition, risk factors, and impact of urbanization, *Circulation*, 104(22): 2746–53.

14   Heart failure

Kathleen Mulligan

Nature of the illness

Heart failure is a complex clinical syndrome in which the ability of the heart to pump is impaired. This impairment can lead to a build-up of fluid in the lungs and other parts of the body, causing breathlessness and fatigue, especially on exertion, and oedema, usually of the ankles and feet. The illness has a high rate of mortality (Levy et al. 2002) and hospital admission (Cleland et al. 2003; McMurray and Pfeffer 2005) and has a major impact on quality of life (Stewart et al. 1989).

There is no simple test for heart failure; diagnosis is based on a detailed history and physical examination, supplemented by further tests (Cowie and Zaphiriou 2002). The guidelines of the European Society of Cardiology (ESC) (Remme and Swedberg 2002; Task Force for the Diagnosis and Treatment of Chronic Heart Failure 2005) specify that a diagnosis of heart failure requires fulfilment of the following criteria:

1   symptoms of heart failure (at rest or during exercise);
2   objective evidence (preferably by echocardiography) of cardiac dysfunction (at rest)

and (in cases where the diagnosis is in doubt);

3   response to treatment directed towards heart failure.

Criteria 1 and 2 should be fulfilled in all cases.

The New York Heart Association (NYHA) classification is widely used to classify severity of heart failure according to how limited patients are due to symptoms during physical activity (see Table 14.1).

Table 14.1 New York Heart Association Heart Failure Classification

Class	Symptoms
I	No limitation: ordinary physical exercise does not cause undue fatigue, dyspnoea or palpitations [patients in this class would have to have objective evidence of cardiac dysfunction and a history of symptomatic heart failure that has been treated to fulfil the diagnosis of heart failure]
II	Slight limitation of physical activity: comfortable at rest but ordinary activity results in fatigue, palpitations, or dyspnoea
III	Marked limitation of physical activity: comfortable at rest but less than ordinary activity results in symptoms
IV	Unable to carry out any physical activity without discomfort: symptoms of heart failure are present even at rest with increased discomfort with any physical activity

Heart failure can be caused by any disorder that damages the heart but the most common causes in Westernized countries are myocardial infarction and hypertension, or a combination of both. Other causes include valve disease, arrhythmias, congenital heart disease and alcoholic cardiomyopathy. Heart Failure may develop suddenly following an acute cardiac event, such as a myocardial infarction, or it may develop more slowly, over weeks or months. Heart failure is a significant public health issue with an overall prevalence of between 1–2 per cent of the adult population in developed countries, increasing with age to approximately 6–10 per cent in those aged over 65 (McMurray and Pfeffer 2005). Prevalence is likely to increase due to improved survival rates (Levy et al. 2002) and a growing elderly population, which is likely to see an associated rise in the prevalence of hypertension and coronary heart disease, two of the main risk factors for heart failure (McMurray and Stewart 2000). Increasing rates of obesity and diabetes could also lead to increases in heart failure (Kenchaiah et al. 2002; Kamalesh and Nair 2005).

The aims of treatment of heart failure are to reduce symptoms, slow progression of the disease and reduce cardiac events and mortality. Treatments include medication, implantable devices such as implantable cardiac defibrillators (IDCs) or biventricular pacemakers, and surgery. Although surgical intervention for heart failure is less widely used than pharmacological intervention, revascularization may improve symptoms in individual patients whose heart failure is ischaemic in origin (Task Force for the Diagnosis and Treatment of Chronic Heart Failure 2001, 2005). Heart transplantation is an option for some patients with end-stage heart failure but is severely restricted by the limited availability of donor hearts. Ventricular assist devices have been implanted while patients have been awaiting transplantation and there is an increasing interest in their use as a long-term treatment (Park et al. 2005). Patients with heart failure are at risk of sudden death due to ventricular arrhythmias and one study has found that an implantable cardiac defibrillator reduced the risk of death by 23 per cent (Bardy et al. 2005). In about 25 per cent of patients with heart failure, there is dyssynchronous contraction between the walls of the left ventricle, caused by abnormal electrical activation. Dyssynchrony may exacerbate cardiac dysfunction and further reduce cardiac output. Cardiac resynchronization therapy has been shown to reduce the risk of death or hospital admission in this group of patients by 37 per cent (Cleland et al. 2005). In practice, implantable devices and surgery are suitable only for a fairly small number of highly selected patients and medication forms the basis of heart failure treatment, particularly diuretics, angiotensin-converting enzyme (ACE) inhibitors, beta-blockers and spironolactone.

Demands of heart failure on the patient

There are many tasks that patients with heart failure need to perform in order to manage their illness. Self-management of the medical aspects of heart failure includes taking medication, self-monitoring to identify early signs of deterioration and making lifestyle changes. Patients usually have to take several medications for their heart failure (Komajda et al. 2003), which may include adopting a flexible diuretic regimen to adjust diuretic dose in response to signs of deterioration. In addition, they often require medication for other co-morbid conditions (Krum and Gilbert 2003). Complexity of the treatment regime may lead to difficulties for self-management which may be compounded by the fact that patients are usually elderly and some may have cognitive deficits (Almeida and Flicker 2001).

Lifestyle changes (Task Force for the Diagnosis and Treatment of Chronic Heart Failure 2001) for patients with advanced heart failure include limiting their sodium and fluid intake (although it should be noted that this advice is based mainly on consensus of opinion rather than research evidence), not smoking and moderating alcohol intake (except where heart failure is due to alcoholic cardiomyopathy, in which case they should abstain). Rest is advised during an acute exacerbation of heart failure but if patients are in a stable condition, they are encouraged to carry out usual daily physical and leisure activities that do not induce symptoms. Exercise training is encouraged in stable patients in NYHA II and III (Task Force for the Diagnosis and Treatment of Chronic Heart Failure 2001).

A significant proportion of people with heart failure do not follow self-management recommendations and a number of studies have suggested that this contributes to poor outcomes. A review of 11 studies published between 1988–2002 (van der Wal et al. 2005) considered non-adherence to medication or dietary recommendations to have contributed to worsening heart failure in between 15–64 per cent of cases. For example, Michalsen et al. (1998) classified 179 patients admitted to hospital for heart failure as 'non-compliant' if they reported taking their medication intermittently or not at all, if their fluid intake was more than 2.5 litres per day or if they regularly added salt to their food. Forty-three per cent reported excess sodium intake, 34 per cent reported excess fluid intake and 23.5 per cent reported poor adherence to medication. Potential factors precipitating the hospital admission were identified in 85.5 per cent of the study sample and non-adherence to medication or diet (excessive sodium or fluid intake) was the leading precipitating factor for hospital admission, considered to have caused 41.9 per cent of cases.

Heart failure can deteriorate rapidly making it essential to identify early signs of problems so that immediate remedial action can be taken. One of the early signs of deteriorating heart failure is weight gain caused by fluid retention; therefore, patients are advised to self-monitor by weighing themselves on a regular basis. In the event of sudden unexpected weight gain it is recommended that they alert a health care professional or adjust their diuretic medication dose accordingly (Task Force for the Diagnosis and Treatment of Chronic Heart Failure 2005). Self-monitoring for signs of fluid retention can also include checking ankles for oedema. It would appear, however, that many patients do not monitor for signs of deterioration and when symptoms such as breathlessness become worse patients often delay before seeking medical help. This can result in an admission to hospital which potentially could have been avoided by earlier action. In a study of 181 older adults admitted to hospital for heart failure, Friedman (1997) found that 91 per cent reported experiencing breathlessness for an average of three days and 35 per cent had oedema for an average of seven days before hospital admission. On admission, only 5 per cent reported weight gain as a symptom, suggesting that they had not been monitoring their weight and/or did not recognize weight gain to be an indicator of deterioration. Another study also found delays, with 28 per cent of patients waiting more than five days from the onset of worsening symptoms before seeking medical attention (Evangelista et al. 2000).

The studies outlined above deal mainly with patients' self-management of the medical aspects of heart failure. However, self-management also involves adapting one's life roles, for example learning new ways of performing everyday activities and adapting to changes in social roles. It is clear from studies that have examined quality of life (QoL) in heart failure that patients have reduced ability to perform their life roles. For example, Hobbs et al. (2002) found that, compared to the general population, patients with heart failure had significantly impaired quality of life on all eight dimensions of the Medical Outcomes Study SF-36 measure of generic health-related quality of life – physical functioning, role limitations due to physical problems, role limitations due to emotional problems, social functioning, mental health, energy, pain and overall perception of health. Nevertheless, little research to date has examined how patients adapt their life roles to manage their heart failure. A qualitative study by Stull et al. (1999) found that some patients reported having to adjust to a new lifestyle which was more restricted in the daily activities they were able to perform. Patients interviewed by Pattenden et al. (2007) reported frustration at no longer being able to do what they used to. Some patients expressed anxiety that activity could lead to an exacerbation of symptoms which resulted in them voluntarily limiting their activity levels, sometimes to the extent of becoming virtually housebound. Such restriction may be particulary difficult for younger patients to accept, which may help to explain the poorer quality of life reported by younger heart failure patients.

Self-management also involves dealing with the emotional impact of having a chronic illness. Depression has been found to be common in heart failure although reported prevalence varies, probably due to differences in the assessment and criteria for classification of depression and in the study populations. A meta-analytic review by Rutledge et al. (2006) concluded that clinically significant depression is present in at least one in five patients, ranging from 11 per cent of patients in New York Heart

Association (NYHA) classification I (asymptomatic) to 42 per cent of those in NYHA IV (symptoms of heart failure present even at rest). The review found that depression was associated with a higher risk of death and associated cardiac events. There is little research on anxiety in heart failure but in one study, 18 per cent of heart failure patients attending a community disease management programme were diagnosed with an anxiety disorder (Haworth et al. 2005). Pattenden et al. (2007) found that some patients reported being anxious weeks after an acute episode and several reported anxieties about the future. A link between anxiety and depression in heart failure has also been reported (Freedland and Carney 2000), in that anxious reactions to dyspnoea were found to be more common in depressed than non-depressed patients. Two studies that examined the relationship between mood and self-management behaviour in heart failure, not surprisingly, found that lower mood is associated with poorer self-management. Patients reporting more depressive symptoms have been found to be less likely to exercise (van der Wal et al. 2006) while better mental health and lower neuroticism are predictive of better self-management (Evangelista et al. 2001). These studies suggest that mood may be an important area to address in self-management interventions for heart failure.

Factors that may influence self-management in heart failure

Other factors besides mood can affect self-management behaviour. However, to date, research in this area is fairly limited. Studies indicate that there is not a consistent relationship between demographic factors and self-management, with the possible exception of age. Older age tends to be associated with better performance of at least some self-management behaviours; for example, adherence to medication (e.g. Evangelista et al. 2001; Artinian et al. 2002; Chriss et al. 2004).

Complexity of the medication regime may be an important factor in how effectively people self-manage (Evangelista et al. 2003). Bohachick et al. (2002) compared rates of adherence to ACE inhibitors between those whose prescriptions were for once, twice or three to four times a day and found rates of 90 per cent, 84 per cent and 68 per cent, respectively. More demanding and complex regimens may be more difficult to remember and implement correctly. Simplification of the treatment regime, where possible, is clearly important to facilitate self-management along with the development of strategies to help patients to manage and remember their medication.

Poor knowledge of the rationale and importance of recommended self-management behaviours is common (Ni et al. 1999; Riegel and Carlson 2002). However, among patients with heart failure, in common with other chronic illnesses, there is not a strong relationship between knowledge and self-management. For example, Michalsen et al. (1998) found that levels of knowledge about medication were similar among adherent and non-adherent patients. In a study by Ni et al. (1999), of those patients who considered daily weight monitoring to be important, only 58 per cent weighed themselves daily and 14 per cent weighed themselves once a month or less. While it is important that patients receive clear information about the recommended self-management behaviours, the findings of these studies indicate that interventions to improve self-management will need to go beyond improving knowledge of the recommended behaviours.

Patients may hold misconceptions about heart failure which influence their self-management. For example, Horowitz et al. (2004) found that patients' understanding of their heart failure lacked depth and breadth such that they did not make the connection between the disease and their chronic symptoms and were unable to give an explanation of what caused their heart failure or its symptoms. As a consequence, they did not recognize that they could minimize fluid build-up and detect signs of deterioration through self-management practices. For example, some patients who held an acute model of their heart failure thought they needed to take diuretic medication only when their symptoms became severe. Lack of a coherent understanding of the connection between the disease and its symptoms meant that signs of deterioration such as weight gain, breathlessness or oedema were not necessarily followed by an appropriate response. Few patients self-monitored for signs of deterioration, by regular weighing for example, but took action only once their symptoms had become severe enough to require emergency medical care. Horowitz et al. concluded that patients mostly held a model of heart failure as an acute condition with episodic exacerbations rather than a chronic condition requiring continuous monitoring and self-management.

Patients' beliefs about the value of their treatment are also important. Van der Wal et al. (2006) found that patients who perceived benefits from their diet and medication were more likely to perform recommended health behaviours. In a clinical trial of beta-blockers, lack of belief at baseline that the study medication would make them feel better was a strong predictor of withdrawal from the trial (Ekman et al. 2006). These studies highlight how the beliefs patients hold about their heart failure and its treatment may influence self-management. Therefore self-management interventions in heart failure should have as one of their goals the modifying of potentially unhelpful beliefs.

Beliefs about self-efficacy; that is, confidence that one can perform a behaviour, have been found to be important in self-management of other chronic illnesses. A positive relationship between self-efficacy and self-management behaviour has also been found in heart failure (Ni et al. 1999, Joekes et al. 2007; Schweitzer et al. 2007) suggesting that strategies that help to enhance self-efficacy may also be an important component in self-management interventions.

The studies outlined above indicate that cognitions and beliefs may be important in self-management of heart failure. Research in this area is nevertheless at a very early stage with relatively little known about the beliefs that patients hold about their heart failure or their ability to manage it. This area requires further exploration to improve our understanding of the role of cognitions and beliefs in self-management of heart failure and how they can be targeted in interventions.

Interventions to improve self-management of heart failure

Over the past 10–15 years, management of heart failure has undergone a significant change with the widespread introduction of disease management programmes

(Bruggink-Andre-de-la-Porte et al. 2005; Gonseth et al. 2004; Gustafsson and Arnold 2004; Gwadry-Sridhar et al. 2004; Holland et al. 2005; McAlister et al. 2001; McAlister et al. 2004; Philbin 1999; Phillips et al. 2004; Phillips et al. 2005; Rich 1999; Roccaforte et al. 2005; Whellan et al. 2005; Windham et al. 2003). Facilitating behaviour change to enhance self-management is, however, a fairly undeveloped part of these programmes. Although most include a patient education component geared towards improving patient performance of recommended self-management behaviours, it is not their main focus. The primary aim of the programmes is to improve the delivery of clinical care, usually through optimization of heart failure medication and frequent follow-up by a health care professional, typically a heart failure nurse specialist. The education component usually follows a traditional didactic approach of providing information and advice, although this may be accompanied by charts to help patients to remember their medication and to facilitate self-monitoring. Change in self-management behaviour is rarely measured therefore it is not known if the programmes have any effect on self-management nor if any impact on health outcomes, for example, hospitalization, is due to a change in self-management behaviour. These interventions therefore do not tell us if improving patient self-management can help to improve outcomes further for heart failure patients, over and above what has been achieved by improving delivery of care with more intensive disease management programmes.

Advice regarding physical activity is a further common component of traditional heart failure programmes, although typically independent of behaviour change strategies. Randomized trials have shown that regular exercise can safely improve peak oxygen uptake and strength (McKelvie et al. 2002), symptoms (Corvera-Tindel et al. 2004) and quality of life (Belardinelli et al. 1999) and it is encouraged in stable patients in NYHA II and III. Exercise training forms one of the recommended core components of rehabilitation programmes for heart failure (Corra et al. 2005), along with education and psychological support. These recommendations appear to recognize the need for broader interventions in heart failure.

To date, only a small number of interventions have adopted a broader self-management approach, in that they included components other than knowledge to facilitate behaviour change. Advice about self-monitoring for early signs of deteriorating heart failure is a fairly standard component but inclusion of strategies to facilitate this behaviour change is more variable. Some provide education but incorporate no behaviour change techniques (e.g. Linne et al. 1999; Gwadry-Sridhar et al. 2005). Others go beyond simple education but use fairly limited behaviour change techniques. For example, Caldwell et al. (2005) included discussion of potential barriers to performance of recommended behaviours and De Walt et al. (2004, 2006) included an action plan for diuretic adjustment based on daily weight and a brainstorming session about ways to reduce salt intake. Not all studies that focus on self-management behaviour assess behaviour change but those that have generally report improvements in at least some of the behaviours (e.g. Arcand et al. 2005; Caldwell et al. 2005; DeWalt et al. 2006; Jaarsma et al. 1999; Koelling et al. 2005).

More complex interventions include that by Kuehneman et al. (2002) who used problem-solving and goal-setting in a nutrition programme. Participants in this pre-post trial reduced their sodium and fluid intake and reported improved quality of life. Dunbar et al. (2005) conducted a pilot study aimed at reducing dietary sodium. They compared a group who received education with one who, in addition to the education intervention, also received sessions that focused on enhancing family support by developing communication techniques. There was a greater decrease in dietary sodium in the family support group. Shively et al. (2005) developed a behavioural management programme that included self-monitoring, goal-setting and cognitive and behavioural skills. The intervention group reported significantly improved disease-specific quality of life compared to the control group. However, there was no significant difference between the groups in quality of life as assessed by the SF-36 on both the physical or mental quality of life subscales or on general health perceptions. Studies for which intervention descriptions have been published but findings are still awaited include the Heart Failure Adherence and Retention Trial, a group programme that focuses on five self-management skills to help build and maintain self-efficacy (Flynn et al. 2005; Rucker-Whitaker et al. 2006), a group programme which emphasizes goal-setting and the planning of behaviour (Schreurs et al. 2003) and an evaluation of the Chronic Disease Self-Management Programme (see Chapter 5), led by a heart failure nurse as well as a lay person (Smeulders et al. 2006).

An important question is the extent to which studies that have focused on self-management behaviours succeed in improving clinical outcomes. A meta-analytic review by McAlister et al. (2004) concluded that programmes which 'enhanced patient self-care activities' reduced hospital admissions. This was, however, based on only four studies. A more recent review (Jovicic et al. 2006), which pooled the effects of just six interventions, concluded that this type of study decreased all-cause hospital readmissions and heart failure readmissions but not mortality. Not all interventions report both self-management behaviour and health outcomes. To gain a better understanding of whether these interventions change behaviour and, as a result, improve clinical outcomes, it is necessary to measure both.

A further issue is the impact such interventions have on mood, given the prevalence of depression and anxiety in heart failure. Improvements in patients' ability to manage their illness may be expected to have some beneficial effect on mood. Two of the ongoing programmes outlined above (Schreurs et al. 2003; Smeulders et al. 2006) include sessions that deal with emotions but few other interventions have addressed emotional aspects of heart failure self-management. A Cochrane review of psychological interventions for depression in heart failure published up to 2003 failed to identify a single randomized controlled trial (Lane et al. 2005). A small pre-post study by Kostis et al. (1994) examined an intervention that included components of cognitive therapy and stress management along with exercise and dietary change. Improvements in depression and anxiety were reported at the end of the 12-week intervention. A pilot study ($n = 14$) of stress management training (Luskin et al. 1999) did not report any improvement in depression or anxiety but did find a reduction in perceived stress. Although Mårtensson et al. (2005) assessed change in depression, it is unclear what techniques their intervention included that specifically targeted managing the emotional aspects of living with heart failure. Patients in the control group were more likely to experience moderate or severe depression at the three-month follow-up but by twelve months there was no significant difference between the groups. Cole et al. (2006) piloted a disease management programme for patients with heart failure and depression. In addition to changes in the delivery of clinical care and support services, the intervention included regular telephone calls from a nurse care manager, which were intended to provide self-management support. However, the techniques used by the nurse to facilitate self-management were not reported so it is not possible to tell in what way this aspect of the intervention addressed depression. In summary, the management of the emotional aspects of living with heart failure remain to be adequately addressed and interventions need to incorporate components that can help improve people's ability to cope with their illness.

Heart failure self-management in the health care system

Integration of heart failure self-management into the broader health care system has been tried in one programme in the USA. Based on Wagner's chronic care model (Wagner et al. 1996) the Chronic Illness Care Breakthrough Series Collaboratives involve health care teams to implement changes in the delivery of care (Glasgow et al. 2002). Self-management support is an important feature of the model and the programme includes skills development for staff in collaborative goal-setting, problem-solving, group facilitation and counselling skills. Nine of the fourteen participating health care teams provided self-management data for heart failure, which showed that self-monitoring of weight increased from 19 per cent at baseline to 93 per cent at follow-up.

Another important issue for translating self-management into the broader health care context is that most interventions have been delivered by heart failure nurse specialists. Currently, nurses and most other health care professionals do not receive training in facilitating behaviour change (Whitehead 2001). If interventions that adopt self-management techniques are to become more widespread in heart failure, then it is essential that the staff delivering the interventions receive training in the techniques required to encourage the development of self-management behaviours (see Chapter 6).

Conclusion

At present, self-management interventions for heart failure are relatively undeveloped; therefore, the efficacy of this approach in improving outcomes for people with heart failure remains unproven. The many disease management programmes that have been implemented typically combine changes in the delivery of care with education in a single package. The implicit model underlying most education interventions is that informing patients about the recommended self-management behaviours will be sufficient to bring about behaviour change. Even studies that appear to recognize that the issue is more complex do not necessarily make use of the extensive literature on health behaviour change and self-management of other chronic illnesses. Existing interventions are mostly limited to dealing with only the medical aspects of the illness. It is important that broader interventions that address all aspects of self-management are developed and evaluated, and it is encouraging that some interventions which are currently undergoing evaluation have adopted this approach.

References

Almeida, O. and Flicker, L. (2001) The mind of a failing heart: a systematic review of the association between congestive heart failure and cognitive functioning, *Internal Medicine Journal*, 31: 290–95.

Arcand, J. A., Brazel, S., Joliffe, C., Choleva, M., Berkoff, F., Allard, J. P., & Newton, G. E. (2005) Education by a dietitian in patients with heart failure results in improved adherence with a sodium-restricted diet: a randomized trial. American Heart Journal, 150 (4) : 716.e1–716.e5

Artinian, N. T., Magnan, M., Sloan, M., & Lange, M. P. (2002) Self-care behaviors among patients with heart failure., Heart and Lung, 31(3):161–172.

Bardy, G. H., Lee, K. L., Mark, D. B., Poole, J. E., Packer, D. L., Boineau, R., Domanski, M., Troutman, C., Anderson, J., Johnson, G., McNulty, S. E., Clapp-Channing, N., Davidson-Ray, L. D., Fraulo, E. S., Fishbein, D. P., Luceri, R. M., Ip, J. H., & the Sudden Cardiac Death in Heart Failure Trial (SCD-HeFT) Investigators (2005). Amiodarone or an Implantable Cardioverter-Defibrillator for Congestive Heart Failure. New England Journal of Medicine, 352 (3): 225–237.

Belardinelli, R., Georgiou, D., Cianci, G. and Purcaro, A. (1999) Randomized, controlled trial of long-term moderate exercise training in chronic heart failure, *Circulation*, 99: 1173–82.

Bohachick, P., Burke, L. E., Sereika, S., Murali, S., & Dunbar-Jacob, J. (2002) Adherence to angiotensin-converting enzyme inhibitor therapy for heart failure. Progress in Cardiovascular Nursing, 17 (4): 160–166.

Bruggink-Andre-de-la-Porte, Lok, D.J., van Wijngaarden, J., Cornel, J.H., Pruijsers-Lamers, D., van Veldhuisen, D.J. and Hoes, A.W. (2005) Heart failure programmes in countries with a primary care-based health care system: are additional trials necessary? Design of the DEAL-HF study, *European Journal of Heart Failure Journal of the Working Group on Heart Failure of the European Society of Cardiology*, 7(5): 910–20.

Caldwell, M.A., Peters, K.J., & Dracup, K.A. (2005) A simplified education program improves knowledge, self-care behaviour, and disease severity in heart failure patients in rural settings. American Heart Journal, 180(b); 983.e7–983.e12,

Chriss, P. M., Sheposh, J., Carlson, B., & Riegel, B. (2004) Predictors of successful heart failure self-care maintenance in the first three months after hospitalization. Heart and Lung, 33 (6): 345–353.

Cleland, J.G.F., Daubert, J.C., Erdmann, E., Freemantle, N., Gras, D., Kappenberger, L., Tavazzi, L. (2005) The effect of cardiac resynchronization on morbidity and mortality in heart faliure. *New England Journal of Medicine*, 352: 1539–1549.

Cleland, J.G.F., Swedberg, K., Follath, F., Komajda, M., Cohen-Solal, A., Aguilar, J.C., Dietz, R., Gavazzi, A., Hobbs, R., Korewicki, J., Madeira, H.C., Moiseyev, V.S., Preda, I., van Gilst, W.H., Widimsky, J., for the Study Group on Diagnosis of the Working Group on Heart Failure of the European Society of Cardiology, Freemantle, N., Eastaugh, J. and Mason, J. (2003) The EuroHeart Failure survey programme – a survey on the quality of care among patients with heart failure in Europe. Part 1: patient characteristics and diagnosis, *European Heart Journal*, 24(5): 442–63.

Cole, S. A., Farber, N. C., Weiner, J. S., Sulfaro, M., Katzelnick, D. J., & Blader, J. C. (2006) Double-disease management or one care manager for two chronic conditions: pilot feasibility study of nurse telephonic disease management for depression and congestive heart failure. Disease management, 9 (5): 266–276.

Corra, U., Giannuzzi, P., Adamopoulos, S., & Bjornstad, H. (2005) Executive summary of the Position Paper of the Working Group on Cardiac Rehabilitation and Exercise Physiology of the European Society of Cardiology (ESC): core components of cardiac rehabilitation in chronic heart failure. European Journal of Cardiovascular Prevention and Rehabilitation, 12 (4): 321–325.

Corvera-Tindel, T., Doering, L. V., Woo, M. A., Khan, S., & Dracup, K. (2004) Effects of a home walking exercise program on functional status and symptoms in heart failure. American Heart Journal, 147, (2): 339–346.

Cowie M.R. and Zaphiriou A. (2002) Management of chronic heart failure. British Medical Journal. 325: 422–425.

DeWalt, D. A., Pignone, M., Malone, R., Rawls, C., Kosnar, M. C., George, G., Bryant, B., Rothman, R. L., & Angel, B. (2004) Development and pilot testing of a disease management program for low literacy patients with heart failure. Patient Education and Counseling, 55 (1): 78–86.

DeWalt, D. A., Malone, R. M., Bryant, M. E., Kosnar, M. C., Corr, K. E., Rothman, R. L., Sueta, C. A., & Pignone, M. P. (2006) A heart failure self-management program for patients of all literacy levels: a randomized, controlled trial. BMC Health Services Research, 6: 30.

Dunbar, S. B., Clark, P. C., Deaton, C., Smith, A. L., De, A. K., & O'Brien, M. C. (2005) Family education and support interventions in heart failure: a pilot study. Nursing Research, 54 (3): 158–166.

Ekman, I., Andersson, G., Boman, K., Charlesworth, A., Cleland, J.G.F., Poole-Wilson, P. and Swedberg, K. (2006) Adherence and perception of medication in patients with chronic heart failure during a five-year randomised trial, *Patient Education and Counseling*, 61(3): 348–53.

Evangelista, L., Doering, L.V., Dracup, K., Westlake, C., Hamilton, M. and Fonarow, G.C. (2003) Compliance behaviors of elderly patients with advanced heart failure, *Journal of Cardiovascular Nursing*, 18(3): 197–206.

Evangelista, L.S., Berg, J. and Dracup, K. (2001) Relationship between psychosocial variables and compliance in patients with heart failure, *Heart & Lung*, 30(4): 294–301.

Evangelista, L.S., Dracup, K. and Doering, L.V. (2000) Treatment-seeking delays in heart failure patients, *Journal of Heart and Lung Transplantation*, 19(10): 932–38.

Flynn, K. J., Powell, L. H., Mendes-de-Leon, C. F., Munoz, R., Eaton, C. B., Downs, D. L., Silver, M. A., & Calvin, J. E. (2005) Increasing self-management skills in heart failure patients: a pilot study. Congestive Heart Failure, 11 (6): 297–302.

Freedland, K.E. and Carney, R.M. (2000) Psychosocial considerations in elderly patients with heart failure, *Clinics in Geriatric Medicine*, 16(3): 649–61.

Friedman, M.M. (1997) Older adults' symptoms and their duration before hospitalization for heart failure, *Heart & Lung: The Journal of Acute and Critical Care*, 26(3): 169–76.

Glasgow, R. E., Funnell, M. M., Bonomi, A. E., Davis, C., Beckham, V., & Wagner, E. H. (2002) Self-management aspects of the improving chronic illness care breakthrough series: implementation with diabetes and heart failure teams. Annals of Behavioral Medicine, 24 (2): 80–87.

Gonseth, J., Guallar-Castillon, P., Banegas, J.R. and Rodriguez-Artalejo, F. (2004) The effectiveness of disease management programmes in reducing hospital re-admission in older patients with heart failure: a systematic review and meta-analysis of published reports, *European Heart Journal*, 25(18): 1570–95.

Gustafsson, F. and Arnold, J.M. (2004) Heart failure clinics and outpatient management: review of the evidence and call for quality assurance, *European Heart Journal*, 25(18): 1596–604.

Gwadry-Sridhar, F.H., Flintoft, V., Lee, D.S., Lee, H. and Guyatt, G.H. (2004) A systematic review and meta-analysis of studies comparing readmission rates and mortality rates in patients with heart failure, *Archives of Internal Medicine*, 164(21): 2315–20.

Haworth, J.E., Moniz Cook, E., Clark, A.L., Wang, M., Waddington, R. and Cleland, J.G. (2005) Prevalence and predictors of anxiety and depression in a sample of chronic heart failure patients with left ventricular systolic dysfunction, *European Journal of Heart Failure*, 7(5): 803–08.

Hobbs, F. D., Kenkre, J. E., Roalfe, A. K., Davis, R. C., Hare, R., & Davies, M. K. (2002) Impact of heart failure and left ventricular systolic dysfunction on quality of life: a cross-sectional study comparing common chronic cardiac and medical disorders and a representative adult population. European Heart Journal, 23 (23): 1867–1876.

Holland, R., Battersby, J., Harvey, I., Lenaghan, E., Smith, J. and Hay, L. (2005) Systematic review of multidisciplinary interventions in heart failure, *Heart*, 91(7): 899–906.

Horowitz, C. R., Rein, S. B., & Leventhal, H. (2004) A story of maladies, misconceptions and mishaps: effective management of heart failure. Social Science and Medicine, 58 (3): 631–643.

Jaarsma, T., Halfens, R., Abu-Saad, H. H., Dracup, K., Gorgels, T., van Ree, J., & Stapers, J. (1999) Effects of education and support on self-care and resource utilization in patients with heart failure. European Heart Journal, 20: 673–682.

Joekes, K., van Elderen, T., & Schreurs, K. (2007) Self-efficacy and overprotection are related to quality of life, psychological well-being and self-management in cardiac patients. Journal of Health Psychology, 12 (1): 4–16.

Jovicic, A., Holroyd-Leduc, J. M., & Straus, S. E. (2006) Effects of self-management intervention on health outcomes of patients with heart failure: a systematic review of randomized controlled trials. BMC Cardiovascular Disorders, 6: 43.

Kamalesh, M. and Nair, G. (2005) Disproportionate increase in prevalence of diabetes among patients with congestive heart failure due to systolic dysfunction, *International Journal of Cardiology*, 99(1): 125–27.

Kenchaiah, S., Evans, J.C., Levy, D., Wilson, P.W.F., Benjamin, E.J., Larson, M.G., Kannel, W.B. and Vasan, R.S. (2002) Obesity and the risk of heart failure, *The New England Journal of Medicine*, 347(5): 305–13.

Koelling, T. M., Johnson, M. L., Cody, R. J., & Aaronson, K. D. (2005) Discharge education improves clinical outcomes in patients with chronic heart failure. Circulation, 111 (2): 179–185.

Komajda, M., Follath, F., Swedberg, K., Cleland, J., Aguilar, J.C., Cohen Solal, A., Dietz, R., Gavazzi, A., van Gilst, W.H., Hobbs, R., Korewicki, J., Madeira, H.C., Moiseyev, V.S., Preda, I., Widimsky, J., Freemantle, N., Eastaugh, J. and Mason, J. (2003) The EuroHeart Failure Survey programme – a survey on the quality of care among patients with heart failure in Europe. Part 2: treatment, *European Heart Journal*, 24(5): 464–74.

Kostis, J. B., Rosen, R. C., Cosgrove, N. M., Shindler, D. M., & Wilson, A. C. (1994) Nonpharmacologic therapy improves functional and emotional status in congestive heart failure. Chest, 106: 996–1001.

Krum, H. and Gilbert, R. (2003) Demographics and concomitant disorders in heart failure, *The Lancet*, 362: 147–58.

Kuehneman, T., Saulsbury, D., Splett, P., & Chapman, D. B. (2002) Demonstrating the impact of nutrition intervention in a heart failure program. Journal of the American Dietetic Association, 102 (12): 1790–1794.

Lane, D. A., Chong, A. Y., & Lip, G. Y. (2005) Psychological interventions for depression in heart failure. Cochrane Database of Systematic Reviews, 1: CD003329.

Levy, D., Kenchaiah, S., Larson, M.G., Benjamin, E.J., Kupka, M.J., Ho, K.K.L., Murabito, J.M. and Vasan, R.S. (2002) Long-term trends in the incidence of and survival with heart failure, *The New England Journal of Medicine*, 347(18): 1397–402.

Linne, A. B., Liedholm, H., & Israellson, B. (1999) Effects of systematic education on heart failure patients' knowledge after 6 months. A randomised, controlled trial. European Journal of Heart Failure, 1 (3): 219–227.

Luskin, F., Newell, K., & Haskel, W. (1999) Stress management training of elderly patients with congestive heart failure: Pilot study. Preventive Cardiology, 2: 101–104.

Martensson, J., Stromberg, A., Dahlstrom, U., Karlsson, J. E., & Fridlund, B. (2005) Patients with heart failure in primary health care: effects of a nurse-led intervention on health-related quality of life and depression. European Journal of Heart Failure, 7(3): 393–403.

McAlister, F. A., Lawson, F. M., Teo, K. K. and Armstrong, P. W. (2001) A systematic review of randomized trials of disease management programs in heart failure, *American Journal of Medicine*, 110(5): 378–84.

McAlister, F.A., Stewart, S., Ferrua, S. and McMurray, J.J.V. (2004) Multidisciplinary strategies for the management of heart failure patients at high risk for admission. A systematic review of randomized trials, *Journal of the American College of Cardiology*, 44(4): 810–19.

McKelvie, R. S., Teo, K. K., Roberts, R., McCartney, N., Humen, D., Montague, T., Hendrican, K., & Yusuf, S. (2002) Effects of exercise training in patients with heart failure: The Exercise Rehabilitation Trial (EXERT). American Heart Journal, 144 (1): 23–30.

McMurray, J.J. and Stewart, S. (2000) Epidemiology, aetiology, and prognosis of heart failure, *Heart*, 83(5): 596–602.

McMurray, J.J.V. and Pfeffer, M.A. (2005) Heart failure, *The Lancet*, 365: 1877–89.

Michalsen, A., Konig, G. and Thimme, W. (1998) Preventable causative factors leading to hospital admission with decompensated heart failure, *Heart*, 80: 437–41.

Ni, H., Nauman, D., Burgess, D., Wise, K., Crispell, K., & Herschberger, R. E. (1999) Factors influencing knowledge of and adherence to self-care among patients with heart failure. Archives of Internal Medicine, 159: 1613–1619.

Park, S. J., Tector, A., Piccioni, W., Raines, E., Gelijns, A., Moskowitz, A., Rose, E., Holman, W., Furukawa, S., Frazier, O. H., & Dembitsky, W. (2005) Left ventricular assist devices as destination therapy: A new look at survival. Journal of Thoracic and Cardiovascular Surgery, 129, (1): 9–17.

Pattenden, J.F., Roberts, H. and Lewin, R.J.P. (2007) Living with heart failure; patient and carer perspectives, *European Journal of Cardiovascular Nursing*, 6(4): 273–79.

Philbin, E.F. (1999) Comprehensive multidisciplinary programs for the management of patients with congestive heart failure [see comments], *Journal of International Medicine*, 14(2): 130–35.

Phillips, C.O., Wright, S.M., Kern, D.E., Singa, R.M., Shepperd, S. and Rubin, H.R. (2004) Comprehensive discharge planning with postdischarge support for older patients with congestive heart failure, *The Journal of the American Medical Association*, 291(11): 1358–67.

Phillips, C.O., Singa, R.M., Rubin, H.R. and Jaarsma, T. (2005) Complexity of program and clinical outcomes of heart failure disease management incorporating specialist nurse-led heart failure clinics: a meta-regression analysis, *European Journal of Heart Failure Journal of the Working Group on Heart Failure of the European Society of Cardiology*, 7(3): 333–41.

Remme, W.J. and Swedberg, K. (2002) Comprehensive guidelines for the diagnosis and treatment of chronic heart failure: task force for the diagnosis and treatment of chronic heart failure of the European Society of Cardiology, *European Journal of Heart Failure*, 4(1): 11–22.

Riegel B & Carlson B (2002) Facilitators and barriers to heart failure self-care. Patient Education and Counseling, 46: 287–295.

Rich, M.W. (1999) Heart failure disease management: a critical review, *Journal of Cardiac Failure*, 5(1): 64–75.

Roccaforte, R., Demers, C., Baldassarre, F., Teo, K.K. and Yusuf, S. (2005) Effectiveness of comprehensive disease management programmes in improving clinical outcomes in heart failure patients: a meta-analysis, *European Journal of Heart Failure Journal of the Working Group on Heart Failure of the European Society of Cardiology*, 7(7): 1133–44.

Rucker-Whitaker, C., Flynn, K. J., Kravitz, G., Eaton, C., Calvin, J. E., & Powell, L. H. (2006) Understanding African-American participation in a behavioral intervention: results from focus groups. Contemporary Clinical Trials, 27 (3): 274–286.

Rutledge, T., Reis, V.A., Linke, S.E., Greenberg, B.H. and Mills, P.J. (2006) Depression in heart failure: a meta-analytic review of prevalence, intervention effects, and associations with clinical outcomes, *Journal of the American College of Cardiology*, 48(8): 1527–37.

Schreurs, K. M., Colland, V. T., Kuijer, R. G., de Ridder, D. T., & van Elderen, T. (2003) Development, content, and process evaluation of a short self-management intervention in patients with chronic diseases requiring self-care behaviours. Patient Education and Counseling, 51 (2): 133–141.

Schweitzer, R. D., Head, K., & Dwyer, J. W. (2007) Psychological factors and treatment adherence behavior in patients with chronic heart failure. Journal of Cardiovascular Nursing, 22 (1): 76–83.

Shively, M., Kodiath, M., Smith, T. L., Kelly, A., Bone, P., Fetterly, L., Gardetto, N., Shabetai, R., Bozzette, S., & Dracup, K. (2005) Effect of behavioral management on quality of life in mild heart failure: a randomized controlled trial. Patient Educucation and Counseling, 58 (1): 27–34.

Smeulders, E. S., van Haastregt, J. C., van Hoef, E. F., van Eijk, J. T., & Kempen, G. I. (2006) Evaluation of a self-management programme for congestive heart failure patients: design of a randomised controlled trial. BMC Health Services Research, 6: 91.

Stewart, A.L., Greenfield, S., Hays, R.D., Wells, K., Rogers, W.H., Berry, S.D., McGlynn E.A. and Ware, J.E. (1989) Functional status and well-being of patients with chronic conditions: results from the Medical Outcomes Study, *The Journal of the American Medical Association*, 262(7): 907–13.

Stull, D., Starling, R., Haas, G., & Young, J. (1999) Becoming a patient with heart failure. Heart and Lung, 28 (4): 284–292.

Task Force for the Diagnosis and Treatment of Chronic Heart Failure, ESoC (2001) Guidelines for the diagnosis and treatment of chronic heart failure, *European Heart Journal*, 22: 1527–60.

Task Force for the Diagnosis and Treatment of Chronic Heart Failure, Swedberg, K., Writing Committee: Cleland, J., Dargie, H., Drexler, H., Follath, F., Komajda, M., Tavazzi, L., Smiseth, O. A., Other, C., Gavazzi, A., Haverich, A., Hoes, A., Jaarsma, T., Korewicki, J., Levy, S., Linde, C., Lopez-Sendon, J.L., Nieminen, M.S., Pierard, L. and Remme, W.J. (2005) Guidelines for the diagnosis and treatment of chronic heart failure: executive summary (update 2005): The Task Force for the Diagnosis and Treatment of Chronic Heart Failure of the European Society of Cardiology, *European Heart Journal*, 26(11): 1115–40.

van der Wal, M. H., Jaarsma, T. and van Veldhuisen, D.J. (2005) Non-compliance in patients with heart failure: how can we manage it? *European Journal of Heart Failure*, 7(1): 5–17.

van der Wal, M.H.L., Jaarsma, T., Moser, D.K., Veeger, N.J.G.M., van Gilst, W.H. and van Veldhuisen, D.J. (2006) Compliance in heart failure patients: the importance of knowledge and beliefs, *European Heart Journal*, 27(4): 434–40.

Wagner, E. H., Austin, B. T., & Von Korff, M. (1996) Improving outcomes in chronic illness. Managed Care Quarterly, 4 (2): 12–25.

Whellan, D.J., Hasselblad, V., Peterson, E., O'Connor, C.M. and Schulman, K.A. (2005) Metaanalysis and review of heart failure disease management randomized controlled clinical trials, *American Heart Journal*, 149(4): 722–29.

Whitehead, D. (2001) Health education, behavioural change and social psychology: nursing's contribution to health promotion? Journal of Advanced Nursing, 34 (6): 822–832.

Windham, B.G., Bennett, R.G. and Gottlieb, S. (2003) Care management interventions for older patients with congestive heart failure, *The American Journal of Managed Care*, 9(6): 447–59.

15 Chronic obstructive pulmonary disease (COPD)

Ad A. Kaptein, Margreet Scharloo, Maarten J. Fischer,
Lucia Snoei and John Weinman

The writing of this chapter has been made possible by research grants (nos. 78.22, 83.22, 85.07, 88.54, 90.37, 92.31, 98.15, 03.80, 06.007) from the Netherlands Asthma Foundation and by the Foundation for Research on Psychosocial Stress (SOPS).

> Chronic obstructive pulmonary disease (COPD) is finally moving from obscurity to prominence, and so it should.
>
> (Kiley and Nabel 2007: 867)

Chronic obstructive pulmonary disease (COPD) is one of the diseases of the respiratory tract. Asthma, bronchiectasis, cystic fibrosis, lung cancer, sarcoidosis and tuberculosis are also part of the respiratory disorders domain. Psychological aspects, behavioural interventions and self-management of these disorders have been explored in varying detail (Kaptein and Creer 2002). Asthma, for example, has been researched by psychologists quite extensively (e.g. Kaptein and Creer 2002, Chapter 12). Bronchiectasis, lung cancer, pulmonary fibrosis, sarcoidosis and tuberculosis are waiting to be explored in much greater detail by behavioural scientists (Thompson et al. 2005; Collard et al. 2007; Lavery et al. 2007). COPD has been the object of research by behavioural scientists for some 40 years (Kaptein 2002), but research on self-management of COPD remains less well-established than in many other chronic illnesses.

In this chapter we outline: 1) the definition, epidemiology, and risk factors for COPD; 2) psychological consequences and concomitants of COPD; 3) behavioural and self-management interventions where psychological components are integrated to varying degrees into the medical treatment; and 4) clinical and research opportunities and implications.

COPD: definition, prevalence and risk factors

Over the last decade, medical societies and journals in the respiratory disorders domain have reached consensus about the definition of COPD, culminating in the publication of Standards for the diagnosis and treatment of patients with COPD: a summary of the ATS/ERS position paper. This is a landmark publication as it allows a comparison between COPD patients (and their health care providers) with regard to diagnosis, treatment and the effects of medical management of COPD.

It states:

> *Chronic obstructive pulmonary disease (COPD)* is a preventable and treatable disease state characterized by airflow limitation that is not fully reversible. The airflow limitation is usually progressive and is associated with an abnormal inflammatory response of the lungs to noxious particles or gases, primarily caused by cigarette smoking.
>
> (Celli et al. 2004: 933)

COPD is an umbrella term for a number of conditions, which include chronic bronchitis and emphysema. *Chronic bronchitis* is defined in behavioural terms: 'chronic productive cough for 3 months in each of 2 successive years in a patient in whom other causes of productive chronic cough have been excluded'. *Emphysema* is defined pathologically as 'the presence of permanent enlargement of the airspaces distal to the terminal bronchioles, accompanied by destruction of their walls and without obvious fibrosis' (Celli et al. 2004: 8, CD ROM).

The prevalence of COPD has been studied by using different methods: questionnaire items about respiratory symptoms (cough, sputum production, wheezing and shortness of breath), spirometry (lung function assessment), reported physician diagnosis and expert opinion (Halbert et al. 2006). Mannino and Holguin (2006) conclude that 'most estimates of COPD prevalence in the adult population were in the 5–10% range' (p. 117). Projections of COPD prevalence in the next decades indicate that COPD will become fifth in the rank order of disease burden (Lopez et al. 2006; Murray and Lopez 1996: 4). Women will be increasingly prominent in COPD cases, given their smoking behaviour in the past half century. Among clinicians and researchers in the respiratory domain, there is discontent about the relative importance that others (media, public, funding agencies) attach to COPD given the level of burden of the disease. In a 1999 paper in the *New England Journal of Medicine* the authors clearly demonstrated the disparity between the burden of disease associated with COPD and the funding allocated by the NIH to work on the condition (Gross et al. 1999). Diseases such as AIDS and breast cancer receive disproportionately more money than COPD. This discrepancy is reflected in the support for psychological research and clinical work with COPD patients (Kaptein 2002). This in turn is reflected in the few published papers on COPD, in contrast to AIDS and breast cancer, in journals of psychology as applied to medicine.

The main risk factor for the development of COPD is smoking of tobacco. Other important risk factors include lower socio-economic status, which tends to increase the risk of occupational hazards, and exposure to outdoor and indoor pollution (Celli et al. 2004: 934). Approximately 20 per cent of regular and heavy smokers will develop some degree of COPD, while in those who have developed COPD, some 90 per cent have been, or are still, heavy smokers. Stopping smoking is by far the best action to follow if one wants to reduce one's chance to develop COPD along with reducing the risks of developing other chronic illnesses such as cancer and cardiovascular disorders which make up for a great deal of comorbidity in COPD patients (Rabe 2007).

We will discuss smoking cessation methods later in this chapter. However, health care professionals need to recognize the difficulties in COPD patients giving up smoking. Those who have been enjoying tobacco for some 40 years do not look forward to giving up that habit in response to a request to do so. In 'Pleas from a pulmonary rehabilitation patient' (Berry 2001: 1427), the patient makes the point:

> ... I'll do whatever you say,
> take my medications every day.
> I'll exercise three times a week,
> practice my belly breathing technique.
> Just don't take my cigarettes away.

Physical and psychological impact of COPD

In the early stages of COPD patients do not experience major physical problems. They tend to attribute sensations of coughing and shortness of breath, especially during physical exertion, to their ageing and/or their smoking. In the later stages of COPD, shortness of breath, sputum production, coughing and fatigue become much more prominent. As COPD is a systemic disease, it also impacts on organs and organ systems beyond the lungs. Many patients with COPD also have cardiovascular disorders as a consequence of smoking. Weight loss, pulmonary hypertension, osteoporosis, loss of muscle tissue and sleep disorders accompany COPD in many patients. The disease-specific symptoms and the symptoms connected with the systemic aspects of COPD are quite often associated with avoidance behaviour. As a consequence of the shortness of breath and fatigue associated with COPD, patients tend to reduce physical activity considerably, setting in motion a vicious cycle (Fischer 2007b).

The history of research into the psychological impact of COPD and clinical work with COPD patients goes back nearly 50 years. The first empirical paper by psychologists on patients with 'primary obstructive pulmonary emphysema' was published in 1961 by Webb and Lawton. It described the personality characteristics of a sample of COPD patients. Compared to healthy controls, the COPD patients had higher scores on measures of psychopathology. Later Agle and Baum (1977) used qualitative methods in COPD patients in a rehabilitation setting to assess the psychological make-up of patients with a severe degree of COPD. In a series of publications, they describe how their 'average' COPD patients suffered depression, anxiety disorders, erectile dysfunction and were alcoholics. The authors were psychiatrists, which may have led them to consider psychiatric diagnostic categories, and the patients were in a pulmonary rehabilitation programme. The findings implied that the medical, psychological, and social problems and pathology converge. Nevertheless, the picture that is painted in these early publications of the psychosocial factors associated with 'the average COPD patient' has tended to survive and seems more or less valid today. Hynninen et al. (2005) in a review paper of empirical studies on psychological characteristics of COPD patients, for example, also report high levels of anxiety, depression, and cognitive and neuropsychological problems.

Early behavioural research on COPD patients examined the neuropsychological consequences of prolonged periods of shortness of breath and, probably, reduced levels of oxygenation of the brain. Various major studies confirmed deficits in different neuropsychological functions and processes (Grant et al. 1982; Prigatano et al. 1984). More recently, these findings were confirmed in a study by Crews et al. (2001) who examined 47 patients with end-stage COPD and found clinically notable frequencies of impairment on measures that assess short- and long-term memory (see also Table 3 in Hynninen et al. 2005 for a review of neuropsychological consequences of varying degrees of COPD).

Depression tends to be high in COPD. For example Stage et al. (2003) found 50 per cent to have mild to severe depression using ICD-10 criteria. High levels of depression contribute to the relatively poor quality of life of COPD patients. An additional consequence of depression and of COPD appears to be sexual dysfunction and sexual problems (Köseoğlu et al. 2005; Kaptein et al. 2008). The topic of sexuality in patients with respiratory disorders, and in particular COPD, is under-researched (Kaptein et al. 2008). In contrast to other disease-specific quality of life measures, only one questionnaire on quality of life in patients with COPD (RIQ-QOL) asks about sexuality (Maillé et al. 1997).

If delineating the psychological impact of COPD is the first phase in developing behavioural interventions in COPD, the *second* phase is to explore the relationship between this psychological impact and various other aspects of outcome. The first research group that did this important work in COPD was the 'Denver-group'. They coined the term 'psychomaintenance': 'the psychologic and behavioral perpetuation and exacerbation of physical illness' (Kinsman et al 1982: 435). The researchers developed a questionnaire, based on their work in asthma patients, the Bronchitis Emphysema Symptom Checklist (BESC). In this scale, emotional responses to symptoms of COPD (e.g. fatigue, anxiety, alienation) are assessed, and the research group demonstrated that these responses were related to self-reported disability, which could not be fully explained by 'objective' measures of severity of COPD, as measured with pulmonary function assessment (Kinsman et al. 1983). Other researchers have also independently found similar relations between psychological factors and outcomes in COPD. For example, anxiety, depression and restlessness were found to be significant predictors of survival in female COPD patients with a severe grade of COPD (Crockett et al. 2002).

Medical treatment of COPD

In most countries the general practitioner (family physician) is the medical professional who provides the bulk of care to the great majority of COPD patients. The hospital outpatient clinics of departments of respiratory medicine provide care for only some 20 per cent of the patients and a proportion of the patients need inpatient treatment.

Medical management of COPD has various components. Pharmacological therapy aims to relieve episodes of increased shortness of breath, coughing and respiratory infections. Physiotherapy aims to ameliorate dyspnoea and fatigue via breathing exercises and graded exercise training. A small proportion of patients are referred to pulmonary rehabilitation programmes (see below), in either an outpatient or inpatient setting, with psychological and/or social reasons being the main indication for the referral. Inadequate coping, with resulting disproportionate use of health care services, disconcordance between objective severity of the COPD and subjective burden experienced by the patient, and/or social impediments are quite often indications for referral to these programmes (van der Schoot and Kaptein 1990; Scharloo and Kaptein 2003).

Domiciliary oxygen treatment

This treatment is used only in a very small portion of COPD patients, namely those with hypoxaemia who would die or be severely disabled if they did not receive supplementary oxygen. In a Cochrane review, Cranston et al. (2005) conclude that this type of treatment tends to improve survival only in those patients with severe hypoxaemia and not in other COPD patients. For behavioural scientists this group represents an important area of research as their pathology and associated psychological problems include depression, suicidal ideation and social problems. There do not appear to be any psychological interventions in this area to date.

Lung volume reduction surgery (LVRS)

LVRS is a recent surgical technique applied in patients with a severe grade of COPD. The surgical procedure aims at reducing damaged areas ('dead space') of the lung(s), thereby improving ventilation and reducing dyspnoea, and possibly morbidity and mortality (Fabbri et al. 2006). However, the National Emphysema Treatment Trial Research Group (NETT) concludes that 'LVRS increases the chance of improved exercise capacity but does not confer a survival advantage over medical therapy; ... the functional benefits of lung-volume-reduction surgery came at the price of increased short-term mortality and morbidity' (Fishman et al. 2003: 2059, 2071). It is noteworthy that in this major trial, quality of well-being, shortness of breath and six-minute walk test were important dependent variables.

Lung transplantation

A lack of donor lungs, strict criteria on the recipient and high costs make lung transplantation an option for only a very small minority of the COPD population. Only a few thousand transplantations are performed per year worldwide, of which half are for COPD patients, or for those who suffer Alpha 1 anti-trypsine (an enzyme-related disorder of the respiratory tract, which also leads to COPD). Survival, however, is limited to some 45 per cent at five years after transplantation for COPD (Patel 2006). At the same time, it is important that quality of life scores are comparable between lung transplant recipients one year after transplantation, and healthy controls (Goetzmann et al. 2005). Burker et al. (2005) summarize the studies done on the relationship between psychosocial factors and survival in lung transplant patients. They report that high levels of internal control were associated with a better survival in 100 lung transplant patients. While research on this group of patients, their family and health care providers are important, a review of self-management interventions in relation to lung transplantation is outside of the scope of the current chapter.

Psychological interventions in COPD

A few distinct patterns can be discerned in the psychological and social intervention in patients with COPD. We outline four approaches in the area of psychological–behavioural intervention in COPD patients:

Psychotherapeutic/psychoanalytic approach

Some of the earliest interventional work in this area was by Rosser et al. (1983) who included psychoanalytically inspired psychotherapy treatment conditions in a randomized controlled trial of psychotherapy in 43 men and 22 women with severe COPD. The study is well designed and includes comparison groups to psychotherapy. Patients were randomly allocated to an analytic group, a supportive group, a nurse-led group and a control group. Pulmonary function, patients' and therapists' expectations, breathlessness, exercise tolerance, psychiatric symptoms, anxiety, depression and psychodynamic status [*sic*] were the rather long list of outcome variables. In this carefully done and described study, the group treated by the nurse appeared to benefit most, reflecting little benefit of psychotherapy or a psychosomatic approach. This is one of the very few studies on COPD patients where a psychoanalytic theoretical framework has been applied.

Education of COPD patients

In the earliest attempts to improve the situation of COPD patients, patient education was the only component of 'psychological intervention'. A classic picture of COPD education shows a nurse in front of a blackboard explaining to a small group of COPD patients how lungs function (Neff and Dudley 1971: 12). These interventions did not result in meaningful improvements in quality of life and improved knowledge, if attained, was unrelated to outcome measures (Scharloo and Kaptein 2003; Kaptein and Rabe 2007). Emery et al. (1998) included a patient education-only condition in a randomized controlled design where the effects of education, stress management and exercise were examined. In the patient education sessions, anatomy and physiology of the lungs, medications, interpreting pulmonary function test and understanding arterial blood gasses were discussed. After having presented their main findings, the authors admit that 'greater knowledge may have been associated with increased distress' (p. 238). In a systematic review, Blackstock and Webster (2007) stated that 'didactical educational intervention for the COPD population appeared to have minimal effect on health outcomes including quality of life, health care utilization, exercise capacity or lung function and is therefore not the education delivery method recommended' (p. 703).

Self-management interventions

Self-management techniques represent a next phase in psychological interventions in COPD patients. In this chapter this includes studies where patients are taught skills regarding symptom perception, symptom management, preventing exacerbations, general health measures and some explicitly psychological techniques such as monitoring of self-statements, coping with anxiety, depression and feelings of social isolation. Bourbeau (2003) provides a comprehensive and critical evaluation of disease-specific self-management programmes in patients with advanced COPD. In it, he conceptualizes 'self-management' as

> engaging in activities that promote health, build physiologic reserves and prevent adverse sequelae; interacting with healthcare providers and adhering to recommended treatment protocols; monitoring both physical and emotional status and making appropriate management decisions on the basis of results of self-monitoring; and managing the effects of illness on the patient's self esteem, ability to function in important roles, and relationships with others.
>
> (Bourbeau 2003: 312–13)

Specifically, in studies of self-management in COPD, the programme components that were examined in this review included education about lungs and medication; smoking cessation skills training; energy conservation training; relaxation and managing stress; nutrition information in order to eat more healthily; managing COPD symptoms and exacerbations; training in using action plans to abort or reduce exacerbations. The general findings of this review

> 'reveal new evidence that disease-specific self-management can improve patients' health status and reduce physician visits and hospital use ... . However, there are still many unanswered questions that need to be addressed with respect to the specific components of effective education for patients with COPD, methods to adjust self-management programs to suit the needs of individual patients, and long-term maintenance strategies.
>
> (Bourbeau 2003: 311–12)

Blackstock and Webster (2007) in their systematic review of changes in health outcomes list the following elements of COPD self-management interventions: giving information on COPD, breathing and cough techniques, energy use and relaxation training, information on the use of medications, using an action plan, smoking cessation, diet, self-care, sex and emotions, exercise programmes, travel and leisure, and community support. This review concluded that 'education focusing on self-management showed encouraging results with a tendency for improvements in quality of life and health care utilization, but the results did not reach statistical significance as sample sizes were insufficient to detect an effect' (p. 703).

These more psychosocial definitions of self-management contrast to those in the more medical arena and publications, where self-management intervention is usually conceptualized more narrowly as teaching the skills of recognizing potential exacerbations and managing such an episode via medication, monitoring of pulmonary function by the patient, and providing patients with an action plan that specifies which medication to take under which circumstances, and when to consult a physician (Gallefoss 2004).

The benefits of the broader conceptualization of self-management is illustrated in one of the most thorough self-management intervention studies in COPD. Atkins et al. (1984) applied a randomized control design with five experimental conditions in a sample of COPD outpatients: behaviour modification, cognitive modification, cognitive-behavioural modification, attention control and no-treatment control. Cognitive-behavioural therapy pertained to combining physical rehabilitation with an intervention where 'individuals are trained to become aware of their own negative and maladaptive thought, feelings, and behaviors, and to replace them with more positive cognitions' (p. 594). Negative self-statements were substituted with more appropriate positive and goal-oriented self-statements; for example, 'This walking is uncomfortable, but I can handle it. Soon I will be able to walk farther' (p. 594). On the major outcome variables, quality of well-being and exercise capacity, the cognitive-behavioural condition was superior to the other conditions.

These findings were replicated by Lisansky and Clough (1996) on a cognitive-behavioural educational programme who reported improvement on the Cognitive Error Questionnaire following an eight-week cognitive-behavioural programme. This improvement was associated with improvements in function as measured on the Sickness Impact Profile (Bergner et al. 1976).

Monninkhof et al. (2002) used the Cochrane review methodology in evaluating the efficacy of COPD self-management educational programmes on health outcomes and use of health services. This in itself demonstrates that the area of self-management has developed quite substantially over the past decades. Their conclusions, however, are sobering:

> There is insufficient evidence to determine whether self-management education for people with chronic obstructive pulmonary disease (COPD) is effective, and more research is needed. Further research on the effectiveness of self-management programmes should be focused on behavioural change evaluated in well designed randomized controlled trials with standardized outcomes designed for use in COPD patients, and with long follow-up time so that definite conclusions can be made.
>
> (Monninkhof et al. 2002: 2)

It is important to point out, however, that in the 12 papers that form the basis for this Cochrane review, self-management or self-management education is not defined unequivocally. Education in the traditional sense of the word (e.g. teaching patients about lung pathology) was included as an intervention element in the Cochrane review, as was coping skills training and stress-management. More research is certainly needed where intricate self-management intervention techniques are examined for their effects on psychological, social and medical outcomes (Kaptein and Dekker 2000; see also Newman et al. 2004).

Research has begun to explore the psychological determinants of self-management skills in COPD patients. Dowson et al. (2004), for example, demonstrated how anxiety, depression, alcohol use and illness beliefs inhibited self-management in COPD patients suffering from an exacerbation of their illness. In a way, these studies emphasize the relevance of illness beliefs or illness cognitions as determinants of various outcomes. This study seems to be very relevant, given the work done by Petrie et al. (2002) in patients with myocardial infarction, where successfully changing illness perceptions lead to improvements in outcome, that is, participation in a rehabilitation programme and better rates of work resumption. It is timely now for a new study to be undertaken like the one by Atkins et al. (1984), where illness beliefs are the object of intervention and behavioural outcomes the criteria for effect of the behavioural intervention (Kaplan 1999). In another relevant study in this line of research, Scharloo and colleagues demonstrated how illness cognitions predicted outcome better than 'objective' factors such as pulmonary function in outpatient with COPD (Scharloo et al. 2000, 2007). Illness representations about breathing and breathlessness were examined by Insel et al. (2005). They found meaningful differences in these representations among patients and health care providers, which may be important for intervention research in due course.

Pulmonary rehabilitation

Psychological interventions for COPD patients have been applied as a separate entity in hospital and outpatient settings. In pulmonary rehabilitation programmes, however, psychological intervention approaches make up a part of the comprehensive treatment package. Pulmonary rehabilitation is defined as:

> an evidence-based, multidisciplinary, and comprehensive intervention for patients with chronic respiratory disease who are symptomatic and often have decreased daily life activities. Integrated into the individualized treatment of the patient, pulmonary rehabilitation is designed to reduce symptoms, optimize functional status, increase participation, and reduced health care costs through stabilizing or reversing systemic manifestations of the disease.
>
> (Nici et al. 2006: 1391)

Early pulmonary rehabilitation interventions focused on education and exercise (Neff and Petty 1971). Nowadays, psychologists, physiotherapists, nutritionists, physicians and expert patients use principles of psychological interventions to try and achieve reductions in psychological morbidity (anxiety, depression, fatigue), and improvements in walking distance, social activities, active coping styles and stress management (Troosters et al. 2005). Exercise training, breathing exercises, respiratory muscle training, nutritional interventions and occupational therapy all make up the larger part of intervention techniques in pulmonary rehabilitation programmes. Increasingly, educational interventions, self-management programmes and psychosocial support have become integral components of pulmonary rehabilitation programmes (Troosters et al. 2005).

An extensive Cochrane review on the effects of pulmonary rehabilitation (Lacasse et al. 2006) found empirical evidence for the approach and made some quite optimistic summaries: 'Rehabilitation relieves dyspnea and fatigue, improves emotional function and enhances patients' sense of control over their condition. These improvements are moderately large and clinically significant. Rehabilitation forms an important component of the management of COPD' (pp. 1–2).

Given the complex multidisciplinary nature of pulmonary rehabilitation programmes, it is impossible to tease out the independent contribution that the self-management training or psychosocial support makes to changes in the outcome measures. An attempt to identify studies that very specifically examined the effects of purely psychological interventions on psychosocial outcomes maintains that the effects of this type of intervention are quite substantial (Kaptein and Dekker 2000). The authors found that short, focused psychosocial intervention sessions were associated with improvements in outcome measures such as quality of life, walking distance, anxiety and depression. Getting COPD patients to participate and making sure that they continue their participation in these interventions remains a major problem. However, given the rather positive conclusions from similar interventions in patients with other chronic illnesses, this area warrants further attention (see Newman et al. 2004).

An important related topic in the pulmonary rehabilitation area is adherence to the programme. Non-adherence represents a determinant of negative outcomes, exacerbations and hospitalization (Grant and Sutton 2006). The determinants of non-adherence in COPD are currently a focus for study (e.g. Fischer et al. 2007a).

Additional intervention methods

Public health measures may be by far the best and most effective means to prevent COPD, and other respiratory problems. Laws on prohibiting smoking in confined public places appear to have spectacular results. Menzies et al. (2006) found that 'smoke-free legislation was associated with significant early improvements in symptoms, spirometry measurements, and systemic inflammation of bar workers' (p. 1742). In those patients where smoking tobacco already has done major damage, smoking cessation strategies have been critically reviewed in Cochrane reviews and evidence-based review papers (van der Meer et al. 2001; Wagena et al. 2004). Their findings are summarized as '... the most effective intervention for prolonged smoking cessation in patients with COPD is the combination of nicotine replacement therapy, coupled with an intensive, prolonged relapse prevention programme' (Wagena et al. 2004: 806).

In a recent review on smoking cessation in patients with respiratory diseases, a European Respiratory Society Task Force concluded that 'individual counseling is effective in helping patients stop smoking ... as is group counseling. It is unclear whether group counseling is more or less effective than individual counseling' (p. 399). The components of relapse prevention or counseling often adhere to self-management principles and draw on psychological theory (Lewis 2007). Psychologists are therefore instrumental in the research on this topic and in the clinical application of this knowledge (West 2006; Tønnesen et al. 2007).

Given the quite encouraging reductions in smoking prevalence following smoking bans in public places and increased taxes on tobacco, it is important to note that public health measures may be cost-effective and efficient in achieving a lower percentage of smokers in a society. However, it still is a sobering thought to consider that even after the intense anti-smoking policies in California over decades, 20 per cent of the population are still smoking tobacco.

E-health is a fast growing intervention technique for patients with different (chronic) disorders (see Chapter 7). A recent publication reported a randomized controlled trial of home telecare versus regular care for COPD patients (Whitten and Mickus 2007). The intervention did not produce a great amount of health gain but the study is mentioned here to illustrate the potential new approach of e-health (see also Nguyen et al. 2005).

Discussion

Forty-five years ago the first empirical psychosocial paper on patients with COPD. The first empirical paper on patients with COPD written by psychologists was published about half a century ago (Webb and Lawton, 1961). Papers on COPD patients in major medical journals now routinely mention 'quality of life' or 'psychosocial care'. Nowadays, in COPD the contribution of psychological theory and experts in behaviour change is actively sought in smoking cessation research, patient-reported outcome development, quality of life assessment, and in developing, performing and evaluating behavioural interventions and self-management programmes.

It may be a bit early still to try and write a review on self-management in COPD, as was done for patients with asthma, diabetes mellitus and arthritis (Newman et al. 2004). However, Cochrane reviews do include behavioural programmes and self-management interventions, albeit incorporated into the mix of intervention approaches in pulmonary rehabilitation programmes. Self-management training, with a focus on cognitive-behavioural approaches seems to benefit patients' well-being. The methodology used in self-management intervention studies in COPD has matured, with longer follow-ups, booster sessions to maintain benefits from psychological intervention, randomized controlled trials and adequate statistical power. Studies now tend to involve interdisciplinary collaboration. Research on what exactly constitutes adequate and adaptive self-management behaviour in COPD is called for. Currently, a wide range of behaviours and skills is subsumed under the heading 'self-management', varying from relaxation training to guided imagery to symptom perception or adjusting of inhaled corticosteroids. Developing a taxonomy of self-management in COPD would be useful and enable a clearer identification of the components in studies and interventions (see Chapter 4).

That Cochrane reviews of self-management in COPD have appeared attests to the growth and progress in the area. These reviews indicate that many intervention studies have quite major flaws in various respects and that as a result the findings of individual intervention studies need to be interpreted with caution. They do, however, serve as a benchmark and provide sufficient evidence for behavioural researchers to come up with better intervention studies in the area of behavioural and psychological research on the subject of self-management for patients with COPD.

References

Agle, D.P. and Baum, G.L. (1977) Psychological aspects of chronic obstructive pulmonary disease, *Medical Clinics of North America*, 61: 749–58.

Atkins, C.J., Kaplan, R.M., Timms, R.M., Reinsch, S. and Lofback, K. (1984) Behavioral exercise programs in the management of chronic obstructive pulmonary disease, *Journal of Consulting and Clinical Psychology*, 52: 591–603.

Bergner, M., Bobbitt, R.A., Pollard, W.E., Martin, D.P. and Gilson, B.S. (1976) The sickness impact profile: validation of a health status measure, *Medical Care*, 14: 57–61.

Berry, M.J. (2001) Pleas from a pulmonary rehabilitation patient, *Chest*, 120: 1427.

Blackstock, F. and Webster, K.E. (2007) Disease-specific health education for COPD: a systematic review of changes in health outcomes, *Health Education Research*, 22: 703–17.

Bourbeau, J. (2003) Disease-specific self-management programs in patients with advanced COPD, *Disease Management & Health Outcomes*, 11: 311–19.

Burker, E.J., Evon, D.M., Galanko, J. and Egan, T. (2005) Health locus of control predicts survival after lung transplant, *Journal of Health Psychology*, 10: 695–704.

Celli, B.R., MacNee, W. and committee members (2004) Standards for the diagnosis and treatment of patients with COPD: a summary of the ATS/ERS position paper, *European Respiratory Journal*, 23: 932–46.

Collard, H.R., Tino, G., Noble, P.W., Shreve, M.A., Michaels, M., Carlson, B. and Schwarz, M.I. (2007) Patient experiences with pulmonary fibrosis, *Respiratory Medicine*, 101: 1350–54.

Cranston, J.M., Crockett, A.J., Moss, J.R. and Alpers, J.H. (2005) Domiciliary oxygen for chronic obstructive pulmonary disease, *Cochrane Database of Systematic Reviews*, Issue 4. CD number CD001744.

Crews, W.D., Jefferson, A.L., Bolduc, T., Elliott, J.B., Ferro, N.M., Broshek, D.K., Barth, J.T. and Robbins, M.K. (2001) Neuropsychological dysfunction in patients suffering from end-stage chronic obstructive pulmonary disease, *Archives of Clinical Neuropsychology*, 16: 643–52.

Crockett, A.J., Cranston, J.M., Moss, J.R. and Alpers, J.H. (2002) The impact of anxiety, depression and living alone in chronic obstructive pulmonary disease, *Quality of Life Research*, 11: 309–16.

Dowson, C.A., Town, G.I., Frampton, C. and Mulder, R.T. (2004) Psychopathology and illness beliefs influence COPD self-management, *Journal of Psychosomatic Research*, 56: 333–40.

Emery, C.F., Schein, R.L., Hauck, E.R. and MacIntyre, N.R. (1998) Psychological and cognitive outcomes of a randomized trial of exercise among patients with chronic obstructive pulmonary disease, *Health Psychology*, 17: 232–40.

Fabbri, L.M., Luppi, F., Beghé, B. and Rabe, K.F. (2006) Update in chronic obstructive pulmonary disease 2005, *American Journal of Respiratory and Critical Care Medicine*, 173: 1056–65.

Fischer, M.J., Scharloo, M., Abbink, J.J., Thijs-van Nies, A., Rudolphus, A., Snoei, L., Weinman, J.A. and Kaptein, A.A. (2007a) Participation and drop-out in pulmonary rehabilitation: a qualitative analysis of the patient's perspective, *Clinical Rehabilitation*, 21: 212–21.

Fischer, M.J., Scharloo, M., Weinman, J. and Kaptein, A.A. (2007b) Respiratory rehabilitation, in P. Kennedy (ed.) *Psychological Management of Physical Disabilities. A Practitioner's Guide* (pp. 124–48). London: Routledge.

Fishman A. for the writing committee NETT Research Group (2003) A randomized trial comparing lung-volume-reduction surgery with medical therapy for severe emphysema, *New England Journal of Medicine*, 348: 2059–73.

Gallefoss, F. (2004) The effects of patient education in COPD in a 1-year follow-up randomised, controlled trial, *Patient Education and Counseling*, 52: 259–66.

Goetzmann, L., Scheuer, E., Naef, R., Vetsch, E., Buddeberg, C., Russi, E.W. and Boehler, A. (2005) Psychosocial situation and physical health in 50 patients > 1 year after lung transplantation, *Chest*, 127: 166–70.

Grant, A.R. and Sutton, S.R. (2006) Interventions for adherence to pulmonary rehabilitation for chronic obstructive pulmonary disease. (Protocol). *Cochrane Database of Systematic Review*, Issue 1. CD number CD005605.

Grant, I., Heaton, R.K., McSweeny, A.J., Adams, K.M. and Timms, R.M. (1982) Neuropsychologic findings in hypoxemic chronic obstructive pulmonary disease, *Archives of Internal Medicine*, 142: 1470–76.

Gross, C.P., Anderson, G.F. and Powe, N.R. (1999) The relation between funding by the National Institutes of Health and the burden of disease, *New England Journal of Medicine*, 340: 1881–87.

Halbert, R.J., Natoli, J.L., Gano, A., Badamgarav, E., Buist, A.S. and Mannino, D.M. (2006) Global burden of COPD: systematic review and meta-analysis, *European Respiratory Journal*, 28: 523–32.

Hynninen, K.M. J., Breitve, M.H., Wiborg, A.B., Pallesen, S. and Nordhus, I.H. (2005) Psychological characteristics of patients with chronic obstructive pulmonary disease: a review, *Journal of Psychosomatic Research*, 59: 429–43.

Insel, K.C., Meek, P.M. and Leventhal, H. (2005) Differences in illness representation among pulmonary patients and their providers, *Journal of Health Psychology*, 10: 147–62.

Kaplan, R.M. (1999) Behavior as the central outcome in health care, *American Psychologist*, 45: 1211–20.

Kaptein, A.A. (2002) Respiratory disorders and behavioral research, in A.A. Kaptein and T.L. Creer (eds) *Respiratory Disorders and Behavioral Medicine* (pp. 1–17). London: Martin Dunitz.

Kaptein, A.A. and Dekker, F.W. (2000) Psychosocial support, *European Respiratory Monograph*, 13: 58–69.

Kaptein, A.A. and Creer, T.L. (eds) (2002) *Respiratory Disorders and Behavioral Medicine*. London: Martin Dunitz.

Kaptein, A.A. and Rabe, K.F. (2007) Chronic obstructive pulmonary disease (COPD): chronic bronchitis and emphysema, in S. Ayers, A. Baum, C. McManus, S. Newman, K. Wallston, J. Weinman and R. West (eds) *Cambridge Handbook of Psychology, Health and Medicine* (2nd edn, pp. 631–63). Cambridge: Cambridge University Press.

Kaptein, A.A., van Klink, R., de Kok, F., Scharloo, M., Snoei, L., Broadbent, L., Bel, E.H. and Rabe, K.F. (2008) Sexuality in patients with asthma and COPD, *Respiratory Medicine*, 102: 198–204.

Kiley, J.P. and Nabel, E.G. (2007) Treating COPD, *New England Journal of Medicine*, 356: 867.

Kinsman, R.A., Dirks, J.F. and Jones, N.F. (1982) Psychomaintenance of chronic physical illness, in T. Millon, C. Green and R. Meagher (eds) *Handbook of Clinical Health Psychology* (pp. 435–66). New York: Plenum Press.

Kinsman, R.A., Yaroush, R.A., Fernandez, E., Dirks, J.F., Schocket, M. and Fukuhara, J. (1983) Symptoms and experiences in chronic bronchitis and emphysema, *Chest*, 83: 755–61.

Köseoğlu, N., Köseoğlu, H., Ceylan, E., Çimrin, H.A., Özalevli, S. and Esen, A. (2005) Erectile dysfunction prevalence and sexual function status in patients with chronic obstructive pulmonary disease, *Journal of Urology*, 174: 249–52.

Lacasse, Y., Goldstein, R., Lasserson, T.J. and Martin, S. (2006) Pulmonary rehabilitation for chronic obstructive pulmonary disease, *Cochrane Database of Systematic Reviews*, Issue 4. CD number CD003793.

Lavery, K., O'Neill, B., Elborn, J.S., Reilly, J. and Bradley, J.M. (2007) Self-management in bronchiectasis: the patients' perspective, *European Respiratory Journal*, 29: 541–47.

Lewis, K. (2007) Smoking cessation – making quitting a real option, *Respiratory Medicine* (COPD update) 3: 128–34.

Lisansky, D.P. and Clough, D.H. (1996) A cognitive-behavioral self-help educational program for patients with COPD, *Psychotherapy and Psychosomatics*, 65: 97–101.

Lopez, A.D., Shibuya, K., Rao, C., Mathers, C.D., Hansell, A.L., Held, L.S., Schmid, V. and Buist, S. (2006) Chronic obstructive pulmonary disease: current burden and future projections, *European Respiratory Diseases*, 27: 397–412.

Maillé, A.R., Koning, C.J.M., Zwinderman, A.H., Willems, L.N.A., Dijkman, H.J. and Kaptein, A.A. (1997) The development of the 'Quality-of-Life for Respiratory Illness Questionnaire (QOL-RIQ): a disease-specific quality-of-life questionnaire for patients with mild to moderate chronic non-specific lung disease, *Respiratory Medicine*, 91: 297–309.

Mannino, D.M. and Holguin, F. (2006) Epidemiology and global impact of chronic obstructive pulmonary disease, *Respiratory Medicine* (COPD update) 1: 114–20.

Menzies, D., Nair, A., Williamson, P.A., Schembri, S., Al-Khairalla, M.Z.H., Barnes, M., Fardon, T.C., McFarlane, L., Magee, G.J. and Lipworth, B.J. (2006) Respiratory symptoms, pulmonary function, and markers of inflammation among bar workers before and after a legislative ban on smoking in public places, *Journal of the American Medical Association*, 296: 1742–48.

Monninkhof, E.M., van der Valk, P.D.L.P.M., van der Palen, J., van Herwaarden, C.L.A., Partridge, M.R., Walters, E.H. and Zielhuis, G.A. (2002) Self-management education for chronic obstructive pulmonary disease, *Cochrane Database of Systematic Reviews*, Issue 4. CD number CD002990.

Murray, C.J.L. and Lopez, A.D. (eds) (1996) *The Global Burden of Disease*. Geneva: World Health Organization.

Neff, T.A. and Petty, T.L. (1971) Outpatient care for patients with chronic airway obstruction – emphysema and bronchitis, *Chest*, 60: 11S–17S.

Newman, S., Steed, L. and Mulligan, K. (2004) Self-management interventions for chronic illness, *the Lancet*, 364: 1523–37.

Nguyen, H.Q., Carrieri-Kohlman, V., Rankin, S.H., Slaughter, R. and Stulbarg, M.S. (2005) Is Internet-based support for dyspnea self-management in patients with COPD possible? Results of a pilot study, *Heart & Lung*, 34: 51–62.

Nici, L., Donner, C., Wouters, E., Zuwallack, R., Ambrosino, N., Bourbeau, J. et al. (2006) ATS/ERS Statement on Pulmonary Rehabilitation, *American Journal of Respiratory and Critical Care Medicine*, 173: 1390–413.

Patel, N. (2006) Transplantation in chronic obstructive pulmonary disease. COPD. *Journal of Chronic Obstructive Pulmonary Disease*, 3: 149–62.

Petrie, K.J., Cameron, L.D., Ellis, C.J., Buick, D. and Weinman, J. (2002) Changing illness perceptions after myocardial infarction: an early intervention randomized controlled trial, *Psychosomatic Medicine*, 64: 580–86.

Prigatano, G.P., Wright, E.C. and Levin, D. (1984) Quality of life and its predictors in patients with mild hypoxemia and chronic obstructive pulmonary disease, *Archives of Internal Medicine*, 144: 1613–19.

Rabe, K.F. (2007) Treating COPD: the TORCH trial, p values, and the Dodo, *New England Journal of Medicine*, 356: 851–54.

Rosser, R., Denford, J., Heslop, A., Kinston, W., Macklin, D., Minty, K., Moynihan, C., Muir, B., Rein, L. and Guz, A. (1983) Breathlessness and psychiatric morbidity in chronic bronchitis and emphysema: a study of psychotherapeutic management, *Psychological Medicine*, 13: 93–110.

Scharloo, M., Kaptein, A.A., Weinman, J., Willems, L.N.A., Rooijmans, H.G.M. and Dijkman, J.H. (2000) Physical and psychological correlates of functioning in patients with chronic obstructive pulmonary disease, *Journal of Asthma*, 37: 17–29.

Scharloo, M. and Kaptein, A.A. (2003) Chronic obstructive pulmonary disease: a behavioural medicine approach, in S. Llewelyn and P. Kennedy (eds) *Handbook of Clinical Health Psychology* (pp. 155–79). Chichester: John Wiley & Sons.

Scharloo, M., Kaptein, A.A., Schlosser, M., Pouwels, H., Bel, E.H., Rabe, K.F. and Wouters, E.F.M. (2007) Illness perceptions and quality of life in patients with chronic obstructive pulmonary disease, *Journal of Asthma*, 44: 575–81.

Stage, K.B., Middelboe, T. and Pisinger, C. (2003) Measurement of depression in patients with chronic obstructive pulmonary disease (COPD), *Nordic Journal of Psychiatry*, 57: 297–301.

Thompson, E., Solà, I. and Subirana, M. (2005) Non-invasive interventions for improving well-being and quality of life in patients with lung cancer – a systematic review of the evidence, *Lung Cancer*, 509: 163–76.

Tønnesen, P., Carrozzi, L., Fagerström, K.O., Gratziou, C., Jimenez-Ruiz, C., Nardini, S., Viegi, G., Lazzaro, C., Campell, I.A., Dagli, E. and West, R. (2007) Smoking cessation in patients with respiratory diseases: a high priority, integral component of therapy, *European Respiratory Journal*, 29: 390–417.

Troosters, T., Casaburi, R., Gosselink, R. and Decramer, M. (2005) Pulmonary rehabilitation in chronic obstructive pulmonary disease, *American Journal of Respiratory and Critical Care Medicine*, 172: 19–38.

van der Meer, R.M., Wagena, E.J., Ostelo, R.W.J.G., Jacobs, J.E. and van Schayck, C.P. (2001) Smoking cessation for chronic obstructive pulmonary disease, *Cochrane Database of Systematic Reviews*, Issue 1. CD Number CD002999.

van der Schoot, T.A.W. and Kaptein, A.A. (1990) Pulmonary rehabilitation in an asthma clinic, *Lung*, 168: 495–501.

Wagena, E.J., van der Meer, R.M., Ostelo, R.J.W.G., Jacobs, J.E. and van Schayck, C.P. (2004) The efficacy of smoking cessation strategies in people with chronic obstructive pulmonary disease: results from a systematic review, *Respiratory Medicine*, 98: 805–15.

Webb, M. and Lawton, A.H. (1961) Basic personality traits characteristic of patients with primary obstructive pulmonary emphysema, *Journal of the American Geriatrics Society*, 9: 590–610.

West, R. (2006) Tobacco control: present and future, *British Medical Bulletin*, 77–78, 123–36.

Whitten, P. and Mickus, M. (2007) Home telecare for COPD/CHF patients: outcomes and perceptions, *Journal of Telemedicine and Telecare*, 13: 69–73.

16 Hypertension

Nina Rieckmann, Manuel Paz Yepes and Karina W. Davidson

Definitions and assessment of hypertension

What is hypertension?

Blood pressure (BP) is assessed as the maximum pressure in an artery at the moment when the heart is beating and pumping blood through the body (systolic BP, SBP), and the lowest pressure in an artery in the moments between beats when the heart is resting (diastolic BP, DBP). Hypertension is an arbitrary level of BP defined to differentiate persons who have an increased risk of developing a morbid cardiovascular event. The diagnosis is based on the average of two or more properly measured BP readings on each of two or more office visits. Hypertension is diagnosed if either the systolic or the diastolic BP level is elevated. For adults aged 18 and older a SBP of 140 or above or a DBP of 90 or above is considered hypertension (European Society of Hypertension-European Society of Cardiology Guidelines Committee 2003). For those patients with chronic kidney disease or diabetes, the goal in the USA is now to treat to a SBP below 130 or a DBP below 80 (Chobanian et al. 2003). Since home-based measurements of BP are generally lower, diagnostic thresholds for patients without kidney or diabetic disease measurements have been adjusted to 135/85 (SBP/DBP) or 137/85. The prognostic value of these thresholds, however, has yet to be replicated in large studies (Reims et al. 2001). Home-based values appropriate for diabetic or renal patients are not yet known.

Prevalence

An estimated 691 million people worldwide have high BP, and hypertension is one of the leading causes of morbidity and mortality. In the USA, it is the most common primary diagnosis (35 million office visits as the primary diagnosis). The 1998 Health Survey for England found that 37 per cent of adults over 16 years of age had a BP of more than 140/90 mmHg (Primatesta et al. 2001). Even though most hypertensive patients can be controlled with appropriate treatment, the survey also found that treatment rates among adults diagnosed with hypertension were as low as 32 per cent and only 9 per cent of those with hypertension had controlled BP. Among these, 59 per cent reported that they had received nonpharmacological advice from their physicians.

Risk factors for hypertension

Hypertension is a multisystem disorder with complex pathophysiology involving the cardiovascular, neuroendocrine and renal systems. However, most patients with hypertension have no definable cause to explain it, and the terms *primary*, *essential* or *idiopathic* hypertension are used to define this situation. Nearly 5–10 per cent of the patients with hypertension have a defined cause, and most of these secondary forms are related to an alteration in hormone regulation and/or renal function (Onusko 2003). In those cases a specific treatment to the primary cause should be undertaken. It is those with essential hypertension for whom self-management may be beneficial.

BP can be influenced by diverse causes, such as environmental, socio-economic, psychosocial and genetic factors. Advancing age, male gender, sedentary lifestyle and obesity have been identified as risk factors for developing high BP (Ford and Cooper 1991; Rutledge and Hogan 2002). There are also some diets that negatively affect BP, such as hypercaloric food, saturated fats, alcohol and salt intake, with this last one as a factor that has received the greatest attention (Ascherio et al. 1992; Ascherio et al. 1996; Karppanen and Mervaala 2006). Lower social class (Lawlor and Smith 2005) and psychosocial stress (Rutledge et al. 2002) have also been associated with an increased risk of hypertension, and BP values vary in different populations. The prevalence, severity, and impact of hypertension are increased in African Americans, who also demonstrate a more difficult control of BP compared with other populations (Freeman et al. 1996; Sheats et al. 2005). Hypertension is also a complex genetic disorder. The occurrence of one genetic alteration or a combination of mutations may result in clinically manifested hypertension. Hereditary factors may confer 20–50 per cent of the variation in BP levels (Agarwal et al. 2005; Strazzullo and Galletti 2007).

Prognosis when hypertension remains untreated

Hypertension is considered both a disease condition and one of the major risk factors for heart disease, stroke and kidney disease. Uncontrolled high BP worldwide is estimated to cause 7.1 million deaths. Most deaths due to hypertension result from myocardial infarction secondary to coronary artery disease or congestive heart failure, and a great morbidity is related to this association. It is estimated that for persons above 40 years, the risk for CVD doubles with each 20/10 mmHg rise in BP (Chobanian et al. 2003).

Damage of the central nervous system, like stroke, hypertensive encephalopathy and retinopathy occur frequently in patients with high BP. Stroke can be caused by cerebral haemorrhage, or by cerebral infarction, secondary to the increased atherosclerosis observed in hypertensive patients. Hypertension also causes vascular renal damage with impairment in renal function.

There is no cure for hypertension, but it can be controlled by changes in one's lifestyle and regularly taking the appropriate medication. It is estimated that 50–60 per cent of people who have hypertension would improve their prognosis if they had levels in the healthy BP range.

Assessment of hypertension

There are different ways of assessing BP. The traditional auscultatory method is the most common method employed in clinical settings; it requires some skills and a stethoscope and a sphygmomanometer are needed.

Ambulatory BP monitoring (ABPM) provides the BP measurement over a 12- or 24-hour period as patients perform normal daily activities and during sleep. The monitor can be worn on a belt around the waist, and the cuff around the arm is automatically inflated to take a reading every 15–30 minutes. ABPM is considered the gold standard for assessing BP; however, it is not always feasible and is somewhat inconvenient for the patient (O'Brien et al. 2003; Pickering et al. 2006).

For long-term use and self-monitoring of hypertension at home, simpler and more convenient home BP self measurement devices are available that provide instant readings and that are easy to use, reasonably accurate and inexpensive (Reims et al. 2001; Artinian et al. 2004; Imai et al. 2004). Home-based measurement of BP constitutes an important part of self-management of hypertension: it allows patients to recognize the effects of antihypertensive treatment and lifestyle changes, thus encouraging medication adherence, follow-up clinic visits and active participation in BP control.

Some devices have a printer function or store the readings electronically, which helps to reduce observer and reporting biases. Importantly, home-based measurements should not obviate the need for clinical BP readings and close medical supervision (see Table 16.1).

Table 16.1 Home self-monitoring of blood pressure with self-measurement devices

Recommendations
During diagnosis and initiation of treatment: duplicate BP measurements in the morning and evening for one week.
For long-term observation: every three months BP should be monitored for one week.
Measure: average BP across all readings except the first day.
Treatment target: SBP/DBP <130–135/85 mmHg (or lower if chronic kidney disease or diabetes is present)

Advantages	**Dangers**

Recommendations

- More accurate reflection of 24-hour BP than BP readings in clinical settings
- Instant feedback about treatment success and failure: motivation for adherence
- Induction of patient anxiety
- Potential for self-modification of medication and lifestyle regimens

Management of hypertension

Hypertension control is best achieved with a combination of pharmacological therapy and lifestyle modifications (Pyorala et al. 1994; Erdine et al. 2006). Major lifestyle modifications include weight reduction in obese or overweight individuals, reduced intake of sodium, increased intake of potassium and calcium, the Dietary Approach to Stop Hypertension (DASH) diet (which encourages the intake of fruits and vegetables), regular exercise, stress reduction and moderation of alcohol consumption. These modifications have been shown to reduce BP, and enhance the efficacy of antihypertensive drugs. Antihypertensive medication – if taken as prescribed – is indicated in almost all cases of hypertension and generally yields larger effects on lowering BP when compared to lifestyle modifications (Ebrahim and Smith 1998). However, only 25–40 per cent of patients who are prescribed antihypertensive treatment achieve BP control (SBP <140 and DBP <90 mmHG) (Chobanian 2001). The key to successful hypertension control in all patients, thus, is that they adhere to taking a prescribed dosage of BP lowering medication on a daily basis. Hypertension control is not achieved with a single, one-time intervention, but it requires ongoing, lifelong commitment from the patient (see Table 16.2).

Table 16.2 Challenges to self-management of hypertension

Silent threat
Hypertensive patients do not experience aversive symptoms
Delayed risk
Hypertension is a long-term risk factor for adverse clinical events such as stroke and acute coronary syndromes
Chronic condition
BP control requires lifelong adherence with recommended treatment, which usually consists of a combination of pharmacologic therapy and lifestyle changes
Long-term BP monitoring
Many diseases require infrequent monitoring, but constant monitoring is needed to confirm treatment success

This is complicated by the fact that hypertension is a 'silent' threat to one's health, with no apparent symptoms such as pain or even discomfort. The benefit of achieving hypertension control lies in the reduction of future, possible cardiovascular events, such as unstable angina, MI or stroke, but there is no immediate, perceivable benefit to the patient, such as relief from somatic pain.

Nonpharmacologic interventions for hypertension control include a wide array of measures, such as patient education, provider education, provider feedback and patient reminders. Almost all interventional approaches include some form of patient self-monitoring, the most prominent being teaching patients to measure their BP levels at home, which provides direct feedback to the patient about the success or failure of their lifestyle habits.

Randomized controlled trials studying the effect of interventions to reduce HTN use one or both of the following two outcomes: 1) mean reduction of systolic and diastolic BP; or 2) control of BP (defined as SBP/DBP <130–135/85 or SBP/DBP <140/90).

Self-management interventions in hypertension

Lifestyle interventions

The targets of lifestyle interventions in the prevention and treatment of hypertension are permanent changes in dietary habits (weight loss and sodium restriction), adoption of regular exercise, moderate alcohol intake and smoking cessation. Several meta-analyses have been conducted assessing the effects of lifestyle interventions on hypertension (Ebrahim et al. 1998; Chodosh et al. 2005; Fahey et al. 2005; Dickinson et al. 2006). These meta-analyses vary according to the patient population under investigation (e.g. hypertensives only versus hypertensives and normotensives), quality restrictions on included studies, restrictions on length of follow-up and whether or not included studies allowed variations in antihypertensive medication over time. Despite these variations, there is common agreement that even though lifestyle interventions generally yield lower effect sizes compared to pharmacologic interventions, some are effective in lowering BP, especially in hypertensive populations. The following lifestyle interventions are associated with significant reductions in SBP and/or DBP: diet (especially with an explicit focus on weight loss), exercise, alcohol restriction, sodium restriction and combinations of these interventions. Interventions focusing on dietary supplements (calcium, magnesium, potassium) seem to have no significant effects. Figure 16.1 displays the overall mean differences in SBP from the most recent meta-analysis of 105 trials that quantified the effectiveness of several lifestyle interventions in hypertensive patients.

Maintaining patient adherence to permanent lifestyle changes is the key to any successful long-term BP reduction, and also the greatest challenge to self-management interventions. Most lifestyle interventions appear to have short-term effects only. Dickinson et al (2006) conducted follow-up analyses that showed that effects of all interventions were considerably less marked in trials with a follow-up duration of at least six months; when restricted to those trials, the significant effects on BP reduction were found only for diet and combined interventions.

What are effective strategies to improve patients' adherence to lifestyle changes? A comprehensive review of studies aimed at improving adherence to lifestyle changes for cardiovascular disease in general, and hypertension in particular, found that different techniques are applied in achieving patient adherence, not all of which are successful (Newell et al. 2000). Table 16.3 lists the techniques used for dietary

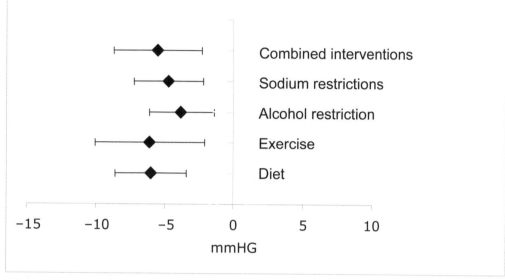

Source: data from Dickinson et al. (2006).

Figure 16.1 Pooled mean reductions in systolic BP from lifestyle interventions

regimens, smoking cessation, exercise regimens, weight-loss regimens and general lifestyle regimens that are strongly or tentatively recommended based on the available evidence.

Table 16.3 Techniques to improve adherence to lifestyle changes in hypertension management

Targeted behaviour	Promising interventions for improving adherence to target behaviour
Dietary regimens (mostly sodium restriction) Smoking cessation	Self-monitoring of urine
	Spousal participation
	Behavioural contracting
	Written educational materials
	Giving audiovisual materials
	Giving a projected coronary heart disease risk assessment
Exercise regimens	Behavioural counselling
	Educational counselling
	Behavioural contracting
	Self-monitoring of pulse rate
	Giving audiovisual material
	Relaxation training
	Giving a projected coronary heart disease risk assessment
	Educational training for partners

Targeted behaviour	Promising interventions for improving adherence to target behaviour
Weight-loss regimens	Behavioural counselling
	Educational counselling
	Self-monitoring of pulse rate
	Relaxation training
General lifestyle regimens	Behavioural counselling
	Educational counselling
	Written educational materials
	Telephone reminders
	Giving audiovisual materials

Note: summary of results from Newell et al. (2000).

For the prevention of hypertension in normotensive people, who have some risk factors that are considered precursors for hypertension and heart disease, such as obesity, sedentary lifestyle and smoking, counselling is a frequently used measure to initiate lifestyle changes. One large study found counselling to be effective in normotensive but overweight people: The Trials of Hypertension Prevention Collaborative Research Group (1997) tested the effects of counselling about weight loss and dietary sodium reduction on lowering diastolic BP, systolic BP, and the incidence of hypertension during a 3- to 4-year period. 2382 normotensive men and women between ages 30–54 years and a body mass index 110–165 per cent of desirable body weight were included in the study and randomly assigned to receive either counselling for weight reduction, counselling for sodium intake, both interventions combined, or usual care. Compared with the usual care group, BP decreased 3.7/2.7 mmHg in the weight loss group, 2.9/1.6 mmHg in the sodium reduction group and 4.0/2.8 mmHg in the combined group at 6 months (all groups, $P < .001$). After 48 months, the incidence of hypertension was significantly less in each active intervention group compared to the usual care group (average relative risks, 0.78–0.82). There was, however, no advantage of the combined intervention over the individual counseling interventions.

Cognitive-behavioural interventions

The short-term increases in BP due to stress are well documented; somewhat weaker and more inconsistent is the evidence that stress influences the development and progression of hypertension (Beilin 1997; Das and O'Keefe 2006), with time urgency and impatience being the most consistent predictors. Nevertheless, patients who report stress are widely recommended some form of cognitive-behavioural intervention to alleviate stress and provide relaxation.

Behavioural strategies include, for example, progressive muscle relaxation, relaxation training and hypnosis. Examples of cognitive strategies are guided imagery, autogenic training, distraction, thought-monitoring, coping self-statements and problem-solving.

Dickinson et al. (2006) analysed pooled BP reductions across interventions focusing on teaching patients some form of relaxation technique (see Table 16.4).

Thirteen of the included trials used physical techniques (progressive muscle relaxation, breathing exercises, yoga), two trials used cognitive-behavioural techniques (talk therapy, meditation and guided imagery), two trials used stress management, four trials used some combination of these and 12 trials used biofeedback. Most trials did not test these interventions exclusively, but combined them with other components such as patient education and BP self-monitoring. Interventions lasted between 4–26 weeks and follow-ups between 8–260 weeks.

Table 16.4 Overview of cognitive-behavioural interventions

Progressive muscle relaxation
Breathing exercises
Yoga
Hypnosis
Meditation
Guided Imagery
Distraction
Problem-solving
Self-monitoring
Stress management
Biofeedback

Notably, this meta-analysis yielded significant BP reductions only in trials that had a control group that did not receive any intervention. In trials where the control group received *sham* interventions, relaxation techniques appeared to have no benefit over the control condition (see Figure 16.2).

An earlier review (Eisenberg et al. 1993) also found that cognitive-behavioural techniques were only efficacious in comparison to no intervention, but not superior to sham interventions. This review subsumed under cognitive-behavioural interventions meditation, relaxation, autogenic training, hypnosis, stress management, imagery and biofeedback. Thus, current evidence suggests that attention alone may improve BP and aid in self-management, but that the active ingredient proposed by cognitive-behavioural hypertension clinical trialists are not needed to achieve BP effects.

Another recent meta-analysis quantified the effects of cognitive self-management interventions in hypertensive older adults: Self-management was defined as *"a systematic intervention that is targeted toward patients with chronic disease. The intervention should help them actively participate in either or both of the following: self-monitoring (of symptoms or of physiologic processes) or decision making (managing the disease or its impact through self-monitoring)"* (Chodosh et al. 2005: 428)

Pooled data from 13 studies conducted between 1977–2003 showed that systolic BP was decreased by 5 mmHg (effect size, –0.39 [CI, –0.51 to –0.28]) and diastolic BP was decreased by 4.3 mmHg (effect size, –0.51 [CI, –0.73 to –0.30]). Out of the 13 studies, 7 were primarily focused on relaxation techniques or anxiety management. These studies alone were found to be effective and yielded no differences in effect size

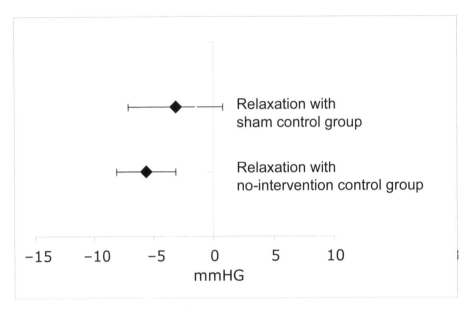

Source: data from Dickinson et al. (2006).

Figure 16.2 Pooled mean reductions in systolic BP from relaxation interventions

from the remaining six studies, which combined lifestyle interventions such as exercise and weight loss programmes with patient education and motivational components to increase self-monitoring. This meta-analysis, however, did not make a distinction between trials that included a no-intervention control group versus trials that included a sham intervention control group.

In an attempt to understand which features of the selected self-management programmes are most responsible for successful BP reduction, Chodosh and colleagues conducted additional subgroup analyses testing the effects of the following programme features: tailored versus generic approaches, group setting versus other settings, interventions providing individual feedback versus no feedback, interventions with versus without psychological emphasis, interventions delivered by physicians versus non-medical providers (Chodosh et al. 2005). However, none of these comparisons yielded significant differences in effectiveness between programmes with versus without any of these features. This is not surprising, as the pooled interventions were extremely heterogeneous and there were often greater differences in the content of an intervention between trials that shared one particular feature (e.g. group setting) than in trials that did not share this feature. These features of self-management for hypertension – group versus other, or tailored versus generic – thus remain interesting candidates to test for their usefulness.

Blood pressure self-monitoring

The development of devices for home BP self-monitoring was accompanied by great expectations. In particular, it was expected that through the availability of immediate feedback about the success of any treatment or lifestyle change, patients would be motivated to sustain these changes and follow the recommendations of their physicians with greater care. Evidence for the efficacy of BP self-monitoring as a stand-alone intervention, however, is not particularly favourable. A meta-analysis of 12 studies comparing home self-monitoring interventions to usual care or no intervention found a significant reduction in DBP of –2.0 mmHG (95% CI = –2.7 to –1.4 mmHG), but no significant reduction in SBP (Fahey et al. 2005). A pooled analysis of four studies assessing BP *control* as the outcome also found no significant effect of home self-monitoring.

Telemonitoring

Some new devices allow the transmission of stored BP data over the telephone. This procedure is called telemonitoring and creates a bi-directional flow of information between health care provider and patient via the telephone. Patients use a toll-free number to transmit their BP readings to a network server provided by a telemonitoring service. The network server generates BP reports and sends the reports to care providers, who use the data to facilitate telecounselling and treatment planning. Such telemonitoring systems have been shown to improve the diagnosis of essential hypertension (Rogers et al. 2002), to reduce mean arterial pressure compared with usual care (Rogers et al. 2001), to improve antihypertensive medication adherence, especially for nonadherent patients, compared with usual care (Friedman et al. 1996), and have been associated with improved quality of life and a tendency towards a more regular treatment regimen (Parati et al. 2004). The possibilities of telemonitoring have yet to be fully explored, but it is likely to become an integrated part of health care in the near future (see Chapter 5). It is a unique tool for patients as it allows them greater control over their care (i.e. 24-hour access to information, feedback and support) and might thus improve motivation in the everyday self-management of hypertension.

Interventions for improving adherence to antihypertensive medication

There is ample evidence that antihypertensive medication is the most effective intervention for lowering BP and achieving BP control (Chobanian et al. 2003; Erdine et al. 2006). However, rates of nonadherence or partial adherence are high (DiMatteo et al. 2002; Mallion et al. 1998), and nonadherence is in part responsible for more than 60 per cent of patients who are prescribed antihypertensive medication who do not achieve BP control.

A review of 38 studies testing 58 different interventions for improved adherence yielded such heterogeneity, that the results were not pooled for a quantitative meta-analysis (Schroeder et al. 2004). Table 16.5 summarizes the results of this review. Most studies did not report changes in BP from pre- to post-treatment.

Table 16.5 Interventions for improving adherence to antihypertensive medication

Type of study	Number of studies with increased adherence rates/ total number of studies	Relative increase in adherence in successful studies
Simplifying dosing regimens	7/9	8–19.6%
Motivational strategies, support and reminders	10/24	Generally small increases in adherence; max. 23%
Complex, multicomponent interventions	8/18	5%–41%
Patient education	1/6	24%

Source: Schroeder et al. (2004).

Are interventions for hypertension based on psychological theories of behaviour change?

In the vast majority of cases, interventions for hypertension are not explicitly grounded in any psychological theory on health behaviour change. Thus, a systematic review of the efficacy of different theoretical approaches for self-management of hypertension is not possible.

Back in 1979, the *Journal of the American Medical Association* published a paper proposing that active participation by the patient is critical to successful management of hypertension, and that physicians should act as 'promoters' of active patient participation aiding in decision-making and problem-solving processes (Working Group to Define Critical Behaviors in High Blood Pressure Control 1979). It was proposed that research should focus on patient attitudes, knowledge and skills and find out under which conditions patients make the decision for control, take their medication as prescribed, monitor their BP on a regular basis, and engage in active problem-solving behaviour when BP control is not achieved. Decades later, the theoretical grounds for this research endeavour are certainly developed, as outlined in Chapter 3 of this book. However, interventions designed to control hypertension have yet to take advantage of these theories and combine existing educational tools about beneficial lifestyle changes with tools designed to help patients not only to initiate these changes, but to also *maintain* them over the years.

Summary and outlook

Uncontrolled hypertension is one of the most prevalent chronic conditions and it is estimated that it is responsible for 7.1 million deaths per year worldwide. Numerous nonpharmacologic interventions have been tested with mixed results. Self-monitoring of BP is a useful tool in hypertension management, but its use alone is not particularly effective in BP reduction and is not associated with increased numbers of patients who achieve BP control. Lifestyle changes appear to lose their beneficial effects over time, except interventions targeting diet and weight loss, and those that pair lifestyle recommendations with other components. Self-management through means of stress reduction, physical relaxation techniques and other cognitive-behavioural strategies are promising approaches, but these interventions do not seem to be superior to interventions that deliver attention alone. Most of these interventions, however, were not grounded in any theory on health behaviour change.

Further, it remains to be tested if the beneficial effects of successful nonpharmacologic interventions are due to increased adherence to antihypertensive medication. It is plausible that the adoption of effective self-management strategies generalizes to improvements in drug adherence behaviour. Thus, more rigorous studies are needed to understand how self-management might exert beneficial, sustained effects on hypertension control: through reduction of stress and relaxation, through reduction of risk factors such as obesity and malnutrition or through improvements in medication adherence. Likely, best results are achieved when all components (adherence to medication, adoption of recommended lifestyle behaviours and effective use of relaxation techniques) are implemented.

Bibliography

Agarwal, A., Williams, G.H. and Fisher, N.D. (2005) Genetics of human hypertension, *Trends in Endocrinology Metabolism*, 16: 127–33.

Artinian, N.T., Washington, O.G., Klymko, K.W., Marbury, C.M., Miller, W.M. and Powell, J.L. (2004) What you need to know about home blood pressure telemonitoring: but may not know to ask, *Home Healthcare Nurse*, 22: 680–86.

Ascherio, A., Hennekens, C., Willett, W.C., Sacks, F., Rosner, B., Manson, J., Witteman, J. and Stampfer, M.J. (1996) Prospective study of nutritional factors, blood pressure and hypertension among US women, *Hypertension*, 27: 1065–72.

Ascherio, A., Rimm, E.B., Giovannucci, E.L., Colditz, G.A., Rosner, B., Willett, W.C., Sacks, F. and Stampfer, M.J. (1992) A prospective study of nutritional factors and hypertension among US men, *Circulation*, 86: 1475–84.

Beilin, L.J. (1997) Stress, coping, lifestyle and hypertension: a paradigm for research, prevention and non-pharmacological management of hypertension, *Clinical and Experimental Hypertension*, 19: 739–52.

Chobanian, A.V. (2001) Control of hypertension – an important national priority, *New England Journal of Medicine*, 345: 534–35.

Chobanian, A.V., Bakris, G.L., Black, H.R., Cushman, W.C., Green, L.A., Izzo, J.L., Jr., Jones, D.W., Materson, B.J., Oparil, S., Wright, J.T., Jr. and Roccella, E.J. (2003) The Seventh Report of the Joint National Committee on Prevention, Detection, Evaluation and Treatment of High Blood Pressure: the JNC 7 report, *Journal of the American Medical Association*, 289: 2560–72.

Chodosh, J., Morton, S.C., Mojica, W., Maglione, M., Suttorp, M.J., Hilton, L., Rhodes, S. and Shekelle, P. (2005) Meta-analysis: chronic disease self-management programs for older adults, *Annals of Internal Medicine*, 143: 427–38.

Das, S. and O'Keefe, J.H. (2006) Behavioral cardiology: recognizing and addressing the profound impact of psychosocial stress on cardiovascular health, *Current Atherosclerosis Reports*, 8: 111–18.

Dickinson, H.O., Mason, J.M., Nicolson, D.J., Campbell, F., Beyer, F.R., Cook, J.V., Williams, B. and Ford, G.A. (2006) Lifestyle interventions to reduce raised blood pressure: a systematic review of randomized controlled trials, *Journal of Hypertension*, 24: 215–33.

DiMatteo, M.R., Giordani, P.J., Lepper, H.S. and Croghan, T.W. (2002) Patient adherence and medical treatment outcomes: a meta-analysis, *Medical Care*, 40: 794–811.

Ebrahim, S. and Smith, G.D. (1998) Lowering blood pressure: a systematic review of sustained effects of non-pharmacological interventions, *Journal of Public Health Medicine*, 20: 441–48.

Eisenberg, D.M., Delbanco, T.L., Berkey, C.S., Kaptchuk, T.J., Kupelnick, B., Kuhl, J. and Chalmers, T.C. (1993) Cognitive behavioral techniques for hypertension: are they effective? *Annals of Internal Medicine*, 118: 964–72.

Erdine, S., Ari, O., Zanchetti, A., Cifkova, R., Fagard, R., Kjeldsen, S., Mancia, G., Poulter, N., Rahn, K.H., Rodicio, J.L., Ruilope, L.M., Staessen, J., van Zwieten, P., Waeber, B. and Williams, B. (2006) ESH-ESC guidelines for the management of hypertension, *Herz*, 31: 331–8.

European Society of Hypertension-European Society of Cardiology guidelines for the management of arterial hypertension (2003) *Journal of Hypertension*, 21: 1011–53.

Fahey, T., Schroeder, K. and Ebrahim, S. (2005) Interventions used to improve control of blood pressure in patients with hypertension, *Cochrane Database Systematic Reviews*, no. CD005182.

Ford, E.S. and Cooper, R.S. (1991) Risk factors for hypertension in a national cohort study, *Hypertension*, 18: 598–606.

Freeman, V., Rotimi, C. and Cooper, R. (1996) Hypertension prevalence, awareness, treatment and control among African Americans in the 1990s: estimates from the Maywood Cardiovascular Survey, *American Journal of Preventive Medicine*, 12: 177–85.

Friedman, R.H., Kazis, L.E., Jette, A., Smith, M.B., Stollerman, J., Torgerson, J. and Carey, K. A telecommunications system for monitoring and counseling patients with hypertension. Impact on medication adherence and blood pressure control. Am J Hypertens. 1996 Apr; 9(4 Pt1): 285–92.

Imai, Y., Ohkubo, T., Kikuya, M. and Hashimoto, J. (2004) Practical aspect of monitoring hypertension based on self-measured blood pressure at home, *Internal Medicine*, 43: 771–78.

Karppanen, H. and Mervaala, E. (2006) Sodium intake and hypertension, *Progress in Cardiovascular Diseases*, 49: 59–75.

Lawlor, D.A. and Smith, G.D. (2005) Early life determinants of adult blood pressure, *Current Opinion in Nephrology Hypertension*, 14: 259–64.

Mallion, J.M., Baguet, J.P., Siche, J.P., Tremel, F. and de Gaudemaris, R. (1998) Compliance, electronic monitoring and antihypertensive drugs, *Journal of Hypertension Supplement*, 16: S75–9.

Newell, S.A., Bowman, J.A. and Cockburn, J.D. (2000) Can compliance with nonpharmacologic treatments for cardiovascular disease be improved? *American Journal of Preventive Medicine*, 18: 253–61.

O'Brien, E., Asmar, R., Beilin, L., Imai, Y., Mallion, J.M., Mancia, G., Mengden, T., Myers, M., Padfield, P., Palatini, P., Parati, G., Pickering, T., Radon, J., Staessen, J., Stergiou, G. and Verdecchia, P. (2003) European Society of Hypertension recommendations for conventional, ambulatory and home blood pressure measurement, *Journal of Hypertension*, 21: 821–48.

Onusko, E. (2003) Diagnosing secondary hypertension, *American Family Physician*, 67: 67–74.

Parati, G., Bilo, G. and Mancia G. Blood pressure measurement in research and in clinical practice: recent guidance. Curr Opin Nephrol Hypertens. 2004 May; 13(3): 343–57.

Pickering, T.G., Shimbo, D. and Haas, D. (2006) Ambulatory blood-pressure monitoring, *New England Journal of Medicine*, 354: 2368–74.

Primatesta, P., Brookes, M. and Poulter, N.R. (2001) Improved hypertension management and control: results from the Health Survey for England 1998, *Hypertension*, 38: 827–32.

Pyorala, K., De Backer, G., Graham, I., Poole-Wilson, P. and Wood, D. (1994) Prevention of coronary heart disease in clinical practice: recommendations of the Task Force of the European Society of Cardiology, European Atherosclerosis Society and European Society of Hypertension, *European Heart Journal*, 15: 1300–31.

Reims, H., Fossum, E., Kjeldsen, S.E. and Julius, S. (2001) Home blood pressure monitoring: current knowledge and directions for future research, *Blood Pressure*, 10: 271–87.

Rutledge, T. and Hogan, B.E. (2002) A quantitative review of prospective evidence linking psychological factors with hypertension development, *Psychosomatic Medicine*, 64: 758–66.

Schroeder, K., Fahey, T. and Ebrahim, S. (2004) How can we improve adherence to blood pressure-lowering medication in ambulatory care? Systematic review of randomized controlled trials. Arch Intern Med. 2004 Apr 12; 164(7): 722–32.

Sheats, N., Lin, Y., Zhao, W., Cheek, D.E., Lackland, D.T. and Egan, B.M. (2005) Prevalence, treatment and control of hypertension among African Americans and Caucasians at primary care sites for medically under-served patients, *Ethnicity and Disease*, 15: 25–32.

Strazzullo, P. and Galletti, F. (2007) Genetics of salt-sensitive hypertension, *Current Hypertension Reports*, 9: 25–32.

The Trials of Hypertension Prevention Collaborative Research Group (1997) Effects of weight loss and sodium reduction intervention on blood pressure and hypertension incidence in overweight people with high-normal blood pressure: The Trials of Hypertension Prevention, phase II. The Trials of Hypertension Prevention Collaborative Research Group, *Archives of Internal Medicine*, 157: 657–67.

Working Group to Define Critical Behaviors in High Blood Pressure Control (1979) Patient behavior for blood pressure control: guidelines for professionals, *Journal of the American Medical Association*, 241: 2534–37.

Part V

Conclusion

17 Conclusion

Stanton Newman and Debbie Cooke

Overall this book has produced the backdrop to self-management in chronic illness by presenting how changes in the population (Chapter 1) and the attitudes of patients to their role in managing their illness (Chapter 2) have led to an increased interest in the role of self-management and a need for interventions to enhance its practice. The evolution of self-management from a variety of different perspectives, professional and lay-led backgrounds has led to a heterogeneity in the way it has developed and been applied. Chapters 3, 4 and 5, respectively, have provided overviews of the theoretical underpinnings of self-management interventions, its common components and different modes of delivery. An important consideration for those who are contemplating the implementation of a self-management intervention is the special training requirements of the individual's responsible for delivery (Chapter 6). The growth of technology in self-management mirrors that in medicine in general, and time will tell the extent to which this increases patient autonomy or creates further dependencies (Chapter 7). Crucial to the further development of self-management is a clear understanding of the existing research base. Chapter 8 considered the design and analysis of research in self-management and Chapter 9, the complex issue of the relationship between different measures of outcome. The final section of the book included chapters that examined the nature of self-management interventions and their evidence base in a range of different chronic illnesses. All these issues influence the likelihood that the practice of health care will change to incorporate self-management. The future of self-management is dependent on how receptive patients, health care systems and the staff working within them are to engaging with self-management. Issues pertaining to this are considered in this concluding chapter.

Predictions of the future of health care abound with some governments of developed countries generating intense political discussion regarding the organization of health care and how to respond to perceptions of the need for change in the way health care is delivered (see e.g. Smith 1997; Commission on the Future of Health Care in Canada 2002). Cost, equity, access and quality are all issues confronting health care systems. Reform in health care is an evolving process determined by demographic, social, political, technological, cultural, economic and political factors (O'Rourke and Immarino 2002). The concepts of patient empowerment and self-management are key drivers of health care reform (Segal 1997; Garson and Levin 2001; Wanless 2002, 2004; Wanless et al. 2007; Harvey et al. 2007). This final chapter considers the implications of such factors for the future of self-management.

Issues relating to the implementation and integration of self-management into routine care

The integration of self-management into routine health care requires consideration of the obstacles that confront any attempt to translate new ways of delivering health care from its research evidence base to its adoption, implementation and integration. The responsiveness and resistance of health care systems, and the people who work within them, to changes in the model and delivery of health care are an important potential limitation to the future of self-management.

The majority of translational research has focused on the introduction of technologies rather than service innovations into routine clinical practice. Service innovations principally involve human capital and have been defined as follows: 'A novel set of behaviours, routines, and ways of working, which are directed at improving health outcomes, administrative efficiency, cost effectiveness or the user experience, and which are implemented by means of planned and co-ordinated action' (Greenhalgh et al. 2004a: 6).

As self-management interventions principally involve changes in the way in which services are delivered by staff, and in some cases lay people, within a health care organization, they accord with this definition.

The evidence base

One of the most obvious barriers to the introduction of any service innovation into routine health care concerns the quality and clarity of the evidence regarding its efficacy (Greenhalgh et al. 2004b). The extent of evidence for the efficacy and effectiveness of self-management interventions was presented in the final section of this book and will not be reconsidered in detail here. In general, however, there are some important issues in relation to the nature, persuasiveness and clarity of the evidence regarding self-management interventions.

In some self-management interventions where positive effects are reported, it is in terms of patient-reported benefits such as quality of life. While patient-reported outcomes are, and have become increasingly important in health care, this type of evidence is often not sufficiently persuasive to those who retain clinical and managerial responsibility for patient care. Many clinicians, managers and policy-makers are likely to be persuaded to initiate changes in practice when faced with an intervention that produces clear clinical benefits which in turn translates into an economic return on investment. Demonstrating clear clinical benefit, in many conditions, requires studies that follow patients for many years. Few studies in self-management have had follow-up periods of sufficient duration to examine whether there is evidence for long-term clinical benefits both in terms of morbidity and mortality. It is also common to use proxy markers of disease progression. An example of this is the use of HbA1c as a surrogate indicator of morbidity and mortality in diabetes. Studies using this as a marker of disease severity have tended to demonstrate only small improvements in this measure which may be statistically but not clinically significant.

Somewhat more persuasive evidence for self-management interventions is provided by findings that indicate changes in health-related behaviour that are assumed to have a clearer relationship with clinical outcome. Examples of these are interventions designed to improve metabolic control in diabetes by targeting behaviour change in relation to exercise and/or diet (see Chapter 10) or following action plans for self-adjustment of medication in asthma (see Chapter 12). While behaviour change has been demonstrated in many studies in the short term, few studies have established clear evidence for enduring changes in behaviour. Maintenance of behaviour change is an important area and one that researchers have repeatedly highlighted as a gap in the field.

Self-management interventions are complex and there is conflicting and often ambiguous evidence relating to their efficacy and effectiveness. This requires constant reframing and interpretation of evidence in different contexts (Ferlie et al. 2001). Conflicting evidence does not support translation of self-management into routine service delivery. In evaluating the evidence base, it is not always clear what demarcates or differentiates a self-management intervention from other chronic disease management approaches. This occurs at two levels. There is no agreed definition of what constitutes self-management. This is compounded by the difficulty of being able to distinguish how an intervention has been labelled from what it actually involved. Many published papers label the intervention as self-management, but on careful reading it is apparent that the intervention constitutes a traditional, didactic educational approach and contains none of the key aspects (e.g. goal-setting, problem-solving) of self-management (see Chapter 4). In some cases insufficient detail is provided about the intervention so that it is not possible to determine whether it contains elements of self-management. The net result is that the term, which is already used in diverse ways, loses any distinctive meaning and any evidence relating to efficacy is attached to interventions that do not embrace any components distinctive to self-management (see Chapter 4).

Even where there is good evidence to support an intervention that gains widespread acceptance, translation into routine service delivery is not always achieved. There is evidence to suggest that complex innovations are less likely to be adopted in organizations (Denis et al. 2002). Application of the Normalization Process Model and WISE (Whole System Informing Self-Management Engagement) Model (see Chapter 7) may help to increase understanding of the factors that lead to the successful adoption and implementation of complex interventions in routine practice (Kennedy and Rogers 2001; May 2006; May et al. 2007a; May et al. 2007b). These offer theoretical frameworks for the evaluation of new interventions within broad social and organizational contexts. Consideration of individual behaviour change domains as outlined by Michie and colleagues will also assist with the adoption of evidence-based practice (Michie et al. 2005). The reasons for problems of uptake into routine service delivery are diverse but some of these are discussed below.

Individual barriers

It is often assumed that self-management is applicable to all individuals with a chronic illness and, to the extent that all individuals are responsible for day-to-day care of their illness, this is true. It may be the case, however, that the application of skills such as goal-setting, problem-solving, and so on is less appropriate for some individuals than others. Although research is limited in this area, it could be hypothesized that individuals who prefer a more paternalistic approach to health care may be less interested in the increased responsibility that self-management advocates. To ensure true patient empowerment, therefore, the needs and desires of the patients should first be elicited and responded to as appropriate (Funnell et al. 1991). In addition, there may be a point when illness becomes so severe that self-management becomes more difficult and a shift towards intensive case management may become more appropriate.

Financial barriers

Perhaps the most important barrier to the introduction of a new form of treatment is lack of evidence on its cost-effectiveness. Few studies on self-management interventions have considered their impact on costs and cost-effectiveness. A systematic review (Loveman et al. 2003) of the clinical and cost-effectiveness of education models for diabetes identified two studies evaluating the cost-effectiveness of self-management interventions (Kaplan et al. 1987; Glasgow et al. 1997). However, the authors of the systematic review argued that these could not be considered a comprehensive assessment of this area. An earlier study that examined the impact on costs was the Arthritis Self-Management Programme, which concluded that it provided clear savings (Lorig et al. 2001). A more recent Cochrane review showed no evidence that lay-led self-management education programmes significantly altered use of health care services (Foster et al. 2007).

The design and measures used in many evaluations of self-management do not always lend themselves to a clear assessment of their economic benefit. Most do not incorporate follow-up periods of sufficient length to enable financial implications to be assessed. Detailed information on the utilization of health and social care resources needs to be gathered over an extended period of time so that these costs can be modelled.

Further, achievement of a positive effect in certain patient-reported outcomes does not always translate into a reduction in costs for the health care organization delivering the self-management intervention. For example, pain control medication in arthritis is frequently treated with over-the-counter medication paid for by the patient. Thus, a self-management intervention that results in reduction in pain and decreased analgesic medication will result in cost savings for the patient rather than the health care system delivering the intervention.

Measures of psychological well-being such as depression and anxiety and also quality of life are commonly reported patient-oriented outcomes in self-management interventions. The level of depression and anxiety reported is often well below the level of clinical diagnosis where referral to a mental health care practitioner is deemed necessary and costs will be incurred. Those interventions that report improvements in measures are often marginal and below any clinical threshold that will involve referral and costs related to health care utilization. Quality of life is often assessed to determine whether participation in the intervention and the constraints it places on behaviour has a negative impact on quality of life or conversely the skills gained improve quality of life. Importantly, however, although it is possible to calculate the effects of the intervention on quality of life (QALY methodology), the translation of quality of life into clear health care savings is not something that is widely applied in self-management interventions.

Some evaluations of self-management have used surrogate markers of behaviour change; for example, self-efficacy as their outcome (see Chapter 3). It is not always possible to determine the relationship of these types of measure to either behaviour or clinical outcome. This means that the possibility of relating such process measures to costs and potential economic benefits of self-management is problematic.

Organizational barriers

In this era of evidence-based health care, there is a somewhat naïve belief that translation of evidence into practice simply requires production of guidelines and endorsement from relevant professional bodies. The movement from guideline development to implementation is more complex and requires change to be effected at a number of levels (Grimshaw et al. 2004). Assuming an intervention can be 'codified' into a guideline, the successful implementation of self-management into routine clinical practice requires change at several different levels: policy, health system and at the individual level of health care professionals' interaction/ communication with people with chronic conditions and/or their informal carers and advocates (Glasgow et al. 2003).

It is essential to consider the extent that a service innovation, like self-management, is compatible with the perceived needs, values, norms and ways of working within the health care organization. While it is not possible to generalize to all health care organizations, a proportion of interventions that have been labelled as self-management are principally information-focused, tend to have less of a behaviour change orientation and do not encourage patient autonomy. As discussed in Chapter 6, the shift towards a self-management-focused approach requires both knowledge and training and is not necessarily easily achieved. This has been identified as a potential barrier to adoption of other human capital innovations in health care (see e.g. Denis et al. 2002; Greenhalgh et al. 2004b).

The successful uptake of a self-management programme is in part dependent on the way in which health care is organized in a particular country. Arguably, there are two diametrically opposed systems of regulation running concurrently in the UK; one where centrally driven top-down planning is implemented and another where decision-making has been delegated to local level (Harvey et al. 2007). Adoption of self-management interventions in this system will be very different to the decentralized system operating in the USA with its division between Federal, State, Health Maintenance Organizations and private care provision.

Gaining widespread adoption of self-management interventions, in a more decentralized system, is more difficult and necessitates a different process that will often involve smaller units of delivery. It is clear that there is a trend by some 'for profit' organizations in health care to attempt to adopt and promote self-management interventions in order to provide them with a competitive advantage in the marketplace. These have sometimes been attached to other health care products (e.g. medication, devices) as an adjunct to the promotion of the product. To the extent that the self-management intervention accompanies such products, which have wide penetration in a particular market, it may be argued that these approaches will encourage the more widespread adoption of self-management interventions. However, these marketing approaches are not necessarily accompanied by research evidence demonstrating the efficacy or effectiveness of the self-management intervention.

The relative power relationships within a health care system may influence successful adoption and uptake of self-management. In the UK context, there is a divide in the delivery of health care and competition for resources between primary and secondary care. Innovations such as self-management require organizational ownership and the need for flexibility in financial arrangements between organizations that may be affected by their introduction. This process is not assisted in the UK by the tension between primary care organizations (purchasers of health care) and the secondary care providers, where issues of costs and the defence of respective budgets is paramount in their transactions.

The UK's Expert Patient Programme (EPP), based on Kate Lorig's CDSMP, provides a good example of the gap between the implementation of policy to support and promote national delivery of self-management and successful adoption (Lee et al. 2006). The public health impact of the roll-out of this national programme has been limited by competing demands and priorities on the organizations responsible for delivery of the EPP as well as by difficulties with recruitment and organization of training courses within Primary Care Trusts. Within this specific context, incorporation of self-management skills training for health care professionals as well as recruitment from both primary and secondary care may overcome these difficulties (see Chapter 6).

Legislation passed by some states in the US mandate a requirement to support self-management education in certain health conditions. The greatest legislative development has been in diabetes (see e.g. Daly and Leontos 1999). Legislation is, however, a broad brush policy regarding the adoption of self-management but does not specify in any detail the nature of the programme or how this should be delivered. This often simply results in relabelling of existing activities. Viewed in a historical context, however, introduction of this legislation recognizes and acknowledges the role of self-management theory and intervention. It is an important step towards the more widespread adoption of self-management.

Conclusion

The development and evaluation of self-management interventions is still evolving. This book has attempted to present the current state of knowledge in this area. Within this chapter the individual, financial and organizational obstacles to the integration of self-management in routine health care have been considered. Overcoming these is part of the challenge of mainstreaming self-management within health care. We have moved from the inception of self-management within traditional patient educational programmes to theoretically based interventions that have been systematically developed and evaluated. We must build upon the existing evidence base so that we can move towards a solid foundation for delivery of appropriately targeted and effective self-management interventions that fit seamlessly within routine care for people with chronic illness.

References

Commission on the Future of Health Care in Canada (2002) *Building on Values: The Future of Health Care in Canada*. Final Report: National Library of Canada (www.hc-sc.gc.ca/english/pdf/romanow/pdfs/HCC_Final_Report.pdf: accessed 29 February 2008).

Daly, A. and Leontos, C. (1999) Legislation for health care coverage for diabetes self-management training, equipment, and supplies: past, present and future, *Diabetes Spectrum*, 12(4): 222–29.

Denis, J.L., Hebert, Y., Langley, A., Lozeau, D. and Trottier, L.H. (2002) Explaining diffusion patterns for complex health care innovations, *Health Care Management Review*, 27(3): 60–73.

Ferlie, E., Gabbay, J., Fitzgerald, L., Locock, L. and Dopson, S. (2001) Evidence-based medicine and organisational change: an overview of some recent qualitative research, in L. Ashburner (ed.) *Organisational Behaviour and Organisational Studies in Health Care: Reflections on the Future*. Basingstoke: Palgrave. 18–42.

Foster, G., Taylor, S.J.C., Eldridge, S.E., Ramsay, J. and Griffiths, C.J. (2007) Self-management education programmes by lay leaders for people with chronic conditions, *Cochrane Database of Systematic Reviews*, Issue 4, No. CD005108.

Funnell, M.M., Anderson, R.M., Arnold, M.S. et al. (1991) Empowerment: an idea whose time has come in diabetes education, *The Diabetes Educator*, 17(1): 37–41.

Garson, A. and Levin, S.A. (2001) Ten 10-year trends for the future of healthcare: implications for academic health centers, *The Ochsner Journal*, 3: 10–15.

Glasgow, R.E., La Chance, P.A., Toobert, D.J. et al. (1997) Long-term effects and costs of brief behavioural dietary intervention for patients with diabetes delivered from the medical office, *Patient Education and Counseling*, 32: 175–84.

Glasgow, R.E., Davis, C.L., Funnell, M.M. and Beck, A. (2003) Implementing practical interventions to support chronic illness management, *Joint Commission Journal on Quality & Patient Safety*, 29: 563–74.

Greenhalgh, T., Robert, G., Bate, P. et al. (2004a) How to spread good ideas: a systematic review of the literature on diffusion, dissemination and sustainability of innovations in health service delivery and organisation. Report for the National

Co-ordinating Centre for NHS Service Delivery & Organisation R&D (www.sdo.lshtm.ac.uk/files/project/38-final-report-pdf: accessed 29 February 2008).

Greenhalgh, T., Robert, G., Macfarlane, F., Bate, P. and Kyriakidou, O. (2004b) Diffusion of innovations in service organisations: systematic review and recommendations, *The Milbank Quarterly*, 82(4): 581–629.

Grimshaw, J.M., Thomas, R.E., MacLennan, G. et al. (2004) Effectiveness and efficiency of guideline dissemination and implementation strategies, *Health Technology Assessment*, 18(6): 1–94.

Harvey, S., Liddell, A. and McMahon, L. (2007) Windmill 2007: the future of health care reforms in England. Discussion paper (www.kingsfund.org.uk/publications/kings_fund_publications/windmill_2007.html: accessed 29 February 2008).

Kaplan, R.M., Atkins, C.J. and Wilson, D.K. (1987) The cost-utility of diet and exercise interventions in non-insulin-dependent diabetes mellitus, *Health Promotion*, 2: 331–40.

Kennedy, A. and Rogers, A. (2001) Improving self-management skills: a whole systems approach, *British Journal of Nursing*, 10(11): 734–37.

Lee, V., Kennedy, A. and Rogers, A. (2006) Implementing and managing self-management skills training within primary care organisations: a national survey of the expert patient programme within its pilot phase, *Implementation Science*, 1: 6.

Lorig, K., Ritter, P., Stewart, A. et al. (2001) Chronic disease self-management program: two-year health status and health care utilization, *Medical Care*, 39(11): 1217–23.

Loveman, E., Cave, C., Green, C. et al. (2003) The clinical and cost-effectiveness of patient education models for diabetes: a systematic review and economic evaluation, *Health Technology Assessment*, 7(22): 1–211.

May, C. (2006) A rational model for assessing and evaluating complex interventions in health care, *BMC Health Services Research*, 6(86): doi: 10.1186/1472-6963-6-86.

May, C., Mair, F., Dowrick, C. and Finch, T. (2007a) Process evaluation for complex interventions in primary care: understanding trials using the normalization process model, *BMC Family Practice*, 8: 42.

May, C., Finch, T., Mair, F. et al. (2007b) Understanding the implementation of complex interventions in health care: the normalization process model, *BMC Health Services Research*, 7: 148: doi: 10.1186/1472-6963-7-148.

Michie, S., Johnston, M., Abraham, C. et al. (2005) Making psychological theory useful for implementing evidence based practice: a consensus approach, *Quality and Safety in Health Care*, 14: 26–33.

O'Rourke, T.W. and Immarino, N.K. (2002) Future of healthcare reform in the USA: lessons from abroad, *Expert Review of Pharmacoeconomics & Outcomes Research*, 2: 279–91.

Segal, L. (1998) The importance of patient empowerment in health system reform, *Health Policy*, 44: 31–44.

Smith, R. (1997) The future of health care systems: information technology and consumerism will transform health care worldwide, *British Medical Journal*, 314: 1495.

Wanless, D. (2002) *Securing our Future Health: Taking a Long Term View: Final Report.* London: HM Treasury (www.hm-treasury.gov.uk/media/A/F/letter_to_chex.pdf: accessed 29 February 2008).

Wanless, D. (2004) *Securing Good Health for the Whole Population. Final Report.* London: Her Majesty's Treasury (www.hm-treasury.gov.uk/consultations_and_legislation/wanless/consult_wanless04_final.cfm: (accessed 29 February 2008).

Wanless, D., Appleby, J., Harrison, A. and Patel, D. (2007) *Our Future Health Secured?* London: King's Fund (www.kingsfund.org.uk/publications/kings_fund_publications/our_future.html: accessed 29 February 2008).

Index

ABPM, *see* ambulatory blood pressure
   monitoring
access 290
ACE inhibitors 242
ACTH, *see* adrenocorticotropic hormone
action plans 49, 84, 85, 101, 103, 105,
   106, 112, 206, 208, 244
action stage 55
active coping 198, 263
active life expectancy (ALE) 17
active listening 103
activities of daily living (ADL) 5, 16, 17,
   18, 19, 20
activity pacing 71
activity-passivity model 28
acute care model 81
acute illnesses 4
adaptive planning 109
adaptive testing 162
adherence 50, 64, 107, 108, 112–14, 170,
   179, 194, 207, 208, 240, 264, 281
ADL, *see* activities of daily living
adjunctive physical therapies 212
adolescents 171–3
adoption 144–5
adrenocorticotropic hormone
   (ACTH) 191, 192
Africa 9
ageing *see* older people
alcohol 67, 240, 263, 273, 276
alcoholic cardiomyopathy 239
ALE, *see* active life expectancy
alienation 258
allocation concealment 141
alternative therapies 212
ambulatory blood pressure monitoring
   (ABPM) 274
American College of Rheumatology 189
American Diabetes Association 136
American Heart Association 225
analgesia 82
Anderson, Barbara 181
angina 70, 224, 227, 230, 274

anonymity 83
antibodies 192
anticoagulants 226
antigens 192
antihyperglycaemic agents 57
antihypertensive medication 275, 281
antiplatelets 226
anxiety 48, 49, 71, 143, 190, 195, 227,
   229, 230, 242, 245, 257, 258, 261, 263,
   293
appraisal 48, 49
arrhythmias 239
arthritis xi, 10, 34, 37, 73, 80, 82, 83, 137,
   189–203, 292
Arthritis Foundation 198
Arthritis Self-Management
   Programme (ASMP) 82, 193, 197, 198
Asia 9
ASMP, *see* Arthritis Self-Management
   Programme
assertiveness training 196
assessment 114, 143, 198–9; *see also*
   evaluation
   reports 57
   standardization of 163
asthma xi, 34, 35, 37, 47, 49, 66, 72, 73,
   122, 124, 194, 204–23, 255
atherosclerosis 224, 274
atrial fibrillation 15
attendance logs 110
attention control 104, 262, 283
attention seeking 104
attitudes 28–44, 47, 52, 282, 290
audio-visual aids 60, 105
audit 110
auditory impairment 30
auscultatory method 274
Australasia 205
Australia
   activities of daily living in 20
   cardiac rehabilitation programme
     attendance 228
   decision-making in 32

provision of advice in 29
self-management models in 36
use of asthma action plans 208
autogenic training 278, 279
autonomy 290, 294

barriers 65, 69, 86, 103, 105, 125, 127,
    145, 244, 291–6
    financial 293–4
    individual 292–3
    organizations 294–5
bathing 19
Behavior Change Consortium 99
Behavioral Risk Factor Surveillance
    System 15
behaviour
    change ix, 47–63, 66–7, 72–3, 84,
        100–2, 105, 107, 111–12, 150, 151,
        244, 262, 282, 292, 294
    healthy 29, 55, 66, 223
    influence on life expectancy 9
    styles 104
behavioural approaches 180
behavioural control 52, 54, 58
behavioural determinants 59
behavioural interventions 193
behavioural measures 159–60
behavioural outcomes 124
behavioural processes 55, 56
behavioural techniques 83
beliefs 54, 58, 70, 105, 143, 148, 179, 228,
    243, 263
BESC, see Bronchitis Emphysema
    Symptom Checklist
beta blockers 226
BGAT, see Blood Glucose Awareness
    Training
biofeedback 279
block randomization 142
blood gasses 260
blood glucose 58, 66, 72, 82, 150, 169,
    170, 171, 173, 174, 179
Blood Glucose Awareness Training
    (BGAT) 174
blood pressure 14, 179, 226, 272–83
blood sugar 35, 171
body mass index 85, 124
booster sessions 72, 88
brainstorming 68, 244
breast cancer 87
breathing exercises 263, 279
breathing retraining techniques 214
breathlessness 204, 238, 241, 243, 260,
    263

bronchiectasis 255
bronchitis 256
Bronchitis Emphysema Symptom
    Checklist (BESC) 258
Burden of Disease Network Project 19
Bury, Mike 20

cafeteria-style theorizing 60
calcium intake 274
caloric intake 148, 150
calorific input 124
Canada
    cariovascular disease in 14
    decision-making in 33–4
    DiSC study in 57
    provision of advice in 29
    self-management models/programmes
        in 36, 79
cancer 9, 34, 87, 257
cardiac rehabilitation 53, 54, 71, 228, 231
cardiovascular disease 4, 10, 13–16, 257
cardiovascular events 272, 275
Caribbean 15, 20
catastrophizing 70, 150, 195
causal model 59
causal pathways 59, 115, 150–2
cause 48, 58, 70, 110
CBT, see cognitive behavioural therapy
CDSMP, see Chronic Disease
    Self-Management Programme
Centers for Medicare and Medicaid
    Services 79
central Europe 9
central nervous system 273
Centre for Disease Control 15
cerebrovascular diseases 12
challenging beliefs 179
change
    behaviour ix, 47–63, 66–7, 72–3, 84,
        100–2, 105, 107, 111–12, 150, 151,
        244, 262, 282, 292, 294
    maintenance 106
    processes 55, 56, 58
    readiness 66–7, 208
checklists 114
CHESS, see Comprehensive Health
    Enhancement Support System
children 4, 122, 123, 207, 211
China 9, 15, 81
cholesterol 86, 225
chronic bronchitis 256
Chronic Care Model 83
Chronic Disease Self-Management
    Programme (CDSMP) 73, 82, 87, 295

chronic obstructive pulmonary disease (COPD) 9, 87, 254–70
classical test theory (CTT) 157–61, 164
clinician–patient relationships 28
cluster randomization 142
coaching 34
coding frames 113
cognitions 243
cognitive accessibility of information 155–6
cognitive-behavioural interventions x, 74, 179, 195, 196, 199, 230, 261, 277–9
cognitive-behavioural strategies 283
cognitive-behavioural therapy (CBT) 74, 173, 230
Cognitive Error Questionnaire 262
cognitive impairment 159
cognitive modification 262
cognitive performance 227
cognitive problems 258
cognitive restructuring 70, 71, 150, 180, 197, 198
cognitive therapy 245
collaborative approach 78
combination treatment 197
common-sense model (CSM) 47, 48, 49, 58, 59
communication 29, 37, 38, 72, 102–4, 110, 111, 125
communication technology 120–31
communication training 71, 196
community-based approaches 37, 80, 197–8, 231–2
community care 109
community resources 72
community self-management programmes 85
co-morbidity 155, 227
Comprehensive Health Enhancement Support System (CHESS) 87
'compression of morbidity' thesis 3
computer-based interventions xi, 182
conceptual modelling 115
conduct disorder 107
confidence 55, 56, 58, 64, 101, 104, 105, 127, 151
conflict 34, 104, 172
conflicting motivations 156
congenital heart disease 239
congestive heart failure 273
consciousness raising 56
consent 127
consumerism 127
contemplation stage 55

continuum theories 58, 60
contract 69
control beliefs 58
controllability 48
controller medications 206
COPD, see chronic obstructive pulmonary disease
coping 36, 48, 58, 173, 196, 197
   self-statements 71, 277
   skills 70–4, 78, 96, 172, 195
   strategies 48, 49, 198
   style 197
coronary artery bypass graft surgery 229
coronary artery disease (CAD) 224–37, 273
coronary heart disease, see heart disease
corrective feedback 106
corticoid releasing hormone (CRH) 191, 192
corticosteroids 265
cortisol 192, 196
cost-effectiveness 90, 126, 199, 200, 293–4
costs 90, 100, 126, 192, 198–200, 289, 293–4
coughing 256, 257
counselling 265, 278
criterion contamination 191
criticism 109
cross-sample comparisons 161
CSM, see common sense model
CTT, see classical test theory
culture 81, 85, 104, 208
cure 110
cystic fibrosis 138, 255
cytokines 192

DAFNE, see Dose Adjustment for Normal Eating
DALYs, see disability-adjusted life years
DASH, see Dietary Approach to Stop Hypertension
data security 127
decisional balance 55, 56
delegation 125
delivery 180–1, 261
demographic change x
demonstrations 102
denial 49
Denver group 258
DEP, see Diabetes Educational Programme
dependencies 5, 19, 198, 290

depression 71, 88, 143–4, 149, 190–1, 196–9, 208, 227, 229, 230, 241–2, 245–6, 258, 259, 261, 263
dermatology 122
developed world
  coronary artery disease in 224, 225
  diabetes in 15
  life expectancy in 8
  population pyramid 10, 11
developing world
  coronary artery disease in 225
  diabetes in 15
  life expectancy in 8
  population pyramid 12, 13
diabetes xi, 5, 10, 14, 15, 34–7, 51, 57, 66, 72, 73, 80, 82, 86, 107–8, 122, 124, 137, 169–88, 239, 292, 293
Diabetes Atlas 15
Diabetes Educational Programme (DEP) 110
diabetes specialist nurses (DSN) 110
Diabetes Stages of Change study (DiSC) 57
diagnostic accuracy 122
didactic approach 65, 78, 81, 103, 106, 179
diet 36, 49, 50, 66, 170, 179, 225, 229, 273, 275–7
Dietary Approach to Stop Hypertension 274
difficulty parameter 160
digital divide 30, 121
disability 3, 16–21, 30, 73, 88, 193, 195, 197
disability-adjusted life years (DALYs) 205, 225
DiSC study, see Diabetes Stages of Change study
disease management programmes 243–4
disease-specific programmes 79, 82
distal outcomes 148–52
distraction 71, 73, 278
distress 49, 261
domiciliary oxygen treatment 259
do-not-resuscitate orders 32
Dose Adjustment for Normal Eating (DAFNE) 173

education 31, 36, 65, 74, 78, 85, 193–5, 198, 208, 212, 229, 244, 260–61, 276
educator experience logs 110
e-health 264
elicitation study 54
email 87, 121

embedded criticism 109
emotional disclosure 194, 195
emotional distress 163, 195, 197
emotional impact 36
emotional representations 48, 208
emotional well-being 173
emotion management 70–1, 101
empathic accuracy 160
empathy 67
employment 191, 192
empowerment 127, 290, 293
enablers 105
enactment 99, 110
energy conservation training 261
England, hypertension in 272
Enhancing Recovery in Coronary Heart Disease Patients (ENRICHD) 230
enjoyable activities 71
ENRICHD, see Enhancing Recovery in Coronary Heart Disease Patients
environmental control 212
environmental re-evaluation 56
EPP, see Expert Patient Programme
equipoise 141–2
equity 290
essential hypertension 273
Estonia 14
ethical issues 127
ethnicity 136
ethnic minorities 30, 80, 205
European Respiratory Society Task Force 264
evaluation
  formal 141–4
  frameworks 127
  of self-management interventions xi, 47, 114, 135
  of telemedicine 123
Evergreen Project 20
evidence base 291–2
evidence-based health care 294
exclusion criteria 142
exercise 49, 50, 83, 124, 150, 179, 198, 210, 228–30, 263, 276, 277
'expansion of morbidity' thesis 4
expenditure 4, 5, 16; see also costs
experiential processes 55, 56
Expert Patient Programme (EPP) 36, 37, 123, 145, 295
exploratory phase 135, 139–41
external validity 100
extravascular immune complex hypothesis 192

FACTS, *see* Families, Adolescents and Children's Teamwork Study
failure of success model 3
Families, Adolescents and Children's Teamwork Study (FACTS) 172, 173, 181
family factors 171–3
fatigue 149, 163, 190, 257, 258, 263, 264
feasibility trials 140, 141
feedback 84, 86, 88, 103, 104, 106, 110, 276
fertility rates 3, 9
fidelity 98–100, 107–15, 180
financial barriers 293–4
Finland
    diabetes in 15
    North Karelia Project 231–2
Five 'As' approach 84–6
flexibility 139
fluid intake 245
fluid retention 241
focus groups 136, 137, 143
follow-up contacts 85
formal evaluation 141–4
Framework for the Development and Evaluation of Complex Interventions 59
France, activities of daily living in 20
functioning 149, 193, 194, 199

General Household Survey 5
generalized programmes 79
General Practice Registry Database (GPRD) 14
generic intervention 136
generic programmes 82
genes 3, 273
Germany 29, 32
Glasgow, Russell 181, 182
Global Burden of Disease study 11, 12
glucose level, *see* blood glucose
glycaemic control 80, 173, 174, 179, 181
goals 50, 51, 66, 67, 70, 99, 100, 101, 102, 105, 114, 125
goal setting 51, 85, 86, 101, 103, 105, 107, 112, 114, 125, 179, 180, 244, 291, 293
GPRD, *see* General Practice Registry Database
Grave's disease 169
Grey, Margaret 172
group interventions x, 82–3, 102–5, 112, 138, 149, 173, 174, 179, 181, 195, 198, 265

guidance-cooperation model 28
guided imagery 265, 278
guided self-management 206, 212, 213, 215, 216

Hamilton, Walton H. 28
hard-to-reach populations 78
headache 87
Health Belief Model 123
health care utilization 5, 6, 261
health education leaflets 31
health literacy 29–31
healthy behaviours 29, 55, 66, 223
heart attacks 70, 227; *see also* myocardial infarction
heart disease xi, 4, 13–16, 272
heart failure 10, 12, 14, 88, 238–53
Heart Failure Adherence and Retention Trial 245
heart transplantation 239
helping relationships
    counter-conditioning 56
helplessness 196, 197
Helsinki Ageing Study 14
HIV/AIDS 87, 256
homebound patients 88
homework assignments 149, 150
hospitalization 10, 11, 14, 36, 190, 197, 209, 230, 244
hostility 109
HPA axis, *see* hypothalamic-pituitary-adrenal axis
human capital 291, 294
humour 104
hypercaloric food 273
hypercholesterolemia 224
hyperglycaemia 169, 171
hyperlipidemia 226
hypertension 5, 14, 15, 224, 225, 239, 257, 272–86
hypertensive encephalophathy 273
hypnosis 278, 279
hypoglycaemia 170, 171, 174
hypothalamic-pituitary-adrenal axis (APA axis) 191
hypothyroidism 169
hypoxaemia 259

IADL, *see* Instrumental Activities of Daily Living
ICHAs, *see* interactive health communication applications
ICS, *see* inhaled cortico-steroids

IDCs, *see* implantable cardiac defibrillators
idiopathic hypertension 273
illness beliefs 228, 263
Illness Perception Questionnaire (IPQ) 49
illness-specific intervention 136
imagery 279
impatience 278
implantable cardiac defibrillators (IDCs) 239
implantable devices 239
implementation 69, 70, 73, 144, 145
implementation intentions 69–70, 73
in absentia health care 120, 121
inclusion criteria 142
India, hypertension in 15
individual barriers 292–3
industrialization 4
infant mortality 7
inflammation 199
information 29–31, 38, 48, 65, 66, 73, 74, 78, 155–6
informational phase 121
inhaled cortico-steroids (ICS) 206
inhalers 35, 206, 207
Instrumental Activities of Daily Living (IADL) 5, 16, 17, 18, 19
instrumental phase 121
insulin 57, 169, 170, 171, 172
interaction with physicians 198
interactive health communication applications (ICHAs) 120–31
interactive phase 121
INTERHEART study 15
Intermediate Care Diabetes Service 110
internal validity 100, 141
Internet 30, 31, 79, 86–7, 90, 121, 123, 127, 138, 173
interpersonal cues 125
interpersonal dynamics 83
interventional phase 121
intervention modelling 138–9
intrapsychic processes 150
inverse information law 31
inverse social gradients 225
IPQ, *see* Illness Perception Questionnaire
IRT, *see* item response theory
isolated populations 126
Italy 14, 20
item characteristic curves 160, 161
item response theory (IRT) 157, 160–2, 164

Japan 7

joint protection 198
judgements 155, 156

Kaiser Permanente 36
keto-acidosis 173
kidney disease 273
knowledge 102–3, 125, 148, 259–60, 282

labour market participation 5
lapses 106
late-life depression 197
Latin America, hypertension in 15
lay information 48
lay leaders xi, 79–82, 138
lay teachers 198
life expectancy 3, 4, 6–9, 225
lifestyle 29, 35, 47, 64, 73, 150, 229, 231, 240, 241, 274, 275–8, 283
limiting long-standing illness (LLI) 6, 19, 20
lipids 226, 230
literacy 29–31
literature reviews 136
LLI, *see* limiting long-standing illness
longitudinal designs 198
Longitudinal Study of Aging (LSOA) 17
long-standing illness 19, 20; *see also* limiting long-standing illness
long-term implementation 144–5
Lorig, Kate 295
lower extremity impairment 196
LSOA, *see* Longitudinal Study of Aging
lung cancer 255
lung transplantation 259–60
lung volume reduction surgery (LVRS) 259
LVRS, *see* lung volume reduction surgery

macro-vascular complications 169
maintenance 55, 145, 195, 196
malpractice 127
management education programmes 36
management skills 74
manuals 108–9, 113, 182
marginalized populations 89
mastery 51, 68, 69, 103
Mauritius 231
measurement 152–3, 160–1
mediation analysis 59
medical management 205
Medical Outcomes Study 241
Medical Research Council (MRC) 59, 135, 139, 140, 144, 145
Medicare 11, 14, 16

Medicare Beneficiary Survey 4
Medicare Current Beneficiary Survey 17
Medicare Health Support 36
Medicare Modernization Act 36
medication 36, 47, 49, 50, 64–6, 70, 124, 198, 207–8, 227, 228, 244, 260
meditation 279
menorrhagia 34
mental health status 227
meta-analyses 78, 82–3, 137, 182, 191, 214, 231, 241, 245, 276, 279–80, 281
methodological issues 181–2
MI, *see* myocardial infarction
microalbuminuria 51
micro-vascular complications 169, 174
mini action plans 105
minor illnesses 29
misspecification problems 150–1
mobile phones 121
mobility 153, 199
modelling 51, 83, 105, 106, 115, 138–9
Model of Action Phases 69
modes of delivery 112
mood 64, 194, 242, 245
Moore's law 121
morbidity 290
mortality 7, 8, 224–5, 231, 291
motivation 66, 67, 84, 104, 125, 156
motivational cards 110
motivational interviewing 67, 84, 85, 86, 88
MRC, *see* Medical Research Council
Multidimensional Diabetes Scale 51
MULTIFIT 230
multi-item assessment 156–7, 163
multi-site trials 143
mutual participation model 28
myocardial infarction (MI) 49, 71, 224, 231, 239, 273, 275; *see also* heart attacks

National Arthritis Action Plan 193
National Cancer Institute 84
National Emphysema Treatment Trial Research Group (NETT) 259
National Health Interview Survey (NHIS) 14, 16
National Heart, Lung and Blood Institute Cardiovascular Study 11
National Institutes of Health (NIH) 162, 225
National Long Term Care Survey (NLTCS) 16, 18

National Occupational Standards for the Practice of Public Health 101
National Population Health Survey 14
needs analysis 136–7
negative thoughts 71
Netherlands 14
NETT, *see* National Emphysema Treatment Trial Research Group
neuropsychological problems 257
neurorehabilitation xi
newsletters 57
New York Heart Association (NYHA) classification 239, 240, 241–2
New Zealand 29, 49
NHIS, *see* National Health Interview Survey
NHS Direct 37
NHS HealthSpace 37
NIH, *see* National Institutes of Health
NLTCS, *see* National Long Term Care Survey
nontraditional treatments 198
Normalization Process Model 125, 292
normative beliefs 58
north America 205
North Karelia Project 231–2
no-treatment control 262
nutrition 198, 231, 261
NYHA, *see* New York Heart Association classification

obesity 9, 15–16, 127, 210, 239, 273, 275, 278
observable variables 154
observation 135, 143, 154–5, 160
occupational hazards 255
occupational illnesses 4
OECD, *see* Organization for Economic Co-operation and Development
oedema 243
older people x, 3–27, 30, 32, 38
on-the-job training 105
open-ended questions 103
operant theory 109
ordering effects 158
organizational barriers 294–5
Organization for Economic Co-operation and Development (OECD) 6
osteoarthritis 88
outcomes 67, 140, 143, 148–65, 179, 205, 260
outpatient service utilization 190
over-the-counter preparations 34, 293
ownership 38

oxygen uptake 244

pain 36, 47, 71, 73, 88, 149, 163, 190, 193, 195–6, 198, 293
pairing 104
panic 229
paraphrasing 103, 112
participant receipt 110
participation 31–4, 38
participatory methods 103
partnership approach 32
paternalism 35
pathology 122
Pathways to Change (PTC) 57
patient-centred approach 65, 217
patient education, *see* education
patient-reported benefits 291
patient-reported outcomes 126
Patient Reported Outcomes Measurement Information System (PROMIS) 162–3
peak expiratory flow meters (PEF meters) 204
peak flow 47, 66, 72
peer relations 171, 172
person-to-person delivery 138
persuasion 51
physical activities 150, 170, 226
physiological parameters 148, 151
piloting 140
plaque 224
Poland 33
population pyramids 10, 11, 12, 13
population trends 3–27
positive reinforcement 106
potassium intake 275
power relationships 295
pragmatic phase 135
praise 104
pre-action stage 57
precontemplation stage 55
preparation stage 55, 67
pre-post assessment 137, 245
prescribed medicines 34
preventer medications 206, 207, 208, 209
primary obstructive pulmonary emphysema 257
printed material 112
privacy 83
ProActive programme 109, 113
problem definition 68
problem formulation 68
problem orientation 68

problem solving 51, 68, 72, 73, 78, 83, 84, 85, 101, 104, 172, 179–81, 196, 244, 278, 292, 293
process assessment 143
processed foods 231
professional leaders 80–2
programme composition 79
programme setting 79–80
progressive muscle relaxation 278, 279
PROMIS, *see* Patient Reported Outcomes Measurement Information System
prompts 110
protocols 108–9
providers 112
proximal outcomes 148–52
proxy markers 291
proxy reports 159
proxy variables 154
pseudo-patients (fake patients) 113, 114
psychoanalytic approach 259
psychoeducational interventions 212, 214, 216
psychological morbidity 214, 263
psychomaintenance 258
psychopharmacological interventions 197
psychosocial factors 174, 199, 209, 212–15, 264, 265, 273
PTC, *see* Pathways to Change
public health measures 264
pulmonary disease, *see* chronic obstructive pulmonary disease
pulmonary function tests 260
pulmonary hypertension 257
pulmonary rehabilitation 263–4

qualitative approaches 136, 139, 145
quality assurance 98–118
quality of health care 289
quality of life 3, 4, 78, 179, 181, 192, 214, 241, 244, 260, 261, 263, 291, 293, 294
questionnaires 110, 143, 157, 158, 159
quizzes 102

RA (rheumatoid arthritis), *see* arthritis
radiology 122
randomized controlled trials (RCTs) 99, 137, 139, 141, 142, 182, 193, 196, 199, 213, 214, 217, 265, 276
Rasch modelling 160
ratings 114, 159
RCTs, *see* randomized controlled trials
reach 99, 100, 144, 182

Reach, Effectiveness, Adoption, Implementation and Maintenance (RE-AIM) framework 89, 124, 144
readiness to change 66–7, 208
RE-AIM, *see* Reach, Efficacy, Action, Implementation and Maintenance
receptor densities 192
reclassification of products 37
recommendations 59–60
recreation centres 80
recruitment 142–3
referral logs 110
reflecting 67, 103
regulatory procedures 38
rehearsal 106
reinforcement 56, 104
relapse prevention 72, 106, 109, 173
relationships 38, 83, 127
relaxation 71, 73, 180, 195, 196, 198, 212, 214, 229, 261, 265, 278, 279, 283
reliever medications 206, 207
reminders 110, 275
renin-angiotensin-aldosterone system blockers 226
reported variables 154–5
representations 48, 49
rescue medications 206
research xi, xii, 37, 115, 125, 126, 145, 173, 199, 107, 214–16, 209, 263
resentful demoralization 141
respiratory disorders 255
respiratory function 205
respiratory muscle training 263–4
respiratory symptoms 256
respiratory tract 255
retinopathy 273
retooling 81
return to work 49, 50
revascularization 239
reviews 182
rewards 114
rheumatoid arthritis (RA), *see* arthritis
role models 81
role playing 60, 103–6, 110

salient beliefs 54
salt 231, 273
Samoa 15
SAM system, *see* sympathetic-adrenal-medullary system
sample sizes 198
sampling of intervention sessions 113
sarcoidosis 255

satisfaction 125, 126
saturated fats 272
schedule of sessions 60
school failure 107
screening 34
SCT, *see* social cognitive theory
secondary prevention 226, 231
security of information 127
sedentary lifestyle 224, 273, 278
selection bias 126
self-blame 197
self-confidence 38
self-diagnosis 34
self-efficacy 47, 50, 51, 52, 55, 56, 58, 67–9, 123, 124, 143, 151, 174, 179, 180, 195, 196, 199, 208, 215, 229, 245
self-expression programmes 194
self-help 29, 37, 38, 57, 84, 197–8
self-injection 173
self-liberation 56
self-management
    aim of interventions 98
    behaviour change 47–63
    by health care providers 89
    chronic obstructive pulmonary disease, 261–6
    components c, 64–76, 111–12
    courses 36
    definition ix, 47, 64, 261–2
    delivery of interventions 78–97, 108–11
    design 99
    development 99, 135–47
    education 36
    evaluation xi, 135–47, 198–9
    evolution 290
    future xii, 199–200, 290
    guided 206, 212, 215, 216
    implementation 291–6
    importance 3
    in clinical practice 83–6
    in hypertension 276–83
    integration into routine care 291–6
    Internet based 86–7
    legislation supporting education 295
    outcomes of interventions 148–65
    plans 207
    programme 72, 79–83, 197
    readiness 84
    research on xi, xii
    skills 107–8
    socio-cultural context x
    successful uptake 294
    support 35–8, 85

telephone 88, 90
theories x
types of interventions 72–3
self-monitoring ix, 34, 57, 66, 72, 73, 84,
    101, 103, 105, 106, 122, 180, 206, 208,
    213, 274, 276, 280–82
self-re-evaluation 56
self-regulation model 47–50, 70, 105,
    216, 230
self-report 114, 156–9, 163
self-statements 261
self-talk 71
senior centres 80
sensitization 193
sentiments 155, 156
service innovations 291, 294
sexuality 258
SHARE, *see* Survey for Health Ageing and
    Retirement in Europe
shared decision-making 31–4, 38
Sharing Health Care Initiative 36
shortness of breath 256, 257; *see also*
    breathlessness
Sickness Impact Profile 262
side-effects 64
simplified regimens 207
Simvastatin Survival Study 226
smoking 50, 209, 210, 224, 225, 240, 256,
    278
    cessation 55, 57, 226, 230, 261, 265,
        276, 277
    laws prohibiting 263, 264
social activities 262
social adjustment ix, 197
social change x
social class 272
social cognitive theory (SCT) 47, 50–2,
    58, 68, 69, 105, 123, 230
social desirability 156
social difficulties 197
social factors 208
social functioning 49, 163
social isolation 261
social learning theory 179
social liberation 56
social modelling 83
social persuasion 68
social position 224–5
social pressures 171, 172
social problems 172, 258
social support 64, 72, 84, 124, 195, 227,
    228, 230
socio-demographic factors 207, 211
socio-economic factors 17, 200, 207, 256

sociology 20
sociostructural factors 50
sodium intake 245, 275, 277
solution implementation 69
Spain 33
spot checks 113
spriometry 256
sputum 256, 257
stages 54–8, 135
stages of change model 47
stage theories 57, 60
standard care 141
standardization 139, 163
Stanford Arthritis Center 197
Stanford Chronic Disease
    Self-Management Program (CDSMP)
    123
Stanford University 36
stimulus control 56
strategies 86, 148
strength 244
stress 68, 170, 191, 192, 196, 278
    management 70–1, 74, 180, 196, 199,
        229, 245, 260, 261, 262, 279, 283
stroke xi, xii, 273, 275
subjective norm 52, 54
sub-populations 136
substance abuse 107
suicidal ideation 259
sulphasalazine therapy 193
summarizing 103, 111
Summary of Diabetes Self-Care Activities
    Scale 51
Summit Report 85
supervision 106
support
    for self-care 34–5
    for self-efficacy 67–8
    for self-management 35–8, 83–6
    psychosocial 264
    social 64, 84
    telephone 180
Supporting Self-Care 36
Survey for Health Ageing and Retirement
    in Europe (SHARE) 14, 20
Survey of Income and Program
    Participation (SIPP) 17
Sweden, high blood pressure in 14
Sweet Talk 123
Switzerland 32
sympathetic-adrenal-medullary system
    (SAM system) 191, 192
symptom-based plans 209
symptom experience 149, 227

symptom management 261
symptom monitoring 209
symptom perception 261, 265
systemic education approach 181
systolic blood pressure 86

Taiwan 20
target behaviours 68
Task Force on Community Preventive
    Services 80
taxonomies 179
technology
    growth of 290
    interactive 79, 86–8
    lack of influence on life expectancy 9
    life-extending 8
    resistance to 125
Technology Acceptance Model 124
telecare 265
telemedicine 120–31
telemonitoring 122, 280
telephone counselling 57
telephone interventions 138
telephone self-management 88, 90
telephone support 180
temporal factors 191
temptation 55, 56, 58
theories x, 47–63, 100, 137–8, 151, 180,
    281, 212, 215–16, 283
theory of planned behaviour (TPB) 47,
    52–4, 58, 109, 124, 229
therapeutic writing programmes 194
thought-monitoring 278
timeline 48, 50, 70, 110
time pressures 33
time urgency 278
TPB, see theory of planned behaviour
training
    didactic 106
    modelling 106
    of facilitators xi, 140
    of lay leaders 81
    of self-management interventions
        98–118
    relaxation 195
    videos 106
trait anxiety 195
transfats 231
transtheoretical model (TTM) 47, 54–9,
    66
treatment differentiation 99
treatment fidelity 98–100, 106, 111–14,
    180
treatment integrity 99

treatment receipt 99
trial design 141–2, 181–2
Trials of Hypertension Prevention
    Collaborative Research Group 277
triggers (asthma) 47, 71, 204, 206, 207,
    209
trust 125
TTM, see transtheoretical model
tuberculosis 255
Turkey, life expectancy 7

UK
    cardiac rehabilitation programme
        attendance 228
    decision-making in 32
    prevalence of asthma 205
    provision of advice in 29
    systems of regulation in 294
    use of asthma action plans 208
underserved populations 182
unexpressed thoughts 160
USA
    cardiovascular disease in 14
    deaths from coronary artery disease 22
    decentralized health care system 294
    decision-making in 33
    health literacy in 30
    hypertension in 272
    legislation in 36, 295
    life expectancy in 8
    obesity in 9, 15–16
    provision of advice in 29

validity 100, 141, 152
values 34, 150
valve disease 239
variable-measure correspondence 153
variables 152–8
verbal cues 110
verification 69
vicarious experience 68
vicarious learning 51
visual impairment 30, 174
voluntary organizations 38
voluntary participation 198
volunteers 81

waiting times 125
walking distance 263
Wanless report 5
warmth 109
Watch, Discover, Think and Act 122
web-based interventions 86–7, 182

weight control 224, 226, 241, 243, 257, 275–7
weight loss 148, 150, 179
wheezing 255
Whole System Informing Self-Management Engagement (WISE) 125, 291
WISE, *see* Whole System Informing Self-Management Engagement

wish-fulfilling fantasy 197
work-books 138
World Health Organization (WHO) 13–16, 225, 226

Xenical 127

yoga 279

LEADERSHIP FOR NURSING AND ALLIED HEALTH CARE PROFESSIONALS

Veronica Bishop (ed)

The aim of this book is to empower would be leaders of nursing and allied health professions to be effective. Leadership in nursing and those health care professions allied to medicine has rarely been a highly visible clear cut business, and certainly many consider that, particularly in the UK, within the past decade a severe erosion of power bases within the professions has occurred.

To strengthen leadership within the professions allied to medicine (PAMs) it is necessary to understand policy and professional contexts, and to review activities across the Atlantic and across Europe, now a growing entity with major implications for healthcare and nursing.

This text examines differences between leadership and management, inspirational education to support would be leaders, and a major UK programme to promote politically aware leaders. The importance of collaboration in achieving standards and quality without loss of identity of one's discipline, or of the core values that make working in healthcare a challenge well worth accepting are examined.

Veronica Bishop asserts that it is time for us to take stock, to promote and support our articulate and strategic thinkers, and to let them shine. Experts from a wide breadth of countries and knowledge have come together in this book to help to achieve this.

Contents: *What is leadership? – Leadership and management: Is there a difference? – Leadership challenges: Professional power and dominance in healthcare – Leadership for the allied health professions – Developing political leaders in nursing – Education for leadership: Transformatory approaches – Clinical leadership and the theory of congruent leadership – Pulling the threads together: Grasping the nettle.*

2009 224pp
978-0-335-22533-0 (Paperback) 978-0-335-22532-3 (Hardback)

EXCELLENCE IN DEMENTIA CARE

Research into Practice

Murna Downs and Barbara Bowers (eds)

'Dementia care has come of age with this book. It is an impeccably crafted collection of papers from eminent experts on both sides of the Atlantic. The book demonstrates confidence, based on both research evidence and well-grounded good practice, and a solid set of shared values both explicit and implicit. The contributors are refreshingly candid about debates and controversies. This book is authoritative and readable which makes it useful to a wide audience. It will provide knowledge, *encouragement and motivation to a hard pressed workforce.'*

Mary Marshall OBE, Emeritus Professor, University of Stirling, Scotland

This landmark textbook draws on the extensive knowledge of researchers, practitioners, and professionals in the care of people with Alzheimer's disease and other dementias. It is informed both by a profound respect for people with dementia and a commitment to including them in decisions about their care and lives. While focusing on care for people with dementia, this core text also addresses the most pressing concerns of families by promoting practices and services that recognise the full humanity of their relative with dementia. In addressing the many complex issues related to offering support to people with dementia and those who care for them, this timely textbook is unique in emphasising strategies for creating sustainable change in practice. The book includes examples from a range of countries, drawn from research, practice wisdom and, most importantly, from the experience of people with dementia and their families.

This key text offers valuable insights about how to:

- Provide competent and compassionate care for people with Alzheimer's Disease and other dementias
- Build systems to provide effective care
- Encourage collaboration among multi disciplinary professionals and users and carers
- Support those caring for people with dementia
- Ensure those with dementia maintain dignity, well-being and meaningful participation in life

Excellence in Dementia Care is a vital resource for those working with people with dementia. It provides an accessible yet sophisticated overview of the knowledge, skills and attitudes required to achieve excellence. It is an essential handbook for those responsible for training, education and skills development in dementia care.

Contents: *Contributors – Foreword – Preface – Acknowledgements – Introduction – **Part 1: Principles and perspectives** – Prevalence and projections of dementia – Toward understanding subjective experiences of dementia – Ethnicity and the experience of dementia – A bio-psycho-social approach to dementia – Flexibility and change: The fundamentals for families coping with dementia – Towards a person-centred ethic in dementia care: Doing right or being good? – Being minded in dementia: Persons and human beings – **Part 2: Knowledge and skills for supporting people with dementia** – Assessment and dementia – Supporting cognitive abilities – Working with life history – The language of behaviour – Communication and relationships: An inclusive social world – Supporting health and physical well-being – Understanding and alleviating emotional distress – **Part 3: Journeys through dementia care** – Diagnosis and early support – Living at home – Care of people with dementia in the general hospital – The role of specialist housing in supporting people with dementia – Care homes – End of life care – Grief and bereavement – **Part 4: Embedding excellence in dementia care** – Involving people with dementia in service development and evaluation – A trained and supported workforce – Attending to relationships in dementia care – Leadership in dementia care – Quality: The perspective of the person with dementia – Reframing dementia: The policy implications of changing concepts – The history and impact of dementia care policy – Index.*

2008 640pp
978-0-335-22375-6 (Paperback) 978-0-335-22374-9 (Hardback)

THE PRESCRIPTION DRUG GUIDE FOR NURSES

Sue Jordan

'This book is exceedingly timely. I am certain it will be invaluable to both undergraduate and post graduate student nurses, and, also act as a continuing reference source. Thoroughly recommended.'

Molly Courtenay, Reading University, UK

'Sue Jordan has combined her deep understanding of her own discipline with her long experience of teaching nurses, to produce just the right type and level of information that nurses need, in a format that they will find relevant to their practice and easy to use. This book will be an essential reference resource for every ward bookshelf.'

Professor Dame June Clark, Swansea University, UK

This popular *Nursing Standard* prescription drug series is now available for the first time in book format! Organised by drug type and presented in an easy-to-use reference format, this book outlines the implications for practice of 20 drug groups.

Each drug group is presented in handy quick check format, and covers:

- Drug actions
- Indications
- Administration
- Adverse effects
- Practice suggestions
- Cautions/contra-indications
- Interactions

Contents: *Preface – Using this book – Abbreviations used in the text – Introduction – Laxatives – Controlling gastric acidity – Diuretics – Beta blockers – ACE inhibitors – Vasodilators (calcium channel blockers and nitrates) – Anticoagulants – Bronchodilators: Selective beta2 adrenoreceptor agonists – Corticosteroids – Antipsychotics – Antidepressants: Focus on SSRIs – Anti-emetics – Opioid analgesics – Anti-epileptic drugs: Focus on carbamazepine and valproate – Antibacterial drugs – Insulin – Oral anti-diabetic drugs – Thyroid and anti-thyroid drugs – Cytotoxic drugs – Non-steroidal anti-inflammatory drugs (NSAIDs) – Idiosyncratic drug reactions – Glossary – References – Bibliography/Further reading – Index.*

2008 192pp
978-0-335-22547-7 (Paperback) 978-0-335-22546-0 (Hardback)

THE HANDBOOK FOR ADVANCED PRIMARY CARE NURSES

Rebecca Neno and Debby Price (eds)

'*I believe that* **The Handbook for Advanced Primary Care Nurses** *should be extensively read and that it will prove to be an essential resource for nurses striving to improve public health and patient care in the communities of today and tomorrow. It may, with political will and a skilled and determined workforce help Florence Nightingale's vision come true.*'

Lynn Young, Primary Health Care Adviser, Royal College of Nursing, UK

This important new handbook for Primary Care Nurses is designed to assist senior nurses in developing the understanding and skills required to be effective at both strategic and operational levels. As well as exploring the context of advanced primary care practice, the book provides the tools needed for enhancing care delivery within both primary care and community settings.

The Handbook for Advanced Primary Care Nurses is an accessible guide to working strategically in primary care. It offers practical support across a range of core areas, including:

- Case finding and case management
- Mentorship
- Leadership and management
- Needs assessment
- Interprofessional working
- Prescribing

Neno and Price encourage readers to think analytically about their practice and include activities and reflection points throughout the book to help with this.

This book is the ideal companion both for nurse practitioners undertaking courses at advanced practice level and for professionals working at all levels in primary care.

Contents: *Foreword – Contributors – Introduction – Part 1: Context – Emergence of the advanced primary care nurse – Part 2: Enhancing care delivery – Legal and ethical issues in advanced practice – Case finding – Case management – First contact and complex needs assessment – Non-medical prescribing – Part 3: Enhancing strategic skills – Developing whole systems thinking – Transformational leadership – Developing and sustaining the advanced practitioner role – Developing and sustaining professional partnerships – From involvement to partnerships and beyond Part 4: Developing skills for the future – Commissioning in health and social care – Social enterprise and business skills – Influencing and getting your message across – Part 5: Future directions – The future for advanced primary care nurses – Index.*

2008 224pp
978-0-335-22353-4 (Paperback) 978-0-335-22354-1 (Hardback)

PERSON CENTRED PRACTICE FOR PROFESSIONALS

Jeanette Thompson, Jackie Kilbane and Helen Sanderson (eds)

This valuable text offers a range of practical, person centred and evidence based approaches to tackling challenges faced by professionals working with people with learning disabilities. It helps the reader to analyze issues relating to person centred practice and citizenship and considers the implications of this key government initiative for health and social care professionals.

The authors aim to support professionals in working through this changing agenda, whilst identifying the interface between their own professional practice and person centred approaches to working with people who have a learning disability. The book includes well referenced practical approaches to the subject area, alongside creative and innovative thinking.

In addition, the book also:

- Explores the historical context of learning disability services and how this has contributed to the development of person centred services
- Introduces a range of practical person centred thinking tools that can be readily used within professional practice
- Contains a model to inform the delivery and integration of person centred practice within professional practice
- Considers the contribution of a range of different professional roles to the person centred and self directed support approach
- Evaluates the relevance of person centred thinking and planning to people from different cultural backgrounds and those undergoing the transition from adolescence to adulthood

Person Centred Practice for Professionals is key reading for students, academics and professionals working or training to work with people with learning disabilities.

Contents: *Contributors – Introduction – Exploring the history of person centred practice – Towards person centred practice – Person centred thinking – Person centred partnerships – Person centred approaches to educating the learning*

disability workforce – Person centred approaches to meeting the health needs of people who have a learning disability – Communication – Meeting the needs of people from diverse backgrounds through person centred planning – Person centred transition – People with learning disabilities planning for themselves – Families leading person centred planning – Support planning – Creating community inclusion – Index.

2007 336pp
978-0-335-22195-0 (Paperback) 978-0-335-22196-7 (Hardback)